Doctor, Your Patient Will See You Now

Doctor, Your Patient Will See You Now

Gaining the Upper Hand in Your Medical Care

Steven Z. Kussin, M.D.

ROWMAN & LITTLEFIELD PUBLISHERS, INC.
Lanham • Boulder • New York • Toronto • Plymouth, UK

Published by Rowman & Littlefield Publishers, Inc.
A wholly owned subsidary of The Rowman & Littlefield Publishing Group, Inc.
4501 Forbes Boulevard, Suite 200, Lanham, Maryland 20706
http://www.rowmanlittlefield.com

Estover Road, Plymouth PL6 7PY, United Kingdom

British Library Cataloguing in Publication Information Available

Library of Congress Cataloging-in-Publication Data

The hardback edition of this book was previously cataloged by the Library of
Congress as follows:

Kussin, Steven Z., 1949–
    Doctor, your patient will see you now : gaining the upper hand in your medical
care / Steven Z. Kussin.
        p. cm.
    Includes bibliographical references and index.
    1. Physician and patient—Popular works. 2. Patient education—Popular works.
3. Medical care—Popular works. I. Title.
    R727.3.K88 2011
    610.69'6--dc22
                                        2010052668

ISBN: 978-1-4422-1059-2 (cloth : alk. paper)
ISBN: 978-1-4422-1060-8 (pbk. : alk. paper)
ISBN: 978-1-4422-1061-5 (electronic)

Printed in the United States of America

For Dad

&

Annie, the blood in my heart

Zach and Efrem, the breath in my lungs

One and the selfsame tongue first wounded me,
So that it tinged the one cheek and the other,
And then held out to me the medicine;

Dante Alighieri, *The Divine Comedy*,
Canto XXXI

Contents

Contents

Preface

The Process of Caring

Annie drove us home that night on a December's winter road. We passed homes, dappled in Christmas lights—studies in pointillism fragmenting the monochrome of our central New York winter. I slept undisturbed, insulated in the warmth and quiet of an SUV large enough to forgive the faults of a country road.

Awakened by Annie's warning, I saw but did not register the portent of the two lights shining in our windshield. Christmas lights? No, oncoming headlights—closing fast. Then, the sudden stop. A neck-snapping, inertia-defying, absolute deceleration. The explosion of noise. The vacuum of total silence. The freezing cold. All in a time too brief to measure. Dazed and detached, there was no pain, no fear, no concerns for Annie or myself. I only wondered how it could be possible for things to change so suddenly, so completely.

Then the pain. How could I breathe? Was my chest crushed against the seat belt? The dashboard? Then the panic. I stepped from the car on my ruined leg, the top of my tibia no more than a powder. Breathing at last, I belatedly remembered that Annie was with me. Phone in hand, bleeding from her nose, she had already called 911, and she told me she was okay. But I saw in her eyes that I wasn't. Days later we learned that she wasn't either (nerve damage to her leg). Few people escape this type of accident unscathed. The teenager in the other car was medevacked to a destination unknown. She lived. She lives. That's all I know.

I knew my leg was broken before the ambulance got the call. I was, and am, a doctor. Without the need of advanced diagnostic skills, the facts were clear. Bone edge pushed up under the skin beneath my right knee. My hands were swollen and had already taken on a mottled lividity. They too were broken. From the car to the ambulance to the emergency room, as the world went by horizontally, I was nothing more than a package. Not just any bundle, but a special delivery package that was treated as gently and urgently as a fragile but overdue birthday gift.

Now it was my turn to lie on a stretcher in the emergency room. I remember that my eyes fixed on the gypsum tiles on the suspended ceiling above me. I absently counted the small holes on those stained tiles. I counted the dimples on patterns I created: concentric circles, diagonals, triangles, and rhomboids. Yes, yes, I was stoned. I lay there with a false spiritual fillip empowered by morphine and lingering shock. This was my first patient-oriented perspective on hospital life—lying down, strung out, looking up and counting.

I was still sufficiently sensate to be aware of, and comforted by, the fact that, because I was a doctor, everybody who was about to attend to my care was going to be careful, mannered, and responsive to my questions. Not so for my "litter" mate next door. My separation from him was far greater than the flimsy curtain that hung between us.

The motor vehicle accident that put me on that gurney was not a threat to life and limb—just my limbs. But it did end my thirty years in clinical practice. I underwent several surgeries and spent months in a wheelchair with both hands and one leg immobilized, followed by a prolonged rehabilitation. During those months I replayed my very bad ride on that winter road and my very privileged ride on the rails of a medical system that received me as an equal.

My doctors were, or became, friends; yours, most likely, won't. Each of my physicians was chosen by me, decisions empowered by my long experience with them and the certain and comfortable knowledge of their professional and personal lives. You are not likely to have that opportunity. Despite even these advantages, mistakes were made. Most were harmless; one wasn't. I recognized the errors that you wouldn't. (Nor would it be as likely that you'd be informed of them.) Most medical mistakes will fly beneath your radar, affecting your recovery but not preventing it.

Imagine sitting on a gurney in the emergency room, sick, in pain, and frightened. You look to the door, wondering about the doctor you haven't yet met. It's no exaggeration to say that as that stranger walks into your life, your life falls into his hands. The overly sanguine err when they mistake a medical degree as sufficient entitlement for their care. The suspicious feel justified in their knowledge of the near ubiquity of medical error and the institutional apathy that can make a healthy person sick or a sick one dead. They are aware of the fact that hundreds of thousands die, or are injured, each year from preventable error and infection. They know that multiple hundreds of thousands more suffer risk, anxiety, pain, and expense for the unnecessary or unproven.

Imagine, then, that the door opens and the doctor enters. Imagine that the stranger you expected turns out to be a family member or trusted friend. Your relief would be palpable. I have seen that exhalation of relief, seen the distress dissipate, seen the softening of the features on the faces of my relatives and friends when I arrived to attend, supervise, observe, or give advice about their care.

For them everything changed at that moment. They were no longer alone. They knew that whatever else happened they had access to a person who would be a valuable resource, someone who cared about them, as well as for them; someone without a personal or financial agenda; someone who would always, and only, act on their behalf without conflict of interest. The trust that inevitably followed was the first step toward recovery.

When I reflected upon how different it is for the vast majority of people who are denied this reprieve, the idea for this book was born.

You might wonder what it's like to be a doctor who suddenly becomes a patient.

I was always treated with respect.

My opinions were sought after and judged to be important.

My questions were straightforward, frank, and occasionally challenging.

The answers were thorough and thoughtful.

Alternative treatments were discussed.

I asked my surgeon if there were other orthopedists better able to repair my fractures than he. If there were none locally, were there others to whom I could be transferred in the central New York region? He answered without rancor.

My consent for surgery was based on a valid assessment of its risks and benefits.

In the weeks of my recovery and rehabilitation I saw my doctors several times a day. They often dropped in just to say hello.

The nursing staff was kind, understanding, and respectful of my privacy. They preserved the remnants of my dignity with grace, even charm. If I needed a blanket or a pain medication it was brought to me as quickly as possible.

In other words, in many ways, I still have no idea at all of what it's like to be a patient.

I hope that this book will re-define for you the idea of patienthood, so that your time as a patient, or as a healthy consumer of medical services, can be like mine. I hope to make your belief in your doctors and hospitals as rational as my own. I hope to make the care you receive as attentive and considerate as it was for me. I have reason to be hopeful. The trajectory of my life has provided a unique perspective on both the process of care, and a philosophy of medical care.

consent. At no time in our lives will we be so detached, distracted, and deprived of our faculties. This occurs at a time when there is little room for error when choosing whom to trust.

Ninety million Americans are living with serious illnesses such as cancer, heart disease, diabetes, Parkinson's, the effects of stroke, and Alzheimer's. This number will more than double over the next twenty-five years, ensnaring both the invincible baby boomers and the cynical Gen-Xers.

Before medicine became confused with science and doctors with scientists, the patient-doctor relationship was a nuanced, subjective collaboration of partners. As doctors have progressed in their knowledge, they have stepped back from their role as healers. Their humanity, even decency, has been replaced by a detached, clinical scientific bearing. Doctors today solve problems. They don't tend to the many other needs of the ill. The sick find themselves without a receptive and sympathetic audience. They lack the words to adequately explain their dilemmas.

You will find little advice on medical conditions in these pages, but you will find the means of obtaining it on your own and the methods that enable you to demand it of your doctors.

As we turn now into the pages of this book's text I am reminded of the three Moirae of Greek mythology, Clotho, Lachesis, and Atropos. Called "The Fates," they may still, with each human birth, spin, measure, and then cut a thread that preordains each life span. We are able now to live on the last few fibers at the end of that thread as never before. In light of this, patients can no longer just passively acquiesce in their health care, or submit to the doctors that attend to it. Patients must take part in and, in fact, be in charge of their medical care and thereby their own destiny. Our penchant for "whistling by the graveyard" may still be understandable. "Whistling by the doctor's office" now carries a steep price.

Acknowledgments

Years ago it was my good fortune to have hired, and then observed the progress of, two associates. Kelly Gassner has served as a transcriptionist, an editor, a psychotherapist, and an unfailingly unflappable ally on this journey. Linda Lovrin, the former business manager of my practice, has been a facilitator, cheerleader, confidante, and friend.

When I started writing this book I thought it unlikely that I would need outside data. Thirty years in medicine seemed a sufficient background from which to draw. Three days later I was on the telephone with Deborah A. Hailston-Jaworski, MLS, director of library services at Faxton–St. Luke's Health Care Center, begging for articles and data. Her assistance shaped and sharpened this book.

Tom and Eloise Cathcart, accomplished authors, supplied friendship and support. Both stayed on my side of the street when they saw me coming.

I have had the benefit of knowing Cynthia Chapple, who both suffered me and suffered with me through the process of writing this book. And no prescriptions were needed!

Dr. Lester Eidelhoch—mentor and friend. He is a role model for the physician and person I have become.

It's all very well and good to write a book, but sooner or later you have to convince someone, other than yourself, that it was all worthwhile. A deep bow then to Suzanne I. Staszak-Silva, senior acquisition editor at Rowman & Littlefield, for confirming what was, to that point, only a hypothesis. She enjoys a seat amongst The Greats in my personal pantheon.

I

WAR: THE BATTLE OF MEDICAL EPISTEMOLOGIES

Each chapter in this book starts with bullet points. More accurately, they are bullet-*dodging* points that preview the lessons, warnings, and suggestions of the ensuing section.

In our first section, "War," you will learn that . . .

- Different doctors use vastly different and mutually incompatible databases to guide their recommendations. Some doctors think they're scientists, others, improv performance artists. It's a WAR between these "geeks" and "poets."
- The difference between the geeks and poets in what they "know" to be true will affect the tenor and quality of your care. Several examples are given.
- There are "must-ask questions" that will inform you whether you have a geek or poet calling the shots. I call these Medical Shibboleths.
- Most physician databases, whether originating from evidence-based medicine (the geeks) or eminence-based medicine (the poets) have been shown to contain biases, conflicts of interest, fraud, and outdated wisdom. You need your own reliable, up-to-date resources to guide your own independent decision making.
- A few extra keystrokes will transform a Google search into a sophisticated, specialized medical search engine.
- Free and subscription professional-grade "doctor-only" sites are accessible financially and intellectually.
- There is a difference between being medically informed and medically educated.

1

- Decision making is crucial—active participants live longer than passive recipients.

Do you get your current events information from the *Boston Globe* or the *National Enquirer*? PBS or *Entertainment Tonight*?

When purchasing a car do you seek guidance from the Insurance Institute for Highway Safety and ConsumerReports.org? Or do you make your decision by watching TV ads or listening to the guy next door?

It's no different for your doctors when they seek information. The quality and reliability of their opinions, in large part, hinges upon the resources they turn to when seeking the data that guides their decisions.

There exist today two fonts for a clinician's source material. The first I call the "New School," which adopts the practices and acknowledges the recommendations of evidence-based medicine, whose goal is to put medicine on firm scientific ground. The second I call the "Old School," which uses information based on a variety of sources that are the distillation of the best practices passed down over the past fifty years. Each uses and trusts widely disparate databases. The tenor and quality of your care depend upon which school your doctor adheres to. Doctors always have questions. In a 1985 study four doctors were followed for a half day. Two hundred and sixty-nine questions regarding patient management came up in just a few hours.[1] A second study found that *each* patient encounter generated up to 1.3 questions.[2] You need to know where your doctor goes and whom he trusts when seeking answers to those questions. Regardless of his databases you need to know if he's up-to-date or behind the times. Has he kept up or given up? In light of this you need your own school, *your* databases, which empower personal decisions. You need "Your School" because your doctors are not engaging in a friendly discussion about divergent databases. For them, it's a war. They are coming at you from two different directions. You have to know if you are going to become collateral damage in their crossfire or wind up a casualty of your own doctor's friendly fire.

Bearded, bespectacled professors in ill-fitting, unkempt houndstooth jackets man their barricades. They are the medical titans, the éminences grises of their day. They stride across their landscape, reducing all to trembling acquiescence. They, members of the "Old School," are now being laid low by Young Turks of the "New School" who refuse the orthodox and embrace new and foreign ways.

The war is the "Battle of Medical Epistemology" or, for a future TV reality show, "The Battle of the Medical Stars." This war might seem a tame and distant fray. It isn't. It is the crusade to protect and advance an all-encompassing approach to medical knowledge. It's not unusual that the quest for "Truth" leads to war. Religions have clashed for millennia over divergent dogmas. Now it's the doctors' turn. From one or the other of these opposing camps will flow the authoritative decrees that will change medical education's theory and practice. Medical schools' curricula, grants, and research and your doctors' books, thoughts, and practices will all be dictated by which of the two schools they ascribe to.

This battle is something you should care about. This fray affects your care today with each decision made in and on your behalf. From colds to cancer, the philosophy of your care, the tests you receive, and the pills you swallow will all be influenced by your doctors' reference material. It's good for you to know what your doctor thinks she "knows" to be true and whether that knowledge is based on evidence or is the proclamation of a contemporary eminence.

The Old School appellation should not evoke notions of the obsolete or outmoded. Old School medical epistemology can maintain intellectual vigor and rigor without divesting itself of comfortable nostalgic feelings. Most patients yearn for a little of the old-fashioned medicine they dimly recall from their youths. No one would or should wish for a return to the "good old days" but certainly a dose of the "good old ways" would be welcomed.

The New School is based on evidence-based medicine. The New School asks for data. It assumes that nothing can be considered valid until medical assumptions, conventional wisdom, and treatments have been subjected to the techniques of the scientific method. It promotes hierarchical criteria for obtaining and then trusting medical knowledge. Foremost and preeminent are randomized controlled trials (RCTs) that are subject to meta-analyses. Okay, we have to get a little technical here. No, don't be afraid. It'll be okay. It will hurt—but just for a few paragraphs.

THE NEW SCHOOL

The New School says, "Show me the beef." The "beef" is the clinically relevant data that arises from scientific research and techniques. The gold standard for these medical truths are RCTs that produce high-quality information that can overthrow unproven treatments and provide new insights on what were previously viewed as settled issues.

An RCT can address the efficacy of anything any doctor can do for any patient—medications, surgery, therapeutics, screening techniques, and diagnostics. RCTs start with a population that is divided into two groups—an experimental (treatment) arm and a control arm. The control group is denied therapy, or given conventional, "sham," or placebo therapy. Except for the treatment there are no differences between the groups. There can be no bias of age, gender, demographics, preexisting conditions, or other variables. Randomization, properly performed, reassures investigators that both groups are the same except for the manipulation performed on one and denied the other. In many RCTs, the patients are unaware of which group they are in. Similarly, the investigators often don't know which patients are in the control or treatment arm. This process is called "blinding." A blinded RCT seeks to eliminate false causality and bias that can occur due to the participants' expectations.

The inquiries are specific, narrow, and highly focused.

For example, a therapy may be tested to determine if it is effective for a single specific condition. It is another question and another study to prove that it is also safe for this condition. Even if the therapy is effective and safe—will a lower dose be as effective? Are there alternative therapies for this questioned condition? If so, separate studies are required to verify their safety and then further studies to determine which treatment is superior.

The New School prefers collective data. There are many RCTs that study one question. If they are deemed of "high quality," they are put into large pools and subjected to what is termed a meta-analysis. This process serves to dilute the effect of any individual RCT. Meta-analysis "averages out" problems in study size, statistical methods, and issues of blinding and randomization. Properly performed, meta-analyses are thought to provide a better summary of the data than those coming from a single small study.

Less reliable evidence comes from "observational studies." A cohort study is a forward-viewing (prospective) observational study. In a cohort study, subjects with an exposure of interest (e.g., high blood pressure, smoking, or use of hormone replacement therapy) and subjects without that exposure are identified and then followed into the future to determine their outcomes (e.g., strokes, cancer, or other diseases). Case controlled studies are also an observational technique. These investigations look backward (retrospective). A group of subjects with a certain disease (e.g., lung cancer) and a group without the disease allow investigators to look back in time via chart reviews and questionnaires to find exposures to putative risk factors (e.g., tobacco) that might have caused the disease in question. Some observational studies are given some, but reluctant, credibility if they are performed within the rigid standards of acceptance established by the arbiters of evidence-based medicine.

Case reports and case series are not accepted as evidence. These are descriptive studies that report on a single patient's or series of patients' experience with a specific disease. These are felt to be anecdotal, reporter dependent, and unscientific.

Finally we come to a tier of information that is so low on the hierarchy of acceptable evidence that it is derided by New School purists. Panels, colloquia, textbooks, strong beliefs, heuristic techniques, conventional wisdom, and untested data are never referenced. Doctors' personal experiences don't count. They are New School poison. Not only does the New School think that these resources fail to inform or reveal clinical truths, they're seen as the *cause* for many of the casual practices that plagued medical progress until the 1990s. Old School promotes "voodoo" and "witchcraft." Its practitioners have been described as "neo-shamanistic."

When the "best research" leads to the "best evidence," the "best guidelines and algorithms" will follow. The best advice inevitably follows.

The New School relies on algorithms which are a set of rules for solving a problem in a finite number of steps. Solutions lie in prescribed pathways set down by evidence-based guidelines. Medical algorithms are precise sets of rules that demand step-by-step adherence in order to solve clinical problems. A map is an accessible model for understanding algorithms. Maps provide many ways of getting to a destination. Evidence-based medicine's clinical algorithms give doctors specific and inviolate routes that get patients and their doctors to a destination. No detours or individual choices are allowed. Guidelines do not allow the contamination that arises from consensus views or individual judgment. It is only within the last fifteen years that guidelines have become based on evidence and are, by many, considered sufficiently sound that consensus-based methods are felt to be inappropriate and personal preferences are forbidden. Guidelines prevent doctors from flying by the seat of their pants or making it up as they go along. Guidelines encourage uniformity in medicine's practices and promises superior results.

New School Weaknesses

Medical practice is a complex and occasionally chaotic experience. When practiced best, it's a highly personal one—for patient and doctor. The reductionism that proposes medical care is a science providing definite answers revealed by RCTs flies in the face of doctors' sensibilities and their DNAs' demand for autonomy. Medicine qua science is intuitively impossible and ultimately undesirable. Each party in a medical transaction is unique and each clinical narrative is novel. In 2010, William E. Doll, Jr., Ph.D., hit the target poetically, writing that, "The 'throbingness' of life, the dynamic interplay of events, and the messiness of personal experience, draws more on metaphor than model."[3] Every patient-doctor conversation is driven by the very certainty of uncertainty. If all that is known in medical care were scientifically proven facts, then all our conversations would be brief and end with "take it or leave it." When it comes to medical transactions, your cellular provider will never tell you "There's an app for that."

In *Against the Gods: The Remarkable Story of Risk*, author Peter Bernstein quotes Nobel Laureate Kenneth Arrow. "Our knowledge of the way things work in society or in nature comes trailing clouds of vagueness. Vast ills have followed a belief in certainty."[4]

Evidence-based medicine was born in the universities and professors were its midwives. Despite the promise of academic detachment, RCTs are frequently contaminated by design flaws, ethical lapses, bias, conflicts of interest, suppressed data, political agendas, and outright frauds. In 2010 it was revealed that the United States leads the world in retracted journal articles and its scientists were cited as the most prone to engage deliberate fraud.[5]

John Ioannidis, a respected epidemiologist, stated in 2005 that "[t]here is increasing concern that in modern research, false findings may be the majority or even the vast majority of published research claims."[6] Despite the fact that some RCT findings are deemed insignificant, they are nonetheless lauded as being "worthy of note." Only 1 percent of RCT's clinical trials are even monitored by the FDA. RCTs sponsored by drug companies have taken away the reassurance that studies' designs are sound, properly conducted and that its results are properly interpreted and reported. According to the editor of *PLoS Medicine*, a respected online periodical, "journals may increasingly become close to works of fiction, telling stories dictated by various lobbyists than works of science."[7]

RCTs are exercises in human experimentation. All, even legitimate ones, are performed without any intent to treat or benefit its subjects. Although a successful trial may provide information that will help its subjects and others, most offer no viable solutions and are never reported or published. In 2011 it was revealed that the trials for which you were put at risk are not even mentioned in subsequent, almost identical trials.[8] You wasted your time and the new trial's participants may be wasting theirs. When ethical and rigorously performed, they are a necessity. Sadly, in today's climate you're not going to be safe if you participate in one. Doctors recommending them to you may be guilty of Hippocratic hypocrisy. When a clinical trial is tainted it performs interventions that are not in its subjects' interests and can subject its participants to harm and death. In 2010, a *JAMA* article warned, "The ethical appropriateness of clinical research depends on protecting participants from excessive risks. Yet no systematic framework has been developed to assess research risks, and as a result, investigators, funders, and review boards rely only on their intuitive judgments."[9] It seems that every month a trial's result, investigators, sponsors, or for-profit institutional review board are called into question, investigated, fined, or even prosecuted.

You or a family member may be a current or future subject in human trials.[10] One-third of all federally financed trials of cancer drugs and treatments involved community hospitals and private practitioners. When drug and device companies are included then the majority of *all* trials are carried out in local hospitals and offices. Doctors become bounty hunters when they're paid to recruit their patients.[11] Issues of unethical conduct, informed

consent flaws, non-disclosure, and defects in human experimental protocols characterize many of these studies.[12] These trials today involve tens of
thousands of patients and thousands of physicians. For now, they're not
for you. People suffering from incurable diseases that have no successful
therapies or those who have run out of options on traditional agents may
want to join a clinical trial. By doing so, desperation may yield to a measure of hope. For others it might serve as an attempt to advance scientific
knowledge for the benefit of others. Who would object to trials in these
tragic but uncommon scenarios? Most trials do not pit patients against
inevitable fates. The vast majority test new therapies for nonfatal diseases
that already have potent medicinal or therapeutic interventions (arthritis,
hypertension, angina, diabetes, inflammatory bowel diseases, etc.). These
are the ones to avoid.

Flip-flops: All of us are familiar with and frustrated by the radical shifts
in opinion that come from clashing RCTs and dueling meta-analyses. Over
time these flip-flops have made a mockery of both medicine and science.
No two clinical trials are the same and the clinical states they study are similarly unique. When two or twenty trials study the "same" clinical state, or try
to "answer" the same question, they're bound to disagree. Valid scientific
insights are expected to endure. Yes, knowledge is relative and paradigms
shift, but the New School offers advice and guidelines that are toppled so
quickly, radically, and unapologetically, we find ourselves reeling from
one truth to the next, bereft of answers to important questions about diet,
lifestyles, preventive strategies, screening techniques, and the efficacy of
medical and surgical treatments. The New School flip-flops are not course
corrections. They are neck-snapping 180-degree hairpin turns that morph
today's truths into tomorrow's taboos and yesterday's wisdom into today's
witchcraft. Is it any wonder that compliance suffers and recommendations
go unheeded? Who can really blame parents who refuse to vaccinate their
children, however much we disagree? Doctors lose the credibility and trust
that is our sole currency.

Echinacea for colds? Thumbs down in 2002 and again in 2005. But a
big thumbs up in 2007. The year 2010, however, brought another study
and more confusion. The effects of echinacea did not reach significance but
"the trends were in the direction of benefit . . . data are also insufficient to
exclude the possibility of a clinically significant effect."[13] The direction of
benefit? Insufficient to exclude the possibility? This isn't science. It certainly
isn't medicine. My homeowner's policy has clearer language than this. I
hope that answers the question for you. It doesn't for me.

Okay, thanks! Two things can be learned from this. There is no scientific
design that will ever answer this question. And second, the press reported
this study as definitive. The evening national network news hailed it as the
last word. Think so?

Seven hundred thousand coronary artery bypass grafts (CABG) are performed each year.[14] In 2008 the use of an ACE inhibitor (an anti-hypertensive agent) preoperatively was strongly recommended to improve CABG survival rates. In 2009, not only was it a bad idea, it *increased* deaths after CABG surgery.[15]

That aspirin you took to prevent heart attacks? You took them for years. Many of you still do. Well, they're not on the menu any longer. We've been advised to abandon their use—they're too dangerous. Similarly, all of us urged our patients to take folic acid for primary prevention against coronary artery disease. In 2009 it turns out that folic acid offers a 38 percent greater chance of dying from cancer.

Do oral bisphosphonates for osteoporosis cause esophageal cancer? "No!" say the authors of an August 2010 *JAMA* article.[16] "Yes" say the authors of a September 2010 *BMJ* study.[17] What a difference a month makes.

Mammogram anyone? If you're between forty and forty-nine years old there is not a single practitioner who will be able to make sense of the last twenty years of conflicting advice in making a recommendation. For those over eighty we thought we finally had sound advice—no mammograms. Yet the majority of physicians order them anyway, awaiting the next RCT and avoiding the next lawsuit. In 2009, decades of evidence was turned on its head as women ran for the exits in confusion and anger. It's still best to ask your doctor. The issue is so important I made it a Medical Shibboleth in the next section.

Speaking about breasts, I bet a lot of you still perform self-examinations. You remember you were told it was important. Well, now we tell you "Don't touch them, for God's sake. You're forcing us to do too many unnecessary biopsies!"

Decades of evidence told diabetics to keep tight control of their blood sugars to avoid heart attacks, strokes, blindness, kidney failure, and amputations. Millions of lives were made miserable trying to balance blood sugar levels on the head of a pin. All in vain. A 2010 review of thousands of diabetics showed that this practice was not helpful for most clinical endpoints and, in fact, caused more complications than "usual care."[18] Please don't get me started on PSAs (prostate-specific antigen tests). They too will be made the subject of a Medical Shibboleth in the next section.

"On Second Thought": Not only do RCTs clash with each other, sometimes there are multiple interpretations of *one* RCT. These "on second thought" analyses can occur years after the facts were assumed to be in. The Women's Health Initiative (WHI), one of the largest RCTs ever performed, found that hormone replacement therapy (HRT) increased morbidity and mortality for heart attacks, strokes, Alzheimer's disease, breast and ovarian cancer, and deep vein thrombosis. The investigation was carried out by the most respected physicians, statisticians, and epidemiologists. The findings appeared in the most rigorous scientific medical journals. So compelling were the findings and the dangers of therapy, two WHI trials were halted midway out of ethical considerations (although a bit grudgingly). The use of HRT for cancer prevention and postmenopausal symptoms plummeted. Here we are seven years later and it turns out the findings were weak and not statistically significant. The conclusions were described as "distorted," "oversimplified," and just plain wrong.[19] It was all just a "false alarm."

All wisdom has a half-life. Sooner or later most truths are altered or changed by progress and science. It would seem, however, that medical truths would live longer if they were revealed using superior scientific methodology. Not so. A research article in the Annals of Internal Medicine entitled "Truth Survival in Clinical Reports"[20] concludes that Old School maxims based on non-meta-analytic data outlived the truths revealed by New School techniques. The New School's entire premise is based on the fact that the "best evidence" would overturn the non-rigorous, unscientific conventional wisdom, rules of thumb, and the "that's the way we've always done it" attitudes that plagued medicine for fifty years. Not only have many Old School assumptions held up pretty well, the New School routinely overturns their own brand-new ones.

And the guidelines? They are the fruit from the RCT tree. You're ill-served by a doctor who straps on the blinders and shuts off his mind when entering you into mandated mazes of questionable value. Many are marketing tools.[21] Others are drug company advertisements. Many aren't evidence-based at all. In 2009 the American College of Cardiology and the American Heart Association were shocked to find that half of their guidelines were non-evidence-based. In 2011 fewer than half of the guidelines from the Infectious Diseases Society of America were based on high-quality data.[22] *Lancet* reported in 2011 that hospitalized patients with resistant pneumonias who were treated on guideline recommendations had *higher* mortality rates than those who were not.[23]

It's like your GPS. If you use it in your neighborhood, you frequently and fearlessly go off the satellite's chosen route, empowered by your better understanding of your neighborhood's roads, shortcuts, and traffic patterns. The trip is safer as a result. When you are in familiar territory there is no right way to proceed, only different ways. When in uncharted territory no one would deny the value of a GPS.

The federal government, hospitals, insurers, and academicians increasingly demand adherence to guidelines. Some physician reimbursement schemes are already tied to guideline worship. Even malpractice suits may be avoided if you experienced harm while on an algorithm's uneven highway. One observer felt more comfortable on Google than on a guideline.[24]

RCTs are dependent on statistics. Clinical investigations' methodologies, at best, are opaque, but more typically they are totally uninterpretable. We lack the skills to evaluate the validity of studies' assumptions and are not able to interpret the strength of their conclusions.[25] Some few doctors may be able to dive into that deep ocean of probability statistics, risk stratification, correlation coefficients, null hypotheses, and regression analyses. Most, however, go right to the bottom of that ocean. For it is here that the predigested, bite-sized conclusions and recommendations live. Yes, most doctors are bottom readers. This is not a weakness of RCTs per se, but it is a reason evidence-based recommendations are often ignored.

RCTs offer clinical advice in fewer than 10 percent of surgical interventions and even fewer are available to help doctors decide on medical devices. So that defibrillator in your heart may not be the best, but you can bet it's the most expensive. Few guidelines address patients with multiple illnesses and those that exist may cause harm.[26] If your doctor is looking for an answer when treating complex problems she's out of luck. Only 20 percent of the questions for complicated and intersecting conditions offer any guidelines. Fewer than half of the general care questions are answered by evidence-based guidelines or RCTs.[27] Every tailor knows that no one size fits all.

From the famine that exists for important conditions, other diseases offer a feast of suggestions. We don't need the ten guidelines that exist for adult sore throats. We could use one good one for rheumatoid arthritis—there are none. RCTs take years to perform and millions of dollars to complete. The moment an RCT is published academic rivals will cite multiple flaws in the experimental design and methodology and demand that more RCTs be performed.

In the many "what do we do now?" scenarios we can't always act with a "what do we know now?" scientific purity. H. G. Wright in his influential book *Means, Ends and Medical Care* states, "when rules are felt to be self-sufficient and superior to judgment then the cultivation of good judgment as well as the intellectual and moral virtues underlying it languishes."[28] There will be no deus ex machina that arrives to save a New School doctor (and you) in EBM's many uncharted territories.

THE OLD SCHOOL

Welcome back, wayfarers. You've returned from the New School section. You'll be glad to be part of the Old School's more familiar and easy-going ways. The Old School is more personal, experiential, contextual, and patient-centered, and its source material more qualitative and accessible. It is here that emotion, imagination, creativity, and narratives thrive. Goodbye for now to the formulaic, quantitative, dispassionate, and rigid New School demands—what a buzz kill!

Old School doctors listen to experts. So do you when seeking advice. Old School doctors value meetings. So do you. School, church, and community meetings keep you in touch, in the know, and in control. Old School doctors read textbooks, not scientific journals. You like books! You don't like *Popular Mechanics* either. Old School doctors use their experience and heed "gut instincts." You know all about intuition. You read Malcolm Gladwell's *Blink*, right?

Well, the familiar *can* breed contempt. Gladwell's book's title finishes with, *"The Power of Thinking without Thinking."*[29] Well that's not something you'd be happy about if it's your doctor who's not doing the thinking.

Old School source material: It turns out that observational studies are back. Having been banished to the back bench by the New School, they're sitting with the cool kids again. According to the *New England Journal*, "the average results of observational studies were remarkably similar to those of RCT trials."[30] Even the New School anathema of anecdotal evidence can inform. Case reports and case report series are found in our highest impact medical journals and can, when used wisely, provide important information.

RCTs do not deserve the reflexive genuflective submission that many give them. Poorly designed RCTs don't hold any sway over a carefully reported and referenced case study.[31] The existence of an RCT doesn't automatically codify a practice, nor does an "absence of evidence" necessarily preclude one.

How can we turn away from trusted observational studies when so much of EBM is tainted and outdated, and when only 4 percent of all medical services are backed by science?[32]

But many RCTs and their derivative guidelines do come from nonbiased investigators. They are focused, ethical, and use the best methodologies. They are subsequently judged dispassionately by peer groups, are published, and become topics of lively debate. These will inform better than more casual methodologies.

When *many* RCTs agree over time and arise from multiple centers they should both codify the practices they suggest and warn doctors off from those they criticize. "The truth must dazzle gradually" (Emily Dickinson). Erstwhile doctors were bound by experience, habits, and tradition. Worthwhile doctors must know the science but be neither slaves nor open sieves to its lessons. Your doctor becomes dangerous if he ignores New School truths and the valid clinical compasses they provide.

Experience: That experience serves as a source of genuine erudition seems so understandable and unequivocal that ignoring, trivializing, and maligning it raises doubts as to the credibility of those who do. If expertise is not a valid font of wisdom, what do the critics feel a doctor's mind *should* contain? Is it a tabula rasa awaiting the imprint of the latest New School doctrine and then reacting robotically to it?

Experience is the result of the hundreds to thousands of private clinical investigations a doctor runs every year—each office visit is a mini clinical trial. Accumulated over the years they serve as his own meta-analyses. An intellect secure in the understanding that unerring mastery in any endeavor is unobtainable will possess the humility that stimulates research. This mind is open to criticism and will acknowledge errors and correct them without resistance

Experience does not simply dredge up old pathways. Experience is creative; it enables recognition of new associations and can assimilate many seemingly unconnected inputs to synthesize novel constructs and imaginative approaches. Past experiences are malleable and can be shaped and molded to be applicable to a variety of new or variant presentations. This is what patients yearn for—open, honest, self-correcting inquiries that produce results born out of curiosity and humility. These are achieved only partially from the accretion of time. It is most associated with a receptive and gifted intellect. This type of experience is a reliable source of knowledge for others who tap into it and a rationale for activity in your behalf by those who possess it.

Experience is not practice makes perfect, nor is it a byproduct of the sheer volume of cases. Some observers cite a ten-year rule before an activity can be mastered. More recently Anders Ericsson introduced the concept of "deliberate practice." This type of experience confers mastery after 10,000 hours of self-observation, mentorship, and unflinching critical analysis of performance. A doctor's age is not a proxy for his experience, nor does a doctor's youth preclude it. Experience is not self-reverential. A doctor will not claim it as the basis for any action. That's how patients can recognize those with experience. Those who have it don't need to claim it; those who don't, must.

Strong Beliefs: The New School excludes the doctor's strong beliefs from your care. When confronted with a fork in the road or a branch in an algorithm, decisions depend, in part, on non-medical considerations. Philosophic, social, religious, economic considerations, backed by experience and expertise allow for action in the absence of evidence. Off-road excursions over unfamiliar roads become safer as a result. Human elements are subverted by a robotic acquiescence to science. Doctors who turn away from their value systems are automatons, not animated partisans.

Strong beliefs as a rationale for action in your behalf can defy the ability to be referenced, chapter and verse, from a journal, book, or clinical experience. This doesn't eliminate an action's usefulness, but it should stimulate a lot of questions. A doctor's "best shot" is not a substitute for best evidence. New School rigor does prevail here. When we doctors grope around in the dark we are using *your* hand to do the probing.

A Case in Point: A seventy-year-old woman on physical examination is found to have a loud left carotid bruit. The word "bruit" (pronounced broowee) comes from the French word for noise. This sound over the artery suggests obstruction to the flow of blood to the brain. The risk of stroke is increased. The resulting ultrasound demonstrates a 60 percent obstruction to the vessel. Options in this setting are 1) doing nothing; 2) instituting medical therapy including statins and anti-platelet drugs that, in a seventy-year-old, carry their own risks; 3) inserting a carotid artery stent, an invasive but nonoperative procedure in which a stent—a hollow tube left inside of the artery—reestablishes flow. This is done through a direct arterial puncture through the skin; 4) performing a carotid endarterectomy—an operative procedure in which direct exposure of the artery is achieved surgically. The vessel is opened and the atherosclerotic plaque is surgically evacuated.

There is simply no data that will allow a clinician to come to a clear, medically based recommendation. It is not for want of studies. There are dozens. They are conflicting, underpowered, from suspect sources, or relate to nonequivalent states. The literature, for a seventy-year-old with this moderate degree of obstruction, is too narrow in scope to answer specific questions that relate to the patient sitting across the room. Doctors who are trained to distrust their own experience and opinions may send you off for invasive exams reflexively, not reflectively. Some doctors become handmaidens to their consults. Others will do nothing while awaiting the next RCT.

Every doctor every day balances the benefits of avoiding a low-probability medical disaster against the immediate risks of an intervention that might prevent it. The way your doctor balances those risks is driven by experience and, even more importantly, by her beliefs about risk. There are no guidelines for this choice in a seventy-year-old.

Only a general belief born out of past, non-medical personal philosophical attachments and unrelated medical experiences will result in a chosen path. She will inform the family that she is giving an opinion that is her best advice. She can explain her philosophy regarding placing patients at risk for diseases they do not have and may never get when there is an absence of reliable data. Strong beliefs will color her every recommendation to you when the data is, as so often is the case, conflicting.

If your doctor has no dominating beliefs that bridge the frequent gap between data and action then you are in for a bumpy ride, as you will, over time, lurch from decision to decision.

Meetings: National and international conferences offer the opportunity to hear many opinions devoted to one condition. Academicians who have spent their professional lives studying a particular disease fight it out with their counterparts on conference room prosceniums. Some of these fights represent long-standing feuds between battle-scarred opponents from the New and Old Schools. They are more entertaining and cogent and have more potential to actually change practice than does reading their baffling

RCTs' methodologies. These exchanges, however heated, are based on evidence, experience, and the wisdom that make these professors mentors and role models.

Intuition: When your doctor doesn't have the luxury of time you want one who "listens to his gut." An article published in 2009 portrayed it as either a feeling of alarm that says "Something's wrong. Something doesn't fit," even when a tentative diagnosis has been made or, in contrast, a sense of reassurance that says "Everything seems to fit," even in the face of continued uncertainty.[33] Ask your doctor about the role of intuition. Confident doctors will not be afraid to admit to it. Diffident doctors will deny its role in decision making. No doctor should rely solely on intuition but every doctor uses it. There is too much uncertainty in medical practice to deny its usefulness. Daniel Kahnemann won a Nobel Prize in part for his work on decision making. In his Nobel Prize autobiography he wrote, "I am now very impressed by the observation . . . that the most highly skilled cognitive performances are intuitive, and that many complex judgments share the speed, confidence and accuracy of routine perception."[34]

Old School Weaknesses

Some feel that as knowledge increases there comes a time when new information is neither sought after nor felt needed. It is at this point that creativity and innovation taper off. This curse is embedded in the Samuel Johnson trope, "The chains of habit are too weak to be felt until they are too strong to be broken."

Some medical observers have suggested just that. And they paint a convincing portrait of Old School benchwarmers who are satisfied working from their outdated databases. These studies suggest that the longer doctors are from training the worse their performance.[35, 36] Defects in basic medical knowledge, adherence to accepted guidelines, poor performance, and more untoward clinical outcomes suffered by patients were associated with a doctor's age in dozens of studies. I have already noted that age does not confer experience and is not a proxy for wisdom. It may be that some Old Schoolers cocoon themselves from new knowledge by wrapping themselves in a cloak of experience and wisdom. They continuously tap into an endless repository of stale, outdated heuristics and fossilized anecdotes that now, frozen in habits' amber, make up their limited repertoires. Whatever problems EBM suffers, doctors must be current on New School literature—recognizing its weaknesses as well as acknowledging its strengths.

Be wary of the doctor who goes on and on about a case he saw, a therapy he pulled from his hat, or a diagnosis made on a whim, or who frequently and self-reverentially points to his long experience and keen intuition. Even older doctors must either get their "tech on" or just move on.

Ultimately the warm embrace of the Old School's perfumed and yielding arms is the only place an ignorant or lazy doctor can find a home or use quackery as an excuse. Experience does not trump evidence nor do anecdotes exclude analysis. The Old School benefits from its inclusiveness but suffers from its lack of filters. It understands the wisdom of others but underestimates the dangers of individual folly. It values wisdom but bows to "group think." And finally, while accepting the unique, it risks lending credence to a rule's exception.

Textbooks and Informal Sources of Knowledge: It is sad to note that textbooks and "humans" (*any* contact with a colleague) are seen as helpful. It's even more alarming to note that these information sources are not only used more frequently, they're also the most valued. A 2007 review of almost three dozen previous studies that rated doctors' research preferences documented that two-thirds of them ranked textbooks first and human contacts second. Electronic sources and the Internet were distant third and fourth choices.[37] The authors noted that doctors' information technology knowledge and skills were shockingly poor—52 percent had never even heard of the largest evidence-based repository, the Cochrane collaborative. Many doctors are as likely as you to go right to Google.

What image is more iconic than that of a doctor standing in his library viewing the contents of his bookshelves? He reaches for that single textbook he knows will help him on a clinical quest. Blowing the dust from its cover, he sits, opens its pages, and gains wisdom.

Nice, right? Well, no. Outdated and outmoded, the textbook to adherents of the New School is as relevant as parchments from ancient Alexandria's library. And they're right. Information changes too rapidly, new approaches to old diseases arrive daily, and older notions have been found inferior to newer ones. By the time your doctor reads the information much of it is out-of-date.

Textbooks are remnants of a past age. They are fine for scholars and students, but for doctors they stopped being relevant over twenty years ago. A doctor who routinely pulls out a textbook or mentions references to them, even for the most basic issues, is one you are no longer safe with.

In the 2007 study referenced above, the "humans" doctors valued were not always experts—almost anyone who was available fit the bill. This too is dangerous. Yes, experts and experience count—but they must be sought after in places other than the doctor's cafeteria. It is unfortunate that most patients when looking for health-care information use unfiltered Internet resources and general search engines. That this is true for many doctors as well is frightening. Either the Old School has roots too deeply embedded in doctors' psyches or the New School has failed through its arrogance and pretense to take root anywhere in contemporary clinical practice.

YOUR SCHOOL

Medical academicians will argue forever amongst themselves about the value of evidence versus experience. But your own doctor can't allow this dialectic to rage even for a moment when the time is short and the odds are long.

Some doctors have made peace with one or the other school. Others have forged unique philosophies that bridge this Manichean divide. But, for *your* purposes, it's more important that you be able to recognize where your doctor stands on the issues that will determine the tenor and quality of your care.

If you see a New School doctor and experience a problem, you may suffer while the EBM juries are out. You may be in for a long wait with a condition that won't. On the other side of the divide you may have a problem that's leaving you "up in the air." You'll choose the experienced pilot over the aeronautical theorist every time. But that pilot may be an Old School daredevil flying by the seat of his pants. Your doctor should neither a daredevil nor ditherer be. So in the end what matters most is whether your doctors use a database or a divining rod.

If you want to prevent cardiovascular disease and have no risk factors will you get reassurance, a CT angiogram, aspirin, a statin, or folic acid?

You've had a small heart attack. Will you be treated with medication? Which ones? Or will you get a cardiac catheterization and a stent? Will it be a metal or drug-eluting stent? Will you get a coronary artery bypass graft? Will it be at your local hospital or the heart hospital fifty miles away? What screening and prevention technologies will be advised? Which will be discouraged?

Will your doctor obey the "seven-year rule"? It warns that any new drug should be avoided for seven years if there are tried-and-true alternatives. That's how long it takes to assure its safety.[38] Or will you always be the first on your block with the latest and greatest?

Will you be given *any* treatment at all if you have depression, osteopenia, chronic fatigue syndrome, fibromyalgia, Alzheimer's, arthritis, and even some cancers?

Where are your doctor's perimeters beyond which she will not venture without consultative back up? Within these perimeters, what are her parameters? These define the limits of what she will or will not do when investigating a problem. If her perimeters are too easily reached, or her parameters are too limited, you'll become grist for the medical-care mill earlier than necessary. Regardless of where your doctor's thresholds lie, you need your own independent databases to verify that any recommendation is within your own comfort zone. You need these databases to verify every opinion you are given.

When people were asked where they would first go for health information, 49% said their doctors. They really went to their computers. Only 10% first consulted their physician.[39] Don't be ashamed. Just be careful. It's a jungle out there. Between 40% and 60% of all Internet users look for health information online and 75% use the results in decision making.[40] You use the Internet for medical answers more than magazines (30%), television and books (26%) and even more than your own family (40%). I hope the information you're getting is trustworthy. The chances are it's not because 70% of you use general web content. General medical search engines are polluted with spam, and many may be collecting your personal data. The Center for Digital Democracy (CDD) filed with the Federal Trade Commission in 2010 because of these intrusions. Consumers seeking medical information online were profiled, tracked, and served up advertisements and other content based on their searches. Social media conversations may be monitored by health and drug marketers. The CDD accused pharmaceutical and health marketing companies of promoting phony word-of-mouth campaigns to drum up sales. Those free online newsletters may not be just offering information. They may be gathering information too, yours.

Only trusted and trustworthy medical knowledge repositories make your questions sophisticated and focused. Their answers become more nuanced and complete and subject to later verification. Ill-chosen databases demote you and your questions and make independent decisions dangerously misinformed.

Almost 90 percent of you use Google to search for health information online.[41] If so, then "buckle up everyone, it's going to be a bumpy ride." After you've entered your question and hit "search," Google's net is cast far, wide, and deep. That net's mesh and the sophistication of your MeSH (acronym for Medical Subject Heading—a formalized dictionary for medical search diagnoses) determine how many millions of pages percolate up in response to a single inquiry. According to criteria established by *JAMA* for a website's accuracy (authorship, references, currency, and disclaimers), only 6 percent of the top 100 websites produced by a Google medical search diagnosis met all four criteria.[42] So, enter "breast cancer" and think about the reliability of all the pending information while you're waiting the 0.17 seconds it takes to bring the *42 million* responses to your screen. It's an eye-popping, jaw-dropping spectrum. From nursing sites to those nursing grudges. From people whose pets have breast cancer to others with pet peeves about breast cancer. Even breast cancer community sites are populated by some who are out-of-date, out-of-step, out of their minds, or out to make a buck. This cyberscat makes you a subordinate—a third party to your own care. No longer part of the equation, you're now the passive recipient of others' calculations. Google's search algorithms change as mysteriously and frequently as do your fortunes on Wall Street.

Searching a symptom (cough, dizziness, headaches, etc.) remains a dangerous way to get advice–better your Bubbe than Google. In 2010, disease searches have become somewhat helpful. Google Health, MedLine Plus and the Mayo Clinic are amongst the first URLs on view. The other first page choices remain an ad cluttered, Wikipedia infested mess. No, general search sites are not for you.

Sending Google to Medical School: You can turn Google into a sophisticated medical search engine. Only then can it be a first stop for a second opinion. People who Google medical issues are not asking questions, they are not even seeking answers. They are increasingly just asking Google what they should *do*. When Google becomes a specialist, it's transformed into a one-stop shopping mall for many of the best, authoritative medical database portals.

First use medical diagnostic terms. An example: You've just received the devastating news that you have breast cancer. Your doctor tells you (or you are forced to ask) what type of breast cancer it is. It turns out that you have a ductal carcinoma in situ (DCIS). DCIS accounts for 30 percent of all breast cancers. That's your search diagnosis, and a controversial one too. Some medical authorities don't think this should even be *called* a cancer. It's obvious then you've got work to do!

Google "breast cancer": 42,000,000 hits.

Google "ductal carcinoma in situ": 600,000 hits.

You've just blown away almost 99 percent of the stuff you didn't want and never needed. It's still way too much.

Searching with Suffixes: Turn Google into your Doctor Uncle Sam by adding the suffixes that bring the Feds right to your window.

Search for "ductal carcinoma in situ.pubmed" and get 290,000 hits for PubMed, a branch of the National Library Medicine (NLM). Or try one of the following:

.gov: 130,000 hits from various governmental health agencies;

.nih: 64,000 hits from the National Institutes of Health;

.cdc: 23,000 hits from the Centers for Disease Control (CDC).

You want it all to be current information, so continue your suffixation by adding the current year:

.nlm 2010: 8,100 hits, almost all from the National Library of Medicine published within the current year.

Say what you will about our government, but when it comes to health care—insuring it through Medicare, delivering it through the VA hospital administration, or informing the public about it, no one comes close. *No one.* And by changing the search terms we have gone from 42 million hits to 8,000 that are now trusted and carry the full faith and credit of our friendly Feds.

Don't be suffixally challenged. Add the suffix "nyt" and you will get the collections of the *New York Times'* estimable medical writers. Use the suffix "society," for professional societies. The suffix "foundation" brings you the foundations that study and fund research. The suffix .edu will filter through university sites. The suffix .org brings up nonprofit sites. Add "evidence-based" or "guidelines" to further refine your hits. The suffixes force the best medical specialty sites to percolate up while filtering off the spam that simmers just below the surface of your screen. During a general search, many of us go running as fast into Wikipedia as we would into a bank's ATM booth when we feel uncomfortable in a questionable neighborhood.

Don't get asphyxiated under the rubbish. Be sophisticated—get suffixiated. Medlineplus.gov is not just another .gov. It caters specifically to patients' information needs. The sources are reliable, current, and advertisement-free. The entries are written clearly and enjoy the benefits of heft, depth, and breadth. Medlineplus also contains current health news, a medical dictionary, and an encyclopedia. It offers links to medical libraries, organizations that provide disease-specific information, MEDLINE, the National Library of Medicine's database, and other countries' health databases.

The Health on the Net Foundation (http://www.hon.ch/MedHunt/) promises a code of conduct that helps standardize the reliability of medical and health information available on the Internet.

Patients.UpToDate.com (PUTD) is the hands-down, thumbs-up best free public domain site. Its information is regularly updated, generated by medical experts, and free from commercial bias. The thousands of articles offer a broad perspective on medical topics. PUTD offers a condition's biography, its life story, not just the single diary pages the previous websites place before you. The other homepages previously discussed offer long, seemingly endless, lists of articles that may, in the end, prove too disjointed, focused, or erudite, or that simply fail to deliver what you're looking for. PUTD doesn't offer thousands of journal articles to scan through. Instead it is a medical encyclopedia.

The bibliography offers more information about daily medical newspapers, monthly magazines, electronic textbooks, and selected websites that offer risk calculators and gateways to open-access medical journals.

Non-proprietary sites steer clear of controversy. This severely limits the amount and type of information you're allowed to see. It's the unresolved issues, however, that offer the best and most important opportunities to participate in decision making. It's only in debates that different opinions, including yours, count the most. When little is known, even less should be taken for granted. If you are unaware of the most current information, you may assume a matter is settled even though debates are seething and the grounds for action shifting. When you are aware of ongoing arguments, your doctors' actions and their responses to your questions pinpoint where they lie on a spectrum from overly reflective to overtly aggressive.

Proprietary medical sites are subscription-only services. They are most useful and the least expensive when obtained online. These databanks fly under the radar of the lay public. Medical journals range in their offerings from general medical topics to the most esoteric fields of genetics, biochemistry, and molecular biology.

To the laity, these sources are otherwise invisible and anonymous. Protected from your scrutiny, these publications are thought to exist for the cognoscenti alone. It's thought that journals are filled with arcane Masonic mysteries, are restricted to physicians, or are brutally expensive. They are available logistically, intellectually, and financially. I entered several proprietary sites and subscribed as a non-physician. The police did not arrive to handcuff me. I was not led out of my office with my raincoat over my head in the glare of news cameras, only to appear on the nightly news "perp walk" segment.

Free public medical domains do not inform the consumer when it is time to see a specialist. They do not provide information on the morbidity and mortality of invasive and noninvasive diagnostic tests. The specificity or sensitivity of diagnostic procedures are not offered or are incomplete. Informed consent wilts when tests' risks and benefits are not precisely spelled out. No intervention is 100 percent specific or sensitive. Diagnostics' interventions follow a sequence from the most accepted, safe, sensitive, and specific options, to the last-ditch efforts to establish a diagnosis that have none of the happy characteristics mentioned above. Only professional medical journals offer the proper sequencing of investigations. Therapeutics also follow a cascade from the most accepted "drugs of choice" to newer, more controversial, emerging agents whose effectiveness may be superior but for which there is less experience. Only professional literature outlines which therapeutic regimens to use when first-line medications fail or are ill-tolerated, or for which there are contraindications or drug interactions. Surgery and invasive diagnostics are often presented to you as the only possible approach. This is only occasionally the case. Access to the professional literature will first recommend safer alternatives and inform you when it's really time for more risky ventures. You won't get that on public access sites. We will learn that many things in medicinal practice are discretionary, elective, controversial, and sometimes ultimately avoidable. Your education will decrease unnecessary care while improving the chances of getting the timely delivery of appropriate interventions.

Public access sites provide lists. They may inform but they do not educate. The informed state is one in which you are being made aware of information gained by other people's education. It is preassembled, prescreened, and predigested. It is not the process by which knowledge is gained. The professional "subscription only" medical sites offer the possibility of an education. Education produces a critical faculty and the facility to employ it, so that answers to clinical questions are revealed in all their depth and nuance. On *Dragnet* it's Sergeant Joe Friday's "Just the facts ma'am." *Dragnet*, Internet—it's all the same. You get just the "facts" without their histories, mysteries, controversies, and boundaries.

Consider purchasing online access to a professional journal, or, failing the resources or commitment, know that there are free open-access medical publications and articles. Their sites hide in plain sight only to those who know how to find them.

We have addressed the issue of your doctors' sources for information. It is your turn. What do *you* know, how do you *know* it, and *where* did you go to learn it? If all you know is what your doctor and WebMD tell you, your interests are not being maximized. There is in medical care today no shortage of the commercial and the controversial. These are the most cogent arguments to go to get your own education. Sometimes the conclusions you reach independently will be in conflict with your doctors' recommendations and advice.

More often and most desirably you will use this education as the basis for a decision-making partnership with your physician. Knowing that there are *always* alternatives before setting off on a given diagnostic or therapeutic journey is better than finding out about them only after you have reached a dead end or worse, a disastrous denouement. The admission fee is surprisingly modest and allows access to original research, general literature reviews of important and common conditions, and current opinion on controversial ones. You can read case studies, editorials, and news updates from the front lines. Journals offer course material and videos that review and summarize the current state of a variety of common problems. Consensus views are outlined and algorithms are provided.

Homepages offer search engines and e-mail notifications custom-tailored to your interests. Articles relevant to your medical problems can be saved for future reference in a journal's archives. Information can be e-mailed to your family or doctors. These sites link you to hundreds of other similar information fonts and thousands of abstracts. You can do ad hoc searches after a doctor visit or prepare before you go. Research, reviews, searches, opinions, alerts, archives, and links do not confer mastery—just fluency.

The *New England Journal of Medicine*, a weekly online and print journal, is one of the most respected sources for current clinical and experimental information. It's equally important to be reading a journal that is in the vanguard of health-care opinion and practice. It is ninety-nine dollars a year for an online subscription. You will find medical research, review articles, case reports, online seminars, video, and editorials. This, of all the journals that will be mentioned here, will introduce you to technical jargon and the most circumscribed areas of investigation. Do as most doctors do—skip to the conclusion of studies that are of interest to you. Most issues have definitive review articles on chosen topics and search engines to explore its archives. No subscription? Searches on the homepage are free and some allow access to free full-text articles. You can request an e-mailed monthly table of contents which includes several free public-access articles. The same is true for all the following journals.

The *Annals of Internal Medicine* is $192 a year for monthly online access. This and the *Journal of American Medical Association* ($125) have more review articles and opinion pieces and tend to be more accessible for you (and us).

The *Journal of Family Practice* is eighty dollars. It is latitudinarian in scope and accessible to casual readers. Family physicians deal with the broadest range of topics in their practices and this is reflected in their literature. From pimples to pemphigoid, from familiar maternal fears to familial Mediterranean fever, the spectrum covers most issues of interest to you and your family. Its search engine is amongst the best. It links you to online medical encyclopedias, evidence-based medicine journals, and current clinical guidelines.

If you are seeking information for a recommended, but highly elective, surgical procedure, *The Archives of Surgery* is a good resource for $125 a year. You can examine articles related to any surgery. The fee seems a small price to pay when facing an invasive therapeutic or diagnostic intervention. Any given surgery's indications, risks, benefits, morbidity and mortality rates, recovery time, and alternative nonsurgical or minimally invasive approaches require more than the time allowed during a consultation with a surgeon. These consultations are subject to economic, educational, geographic, language, and class biases, to mention only a few. You need trusted dispassionate resources before such important decisions are made or an individual surgeon is chosen. Some surgeries are best done in specialty hospitals; other minimally invasive techniques may not be available locally and, therefore, may not be discussed. Surgeons—honest and skilled—routinely underestimate the risks and recovery time for their interventions.

The gold standard for medical reference is UpToDate.com. This site is not a periodical. It's an online subscription encyclopedia for doctors. All articles offer literature reviews and make consensus recommendations. The references for opinions are cited and can be further investigated by exploring their links with a simple click. UpToDate deserves its name. The topics are timely and are updated frequently. The reviews can be arcane but are more typically accessible. Most end with a suite of recommendations and a summary of current opinion. This is an expensive site at $440 per year. The expense may, for you, be unacceptable. UpToDate is simply the most useful and accessible point-of-care reference in the English language.

For a group subscription, UpToDate can serve as a less expensive access point and axis point around which medical information is shared and evaluated. UpToDate.com offers an all-important all-access one week pass for twenty dollars. Later in this book I will show you how a twenty-dollar transaction on UpToDate may save your life or point the way to care so rare that neither you nor your own doctor even know that it exists.

Or just pay ninety-nine dollars for a year for Journal Watch (jwatch.org). Sign up for weekly e-mail alerts in four primary care and nine specialty care areas. Take advantage of the summaries and insights on twenty key medical topics.

Living in the digital age means that nothing needs to be taken for granted and no action should be taken on faith alone.

It is now time for an Old Testament admonition: "Behold I set before you today a blessing and a curse" (Deuteronomy 11:26). We have discussed the blessings in detail. You will, however, be subjecting yourself to confusion, anxiety, misinterpretations, and a case of advanced cyberchondria. The temptation to call your doctor more than would be tolerated is guaranteed. Receiving a body of knowledge that was never really meant for you is prone to its hazards. There is no reason to avoid these potential pitfalls. The benefits of access to your personal database and your doctor's professional databases far outweigh the risks. But the curse of being subjected to information glut and technobabble will be frustrating. Seeing the five-year mortality statistics for your disease will be unsettling. The danger of self-diagnosis is raised here. Worse yet is self-therapy. It has been demonstrated that medical concerns were *reduced* in 90 percent of readers who used authoritative sources.[43] It is best to use these resources for problems that have been diagnosed by your doctor rather than for conditions you think you may be suffering. Trying to be a doctor by reading his or her journals leads to the same disastrous results as thinking yourself a pilot because you own a flight manual.

The alienation of your doctor is also a possibility. You're all grown up now and you are not peeking at dad's mail. You can inform your doctor of your intention to subscribe to a periodical. Obtain his impression—not his permission. He will be correct when he tells you that misunderstandings and anxieties will arise. At best you will be a highly informed, appropriately confused, and somewhat skeptical consumer of medical advice—at worst, a nervous wreck.

And If You Act Right Now: But wait, there is more! If a subscription is not in your future, let's refer you to all the free stuff.

JAMA and all the Archives (Internal Medicine, Surgery, Dermatology, General Psychiatry, Pediatrics and Adolescent Medicine, Otolaryngology, Head and Neck Surgery, Ophthalmology, and Facial Plastic Surgery) offer free full-text articles six months to a year after they publish their original research articles. PLoS, the public library of medicine, has its open-access site, PLoSmedicine.org.

Shibboleths

A shibboleth is a tool to identify the practices of people within a group. Whether it's a peculiarity of pronunciation, a behavior, or a manner of conduct, a shibboleth distinguishes a particular class or set of persons from others. The word arises from Judges 12:4-6. The Gileadites used their pronunciation of the word "shibboleth" (a stream of water) to test fleeing enemy Ephraimites, who pronounced it as a more sibilant "sibboleth." This dialectical alternative did not bode well for them. They were then slaughtered "forty and two thousand." Language proved the difference between life and death. So it is with medical shibboleths. Your doctor's responses to carefully chosen questions will be weighed using "Your School" to help identify her school. These inquiries pinpoint the databases she uses or rejects and her threshold for testing that will influence your care in every clinical scenario. In other words, now moving to the New Testament, "Ye shall know them by their fruits" (Matthew 7:16).

The toughest decisions in medicine also carry the greatest importance. It's important that a patient's fear of harm must be in line not only with its severity but also with how probable that harm will be and the price that must be paid to avoid it. Your doctor's approach and response to inquiries over PSAs and mammographys are precisely those types of problems and are relevant to every man and woman under a doctor's care. Your doctor's answers reveal his willingness to use information that is still not verified by RCTs or his unwillingness to proceed without them. You'll need the reference material in "Your School" to determine if a doctor's answers are only bowing to a popular treatment of uncertain benefit or if he is guilty of bucking a trend based on a single article or a singular attitude. That's the rationale for shibboleths.

It's better to find out what kind of doctor you have now while you're in the office than later while you are fighting for your life.

The Cancers That Dare Not Speak Their Names: Not all breast and prostate cancers pose a threat. Some pose only minimal risk. The types that pose little threat are the cancers that "dare not speak their names." Laura Esserman and colleagues[44] have suggested that these cancers be renamed. Because once the word "cancer" is heard patients are understandably willing to sign up or lie down for anything. A follow-up alone approach is unthinkable. Despite this, the harms of screening technologies are not appreciated until patients face their complications, expense, anxiety, and finally the diagnosis and therapy of a cancer "that dare not speak its name" and the lifetime of surveillance that follows. Esserman suggests that a diagnosis of IDLE (indolent lesions of epithelial origin) replace ductal carcinoma in situ for "breast cancer" and that a different clinical approach might mirror its now less threatening name. The same is true for prostate "cancers." These lesions may be local areas of severe cellular changes that were never destined to cause harm. Eighty percent of post-mortem exams of men in their seventies spot these innocent microscopic curiosities. If they were diagnosed in their lifetimes they would have faced surgery, chemical castration, or radiation. Better tests are needed to distinguish cancers that threaten from those that frighten. Until then you need to balance your fears against your welfare. Overdiagnosis and unnecessary therapy are epidemic. In 2010 H. Gilbert Welch and William Black concluded that 25 percent of breast cancers detected on mammograms and about 60 percent of prostate cancers detected with prostate-specific antigen (PSA) tests could represent overdiagnosis.[45] That's why the shibboleths we use are the mammogram and prostate talks. These best show whether your doctor is aware of important issues and can discuss subtleties clearly.

Here's an example of a mammogram shibboleth:

Your doctor gives you a brochure and says "Please read this brochure. We will discuss it on your next visit and act according to your wishes."

He continues, "You are facing the doors to two rooms. In room one there are 2,000 women age 39–49 who do not wish to have mammography. Six cancers will occur in a ten-year period and there will be one preventable death for those in this room.

Room two has 2,000 women age 39–49 who *do* wish to have mammography. Six cancers will occur in a ten-year period but there will be NO preventable deaths.[46, 47]

If someone wishes to go from room one to room two the price for prevention must be paid. The price is the cost and inconvenience for the mammographys. Another price is the fifty-fifty chance that a woman's mammogram will be incorrectly interpreted during that ten-year period, leading to more irradiation, anxiety, and expense. There must be recognition of the fact that there will be over 300 biopsies performed in that group of 2,000 in room two and although they will prove negative for cancer, severe anxiety, and more irradiation and expense will result. The last price that's necessary to pay in order to eliminate that one death amongst the 2,000 in room one is the fact that one-third of the surgeries that take place will be, in retrospect, unnecessary—the result of the overdiagnosis and overtherapy.

Please think about these issues. On your next visit we will discuss your feelings and reach a mutual decision."

That's it. That's the issue and those are the tradeoffs. The "two room" scenario is accurate, clear, concise, and accessible. Other doctors will come up with their own examples. But because it is 100 percent certain that *some* discussion will be needed, your doctor better come prepared to talk with you about it in a way that is understandable. If she isn't prepared you're in trouble and will always be in trouble when clear communications are key and decisions are needed. The discussion for older women only requires small changes in this "two room" scenario.

The Prostate-Specific Antigen (PSA) Shibboleth: What's a boy to do? The public not only accepts the need for PSA blood tests, they expect it. PSAs have become a de facto rite of passage for men over forty.

Despite this, the ability of PSAs to prolong life through the early detection of prostate cancer has been questioned for years. When it comes to PSAs, the American Cancer Society, the American Urologic Association, the US Preventive Services Task Force and the National Comprehensive Cancer Network agree on only one thing—doctors and patients must discuss them prior to performing them.

Prostate cancer is both common (over 200,000 diagnosed each year) and harmful (30,000 deaths each year). In light of the possibility of early detection, PSAs are assumed to be necessary. Yet, just as for breast cancer, people often buy in to a preventive technology but unknowingly expose themselves to harm.

Any test or therapy must address seven elements that permit you to make a knowledge-based decision.[48] A discussion of what question the test seeks to answer, the uncertainties that exist over its efficacy, your role in decision making, alternative strategies that achieve the same goal, and the pros and cons of the suggested intervention. There also must be an inquiry regarding your understanding of the discussion, and your consent must be assessed, rather than assumed.

No man over forty should be denied the PSA talk. This is particularly true in light of several studies published in 2009 and 2010 that demonstrated a negligible to nil survival benefit for those who were screened with PSAs and who jumped on the bandwagon for all that followed when their levels were elevated. [49, 50, 51] The studies also revealed the high rates of overdiagnosis and overtreatment that lead to the potentially preventable devastating sequelae of impotence, urinary incontinence, and bowel dysfunction.

If men are made to think that the PSA is a safe, accurate, and effective method to prolong their lives, many, perhaps most, would accept some risk to avoid this feared disease. The fact is PSAs share none of these features.

Every prevention and screening technique balances on one side a great number of healthy people, many of whom will be placed in danger, against a very small number of people who actually benefit from it. When it comes to saying yes to prostate cancer screening, men must decide if they want to be amongst the 1,400 who get tested with PSAs and perhaps be one of the fifty who must suffer the effects of unnecessary invasive treatment and its attendant risk of debility and injury, so that *perhaps* one lone stranger (or you) will get to live longer. It is a cold calculus.

In light of this, it's particularly disappointing that few men are fully informed when they make their PSA decision. For many, no decision is needed—30 percent had PSAs drawn without their knowledge, much less a discussion. In a 2009 study its authors noted that only 1 in 5 men were presented with the pros and cons for PSAs and fewer than half were asked about their preference.[52] Half of those who accepted PSAs walked out of the office unable to answer *any* of three prostate knowledge questions.

The driving force for a patient's acquiescence to testing is the doctor's recommendation that it be done. Seventy-five to eight-five percent of doctors recommend it to their patients and 80 percent of men march off for it. If you have a doctor who even discusses a PSA with you, rather than just ordering one for you, you're already ahead of the game. If, however, you are part of a conversation that fulfills the elements of an informed consent and can then reach an educated decision, whatever it may be, you're with a doctor who is amongst a rarefied few who recognize that you cannot take risks without a complete understanding of what you're getting into. This attitude will be repeated in every clinical dilemma.

The PSA shibboleth is less about the actual facts of PSA screening than it is about the quality of the dialogue that precedes it. So should you get a PSA? My law firm "Lizer/Hassholf" forbids me from offering advice.

Every pill you take and every condition you suffer is subject to controversy. Using "Your School," you will be able to form your own shibboleths.

That's what shibboleths are all about—they distinguish your doctors from others and ensure that your doctor has both a receptive attitude and the cognitive aptitude that merits your trust and care. If your doctor doesn't measure up, you have time to find one who does. Because when it's your turn to be sick—time's up.

II

A MEDICAL DAY

1

The Office

- What is it that doctors *do* all day anyway?
- The myths of "Long waits for appointments = Good doctors" and "Waiting for Doctor Wonderful."
- Medicine as a business—it's your business too.
- How to judge a doctor by her office. When to run for the exits.
- The dangers of being a patient in a solo or a mega-multispecialty practice.
- The preferred office-based delivery system.
- Why do doctors spend most of their time caring for you *before* and *after* your visit and so little time *during* it?
- Patients—the necessity of your company, the complexity of your company, the burden of your company.
- Doctors are increasingly shrugging off traditional medical responsibilities. When does the delegation of duties become a dereliction of duties?
- The role of nurse practitioners and physician assistants—what to expect and what to reject.

We will begin by reviewing doctors' daily dilemmas, routines, and obligations. Even with these legion responsibilities, your doctor shouldn't be forgiven for personal lapses nor judged less severely if she succumbs to self-pity. Sometimes doctors are so busy posing as stricken victims of their heavy schedules that patients tolerate levels of frustration, anger, and even poor results that they might reject out of hand in other transactions. Even when your doctor is more like Dr. Gregory House than Dr. Marcus Welby you still accept it as your due and push on bravely.

31

We must approach our duties with enthusiasm. Our days always begin and end with these assignments. These nonclinical, unreimbursed responsibilities include serving as the referee for staff disputes; sitting in on the myriad meetings with vendors, consultants, and advisors; listening to the preening and keening of the physician staff; chasing away the salespeople and medical office hangers-on who congregate in our public and clinical areas; inspecting workstations; and performing departmental quality assessment reviews.

I will never forget all the hair I pulled out completing the official documents sent to me from insurance companies and various federal, state, and municipal governmental bodies. Their agencies, bureaus, official bodies, governing deliberative boards or review committees demanded patients' data and demographics. The verification of compliance with workplace safety, health codes, privacy mandates, and environmental safeguards were only a pinhole view into a firmament of factual data that had to be delivered on deadlines. The adjudication of the complaints from employee performance reviews; the daily banking and overhead reports; the obligatory six to twelve self-flagellatory apologies made throughout the medical community for transgressions known, unknown, or now forgotten; the "No you can't observe a physical examination; you are our handyman, for God's sake"; hiring, firing, and acting as a lawyer, confessor, doctor, father, taskmaster, and big brother to our dozens of staff.

These duties should be treated as a part of our days, not interruptions in them. If, however, they are treated as chores or obstacles, they become obstacles indeed—to success. This success can elevate the personal and professional lives we lead and, more importantly, ensure the care you expect and deserve. There are ways your doctor can lower her stress level, open her schedule, sneak in a lunch to reboot, and fidget less during your time together.

Daily duties and stressors paradoxically confer a patina of status that only serves to institutionalize deficiencies. For example, it's commonly thought that there is a correlation between the length of time it takes to obtain an appointment and the quality of the doctor you're waiting for. Some doctors buy into this notion and even revel in it. Disingenuously, they complain about their schedules, but do nothing to address the failures that keep them hopping and you waiting. For me the Yogi Berra trope, "the place is so popular nobody goes there anymore," should apply. If a doctor's waiting list for a non-elective visit is greater than two to three weeks, or, for an emergency, more than a few hours, then he should not be your doctor. This phenomenon of "Waiting for Dr. Wonderful" is a fallacy. It's said, "If you have a dog who won't come when called, you don't have a dog." If you have a doctor who won't see you when you call, you don't have a doctor. The fallacy that your doctors are so busy and so care-worn by the many demands thrust upon them—as if they had no choice in the matter—leads to the attitude that you better get in that long line and wait your turn. After all, your doctor is too busy reaching into the void to retrieve patients from their own "event horizons" that border on mortality's black hole. Your heartburn can wait.

This view is further foisted on you by the behavior of the suffering servants' office staff. Just being in his presence should be met with humble and Eucharistic rapture. If your doctor is so burdened by his responsibilities, so busy saving the more deserving, so clinically consumed, so lacking in comportment and calendrically challenged, then do him a favor, lessen his load and move on—it's a deal breaker.

You wait 15.5 days on average for a cardiology appointment, 17 days for an orthopedic surgery appointment, 22 days for a dermatology appointment, 27 days for an ob-gyn appointment, and 20 days for a family practice appointment.[1] Some offices force you to wait several months for an appointment. A few ask you to wait a year. In light of these figures you can determine where your doctors stack up.

Both Kathryn Montgomery and Jerome Groopman published books titled *How Doctors Think*, in 2006 and 2007, respectively. *I* wonder, more prosaically, "How Doctors Have Time to Think?" Doctors do not retreat to a cloister, charts in hand, to muse in abstract fashion about the human condition and their patients' conditions. Interpreting, integrating, and implementing the deluge of data that initiates or continues a clinical investigation is a process that occurs in real time. We respond to input immediately—literally on the fly.

There is no doubt that overextended clinicians make you suffer. Busy and burdened doctors become unhappy. Unhappy doctors can become sloppy. The inevitable medical errors will follow.

Understanding your doctor's daily dilemmas, routines, and obligations is a reasonable starting point for this section. By illustrating how overworked and unhappy a doctor can be, we show that a doctor who can divest herself of some of these obligations is acting in a pragmatic and responsible manner. There are many legitimate avenues available to doctors that allow them to both free up time in your service and enhance the quality of their own lives.

Some doctors, however, have already unburdened themselves using techniques that are harmful to you, ethically questionable, and ultimately impermissible if they are to continue with your care. They are abandoning you at the intersection of clinical responsibility and time management. They take the road that makes their schedules more humane for them, but leave you behind when you need them the most.

We will outline the techniques you can use to become better informed about your doctor. By eliminating the myth of busy doctor = good doctor, you will be better able to evaluate the kind of job your doctor is doing.

Medicine is a business—it's your business too. The list of our quotidian corporate cares may seem to you like dry, uninteresting, irrelevant issues. So what?! That's his problem! That's a reasonable assumption at first, but you must realize that your doctor's organizational and medical skills go hand in hand.

It's important to be familiar with how doctors initiate, organize, and maintain what first must be a business, and then what becomes a medical practice. We're going to teach you how to become a diagnostician of a medical office's strengths and weaknesses through a dissection and analysis of these protocols. This leads to an understanding of your doctors' priorities and strengths; or more sadly, the deficiencies that are reflected in your care.

Successful implementation of a tactical approach to each day leads to the realization of every good doctor's ultimate goal—the delivery of quality care to as many patients as her time and sanity allow.

When you call your doctor you may be happy to receive a 1:00 appointment but less than ecstatic when you finally trudge into the exam room two hours later, missing your children's 3:30 school bus or your 3:00 meeting with the boss.

Unlike airlines or hotels that bump you, a medical office will lump you and dump you. You will be squeezed into an inflexible schedule: you've been lumped. An unmanaged staff wants you out of the way and into a time slot: you've been dumped. It's no problem for them to schedule two patients more per hour than your doctor can handle. It then becomes your problem—and your doctor's. If a physician insists on three patients or ten patients an hour, she should tolerate no more. Overbooking is the failure of physician management or the victory of corporate goals over medical ones. Overbooked physicians, hours behind in the day, deny you the few minutes you expect and the attention you deserve. Manners are the first thing to suffer—the quality of care is the second.

Your doctor's schedule is the cumulative product of his staff's quality, priorities, morale, flexibility, and distribution of skills. All this presupposes his leadership, his demands for accountability, and his accessibility to the staff when guidelines cannot be realistically met.

The physical plan of the office will be conducive to your comfort . . . or not. It will be conducive to patient flow that is efficient, dignified, and private . . . or not. It will be conducive to a doctor's sense of substance, self, and style . . . or not. A calm environment may not lead to idle bucolic reflections, but it will at least avoid distractions and disorder, the handmaidens of medical error. What does the dirt and dust, the frayed yellow paper signs and dead plants, the stained carpets and littered exam rooms mean to you? More importantly, what do they say about your doctor? A lot. How can you tolerate this in a clinical setting? Why should you?

Only 30 percent of physicians' source materials for clinical information or its verification are available during office visits. Textbooks and journals are poorly organized and inadequately indexed. Up to two questions arise for every three patients seen. Forty percent of questions relate to medicinal side effects, 43 percent to medical opinion, and 17 percent to important non-medical logistical issues.[2]

Access to computers is a volitional organizational decision. If your doctor is not wielding a personal computer, Internet notebook, personal digital assistant, or smart phone—leave the office. Their absence implies a haphazard office management, and further, a lackadaisical approach to quality of care. Schedules, the surroundings you move in, and the presence of information technologies are all the result of organizational and fiscal decisions. A long wait, in unpleasant surroundings, culminating in a tentative or hedging response to your questions, may be reflective of a bad business as much as a bad doctor, or worse—both.

The list of medical office obligations may be boring for you but it better not be for your doctor. The unpleasant consequences that result from an office in disarray do not boomerang or backfire—they ricochet. You take the blow.

The speed with which an office staff can move down the evolutionary tree if the primate with the M.D. relinquishes these responsibilities, and fails to control her territory, is dazzling.

The problems an office poses to its physician-manager can be more complex and require more time than the illnesses and complaints that you present with. But, as noted, unless the office runs well, your problems may never be addressed in a timely, private, mannered, and thoughtful fashion. Your doctor's problems can become yours very quickly. The duties that are required are endless, repetitive, unreimbursed, and monumentally unappreciated. That's why so many doctors avoid them. For others these tasks inspire individual creativity, sharpen problem-solving skills, and permit a gratifying control over the work environment, the situations that arise within it, and the people who populate it.

The demands of running a medical practice are changing rapidly in the face of the radically altered medical demographics and the technologies that will continue to evolve over the next decade. The spectrum of practice models available to you now is almost unrecognizable from what was offered only twenty years ago. Those doctors who can adapt to changing circumstances and modify their working environments will look confidently to the next twenty years. You should not be getting 2008 care in 2011.

The Extinction of the Sole Practitioner: The single variable of electronic medical records (EMR), now a federal health-care goal and a purported proxy for high-quality care, will increase the trend, already under way, that shifts care from solo practitioners to group practices. While independent groups will survive, individual practitioners will not. In an aptly titled article, "The Independent Physician—Going, Going . . . ," that appeared in the *New England Journal of Medicine* in 2009, the authors note that "the percentage of U.S. physicians who own their own practice has been declining at an annual rate of approximately 2% for at least the past 25 years."[3]

The independent, self-confident, business-savvy risk takers who are willing to put in the bruising hours of a sixty- to eighty-hour work week, are a vanishing breed. As recently as fifteen years ago, half of the medical practices were single-operator, independent concerns; fewer than a fifth of such medical practices exist today. They cannot fulfill the administrative, financial, and clinical responsibilities of twenty-first-century medicine.

The Rise of Group Practices: While the private, single-specialty, three-to-eight physician group is preferred, the reality is that private multispecialty groups, and managed-care goliaths staffed by disengaged, salaried physicians and overseen by a professional managerial tier, are becoming the default option for most younger physicians. A sea change has occurred in the last three years; a 2010 report noted that hospital-owned practices now outnumber physician-owned clinics. According to a 2010 online "Physician Sentiment Index,"[4] an excessive focus on business and bureaucracy has 59 percent of physicians predicting that the quality of medicine will suffer over the next five years. Seventy-seven percent of doctors feel they spend too much time with payors and not enough time with patients.

Hospitals are hiring their own physician-staffers and establishing neighborhood offices. A 2010 report noted that 50 percent of all doctors hired directly from training are now employed by hospital-owned practices.[5] Just as your choice of specialists is limited in HMOs and multispecialty groups, so, too, will your choice of hospitals be limited when you are in one of these community outreach offices that are hospital satellites. The disconnect between the increasing size of practices and the decreasing choices of patients is beyond dispute.

Only a small number of principals can assure the maintenance of the office's principles. A practice should be the direct extension of the will of its owners. The intentions of its proprietors should be transparent. When too many doctors congregate as partners in a mega-multispecialty practice there will be no collective will or guiding philosophy.

The small, private, three-to-eight member physician single-specialty group is the preferred model for your care. Whether it's primary or specialty care you should seek out the smaller groups that offer only one specialty. Once you are a patient in one of these practices make sure that your care will not be divided between the clinicians but that it will be continuous with one of its members. Everywhere you journey in the medical world there should be doctors who identify you as *their* patient. Few patients, even those hospitalized, can even name their doctors, much less recognize them.

A group of eight cardiologists working together in one office functions better than eight cardiologists each practicing alone, and far better than eight cardiologists that are part of a 200-physician group offering multispecialty work in surgery, gastroenterology, rheumatology, etc. In a smaller single-specialty group there's no distant, detached corporation your doctor can hide behind, or point a finger toward.

You shouldn't have to deal with a monolithic corporate face or apathetic operator on the other end of a 1-800 number when you call to impotently register your complaints. When the care you receive at the office fails to meet your needs, you are the first to know. But you don't want to be the only one. At a small private medical group, deficiencies should become obvious to its owners almost as quickly as they do to you.

If you are not treated with respect, or your voiced complaints are not rectified by remedial actions or explanations, market forces (that's you) should weed out inefficient medical practices. Exercise your consumer powers and seek care elsewhere. Tell your friends about your experience. But managers of large groups or big-box HMOs are more insulated from feedback. They can thrive even in the face of failure.

Smaller, single-specialty groups will seek advice from only the best outside sources. If a medical practice is so large that it can afford its own in-house lawyers, business consultants, and accountants, you can be sure they are not the best available and that you are paying for their lunch.

More importantly, when doctors in that small, single-specialty group refer you to specialists, subspecialists, radiologists, pathologists, and laboratories, the *only* factors determining those referrals should be their quality, their demeanor, and their responsiveness to you and the referring physician. I am as responsible for your results as the subspecialists to whom I refer you.

Multispecialty groups have financial incentives that will keep you in-house for all testing and consults. They will pressure you to stay under their roofs with them. You should avoid this practice model if for no other reason than the following: No single building will *ever* contain within its walls the best of everything medical that your community can offer. Their less-selective hiring practices make this even more likely. Referrals for consultation and testing usually denote a problem that may be, or may become, serious. The reasons for the referral should have nothing to do with your doctor's profit-sharing plan. Keeping you in-house is rule one for multispecialty groups. Doctors in large groups may even refer you to colleagues they know or suspect are impaired in order to avoid referrals outside their building. This is even more of a problem in small solo or two-person groups. In 2010 it was demonstrated that 56 percent of physicians in solo or two-person practices "who were aware of an incompetent or impaired colleague failed to report that colleague."[6]

Smaller, private groups offer care that is more personalized. If you're in a waiting room and the sound of your voice echoes across a cavernous expanse, it may be time to move on. Likewise, the indignity of a receptionist hollering your name across this arena is intolerable. Neither a distinguished jurist nor a hard-working mason should have to suffer a shout of, "Bob— come to the front desk." Not even "Robert," but "Bob." Feel privileged that you're not "Bobby."

Single-specialty groups may offer specialty-appropriate in-house procedures. Endoscopy, dialysis, I.V. therapies, or minor surgery clinics offer flexible scheduling, convenience, ambience, and quality control. They will reflect the institutional persona of the medical office they are attached to.

In a small, single-specialty private practice, if your doctors identify that it's necessary to invest in a new technology or a patient-centered amenity, they need not convince, or receive permission from, partners in competing specialty departments within the group or an outside corporate entity or hospital board. Conflicting departmental needs and general financial constraints are barriers when many interests are vying for the same dollar. The perks associated with a professional management tier that requires catered lunches or junkets to seminars in Maui will not compete with *your* doctor's access to the best information systems and medical devices available.

In 2011 many of you will prepare to make the acquaintance of Accountable Care Organizations (ACO). This reimbursement model offers doctors and hospitals financial incentives to provide good-quality care to Medicare beneficiaries. The real emphasis is on cost controls. If an ACO cuts costs by a certain percentage below a benchmark, providers will receive extra payments. An ACO is just another way to spell HMO (the reviled and now defunct Health Maintenance Organizations). Although ACOs are designed to redistribute hospital and doctor incomes, they may also redistribute (decrease) your access to care, your choice of care, and the quality of that care. Doctors and hospitals currently get paid when they treat you. ACOs will provide incentives for them not to. How to protect yourself? Not in large multi-specialty groups. They will be the first to profit. In 2011 Health Affairs noted that ACOs will find that single specialty groups will be "as hard to absorb as gravel in the digestive tract."[7] It sounds like a single-specialty group is a good place for you to hide out until the dust settles.

Finally, physicians are happier in small private practices. Happier physicians offer you better clinical outcomes. Clinical depression rates run from 9.7 percent to 27 percent for doctors. It was reported in 2011 that 1 in 16 surgeons reported suicidal ideations in the previous year.[8] Suicide rates are 40 percent higher in male doctors than in the general population and over 100 percent higher for women physicians. I have been close with five doctors who have killed themselves. How many people do you know who have gone this route? Fewer, likely. Eighty percent of general practitioners score positively for high stress levels. But despite the fact that the hours are longer and the demands are greater, studies unfailingly demonstrate greater professional satisfaction and higher quality of life indices for those in private practice as compared to managed-care, HMO, or big-box clinics.

However, if your doctor is a poor manager your experience will be the photographic negative of the attributes mentioned above. You will quickly recognize it and correctly assume that it reflects as poorly on his medical abilities as it does his medical management talents. Time for you to move on.

Smaller, more personal, single-specialty practices ask more of their doctors than larger multi-specialty groups that can, and indeed must use a professional management tier. That is why greater numbers of physicians are choosing to avoid the business burdens and instead are migrating to the relatively cloistered, salaried positions in government, hospitals, the pharmaceutical industry, universities, the military, big-box clinics, and private or publicly held, large multi-specialty groups.

Other doctors are making end runs around the work, and the woes, of medical offices' business demands. They create new office paradigms (boutique practices, cash-only policies, refusal of Medicare and other carriers deemed intrusive to their days) that eliminate much of their daily scheduling, telephone, staffing, reimbursement, and insurance hassles.

Good for them; bad for you. In the attempt to avoid business worries, many of these paradigms cater to the wealthy or leave you without doctors who will accept your insurance plans.

Two decades ago, the top ten insurers covered about 27 percent of all insured Americans. Today, four companies—WellPoint Inc., UnitedHealth Group, Aetna Inc., and Cigna Corp.—cover more than 85 million people, almost half of all those with private insurance. As a result, doctors and hospitals have little negotiating power and few options when an insurer rejects a bill.

In 2008, 29 percent of Medicare beneficiaries looking for a primary care doctor had a problem finding one to treat them, up from 24 percent the year before.[9]

The desire to move away from business and management skill sets that are foreign to many of us is understandable. But there's another reason for the shift. Many doctors are now seeking out these sanctuaries to escape the onerous clinical duties for which they have been perennially responsible. Doctors are now employing physician extenders and initiating previously unheard-of practice models. But there are some patient-related therapeutic responsibilities that cannot be safely delegated. Unfortunately, some mandatory clinical obligations are, for some doctors, now thought of as optional. These flights of physician fancy are flights from responsibility. Some clinical responsibilities are immutable, whatever temporal, financial, physical, or psychological burdens they carry.

We previously referred to the increased business demands that have culled the herd of lone physicians. Now there's a new threat decimating their numbers: actual *clinical* duties.

But what *are* the clinical commitments that are chasing doctors from traditional roles? There are three factors, each of which increases the burdens on the other two.

1. In a solo practice the volume of patients needed to sustain its sole practitioner is becoming logistically, financially, and emotionally impossible to maintain. The demands of the chronically ill are too onerous for the solo or micro-group practices. Thus, mega-groups are born. They allow techniques that dilute the one-on-one contact most of you have previously experienced with your doctors.

2. The burgeoning volume of information emerging from the biosciences requires a commitment to mastering new advances. There is no room at the table for the jack-of-all-trades. Medical problems compel you to be shuttled off to those specialists who can devote the time to technologies and information bases specific to their fields. Proficiency in new, more complex tasks, expanding pharmacopoeias, newer invasive techniques, and diagnostic technologies require your old and trusted family doctors to back off and leave you to those best able to advise. In light of the complexity of clinical challenges these specialists, many of whom fancy themselves scientists, often take over your care. Your family physicians, general practitioners, and general internal medicine doctors are increasingly in the dark and marginalized when it comes to your status and progress. Not only have business concerns driven them away, now the clinical ones have, too. If you're healthy they'll treat you. Get sick and you get packed off. You've become too complicated for their care.

3. Not only are your clinical needs more complicated, they generate more data. Much of it is wasteful and the rest arrives in such torrents that it simply can't be managed. The increasing number of patients per physician combined with more testing per patient results in an expanding penumbra of data that follows each patient with each visit. The data continues to flow unchecked between visits as well. The thousands of raw numbers, ratios, serum levels, genetic and immunologic markers, and acute phase reactants all need to be taken in. Try drinking from a fire hose.

Does all the testing make your care better? No. It's more likely to decrease your time with your providers, who, inundated with your lab values and testing results, don't have time for you. So now we see larger groups with more doctors who are less responsible and responsive to you. They are backing away from their individual clinical responsibilities to you by sharing them with more professional and para-professional "prescribers," "health-care professionals," and "providers." Let's deal with these three factors that face your doctor all day, every day:

1) LARGER MEDICAL GROUPS
(THE NECESSITY OF YOUR COMPANY)

With increasing competition, decreasing fees, and higher overhead, contemporary medical practices must increase their patient volume to offset some of these costs and generate new income. This in turn requires greater numbers of doctors.

Larger groups decrease the burden of night, weekend, and holiday call—a benefit that cannot be overestimated. The twenty-four-hour, on-call availability of your physicians carries a lot of psychological and physical costs that affect their clinical skills and your outcomes.

Further, lots of docs in a box can increase the number of specialties a practice offers, ensuring a steady flow of patients from one specialist to the next in the same office. An example of an income-generating specialty, and a service denied to all but sizable multi-specialty groups, is radiology. Ultrasounds, CAT scans, and MRIs and their multiple variants keep patients in the box and, through high levels of use, generate income. This, in turn, lowers the threshold for testing and increases blatantly unnecessary procedures. This is yet another reason to look for a smaller general or specialty practice that offers fewer on-site services. Although the big boxes are convenient, they are also yawning chasms whose debt service and profit imperatives must be seen to at all costs. And this translates into cost to you—both financial and physical. This conflict of interest is called physician self-referral. When you are sent for services owned by the ordering doctor you can never be sure of his motives, particularly when your pain becomes his gain. Large groups with many services have a lot to sell.

Physician self-referral for entire suites of diagnostic radiology testing accounts for most of the large recent upsurge in these services. MRI scans increased by 254 percent between 2000 and 2005 when ordered by physicians who profit from them.[10] When it comes to PET scans, non-radiologist-owned or leased scans grew by 737 percent between 2002 and 2007.[11] CAT scans saw a 263 percent increase between 2001 and 2006 for non-radiologist doctors who owned a machine.[12] When Dr. Phil T. Louker owns an MRI, a PET, or a CT, you're several times more likely to get one and suffer any of their many potential harms.

If you are a patient in the clinic that has a 64-slice CAT scanner, you should be aware that it takes 3,000 studies to pay off its one-million-plus-dollar tab.[13] This machine can, when used to perform CT angiography, screen healthy asymptomatic patients for unsuspected heart disease. This is an easy way for a clinic to get to that magic number, 3,000. There is no convincing evidence that this test provides benefit and, indeed, there is excellent evidence that it adds to your risk. Each scan, delivering the equivalent of up to 600 chest x-rays, increases your lifetime risk of cancer.

The risk, small but real, should make you think twice when, to your doctor, your heart doesn't go "lub dub" but rather "ca ching." CT angiography can double a cardiologist's income.

Despite Medicare's attempt to stop payments for these CT studies when performed for screening purposes, vigorous lobbying efforts prevailed. Expect the thousands of hospitals and hundreds of clinics that today own this cash register to multiply in the years ahead. Expect as a result more unnecessary cardiac catheterizations, coronary artery stents, angioplasties, deaths, and cancer—all in the service of finding a problem you don't have, won't get, or that could have been prevented, diagnosed, and treated in a far safer fashion.

Beware the doctor with a machine! Remember Finagle's Law, which states that "inanimate objects are out to get you." Use your sources (see "Your School" chapter). It is important to note that CTAs are valuable in those patients who suffer known coronary artery disease or who have acute chest pain in the emergency room setting. But the hard, undeniable fact is that a physician who offers you a service from which he profits raises doubt as to its necessity. This problem has led to a 2010 initiative to study the effect of physician self-referral for advanced medical imaging.[14] Unlike many other services, your physician is allowed to refer you for radiological services from which he profits. As of 2011, it is mandatory that doctors who refer Medicare patients to imaging machines they own disclose this fact in writing and provide a list of alternative sites that provide the same service.

Medical necessity is a very subjective affair, easily influenced by non-medical considerations that become more acute the larger the practice and the greater the number of specialty services it offers. The best outcome is when you are the one to profit medically from a procedure, not your doctor financially. You should research the motives and validity behind the choice of any drug, device, or treatment. Access to trusted impartial medical databases is of inexpressible value. They will inform you about the correct sequencing for tests, x-rays, technology, and therapies when it becomes necessary to confirm a doctor's advice by subtracting profit motive from clinical decision making.

A clinic that offers the identical services performed by a hospital is different from a specialty group or hospital that offers only the services its doctors are trained to perform. A cardiology group that offers stress tests is desirable—a cardiology group offering mammograms is not. Some very large multi-specialty medical groups would rotate your car's tires if they could. This is fine if everything they offer is needed and is of the best quality that a community offers. But each of these suppositions alone is dubious, and together, almost an impossibility. The human herding instinct is not always healthy when doctors make up the herd.

2) THE CRUSH OF MEDICAL TECHNOLOGY
(THE COMPLEXITY OF YOUR COMPANY)

"It takes a Medtropolis": High physician population density in a clinic allows for better communication and coordination. Broader spectrums of specialists are available for immediate consultation and advice. It takes a clinic to support a cardiac electrophysiologist. Evolutionary history confirms that people have a natural drive to congregate. Clinics, just like cities, are more interesting places to work, talk, share, and experience the crosscurrents that play out in a variegated community. Congregate medical facilities, like cities, decrease direct exposure to the elements via the mutual protection provided by other doctors and the creation of barriers to outside intrusion. In a medical practice the elements are *you*.

There is undeniable good in this. The explosive life-science breakthroughs make even subspecialists unequal to the task of being up to speed on every issue, much less mastering them. It may take a village to raise a child, but it takes a Medtropolis to appraise a patient.

New medications—their modes of action, novel delivery systems, side effects, warnings, drug interactions—and the monitoring necessary to safely administer them is only one "bullet point" in the spectrum of change in medical sciences. The advances that are overtaking rheumatology, oncology, gastroenterology, cardiology, and surgical subspecialties are so stunning that many subspecialists can't hope to keep abreast of them. They can't develop new skills and techniques fast enough; nor do they have at their disposal the patient populations large enough to implement these new techniques. And, except in the largest medical practices, they certainly can't amass the volume of cases that are needed to confer experience and expertise. This, in turn, leads to increasing referrals to tertiary care centers, or the self-reverentially named "centers of excellence." For example, only a small minority of kidney surgeons currently perform the newest, safest, and most effective surgery for renal cancer. These techniques allow the removal of only part of the affected kidney and are done with a minimally invasive laparoscopic technique. Donor kidneys can now be removed via a patient's bellybutton, leaving no scars. You won't find these services around the block at your solo kidney doctor's office.

Arguments such as these can be made for large clinics. There are others. The typical Medicare beneficiary sees two primary care physicians and at least five, but up to sixteen, subspecialists per year. In light of this, the potential benefits of a large multi-specialty group that has one record room, one pharmacy, one internal mail system, and one hospital to which it refers patients are noted. The resulting improvement in communication and the coordination of care will not overcome the poorer quality of care, overtreatment issues, and the interference of the profit motive, previously mentioned.

If you don't have the best doctor possible, are overtested and then overtreated as you ricochet around inside the building, consulting everyone but the janitor, the enhanced coordination and communications may do nothing more than disseminate the bad news about your recent complication or bankruptcy more quickly.

When I started out in gastroenterology thirty years ago, I never dreamed that I and my colleagues would be called upon to use chemotherapeutics and biologic agents. Immunological modulators that ramp up or tamp down your body's defenses are used daily to fight infection and autoimmune diseases, respectively. Anti-viral therapy did not exist thirty years ago. We now write for them dozens of times each week.

When I was in medical school in the 1970s, my Uncle Harry, a general practitioner, read his medical periodicals on Sunday afternoons. He graduated from medical school in the 1930s. How it was possible for him to keep up, much less understand, the clinical technologies that were, at that time, overwhelming to me? I decided he couldn't.

Now, thirty-five years after medical school, I can feel the stares of twenty-five-year-old medical students wondering the same about me. They can be skeptical with even greater justification, given the complexities of twenty-first-century medicine. Oh, Uncle Harry, now long gone, I finally understand your helpless smiles when I looked to you for solutions to clinical problems.

English professors lose half the value of their knowledge in twenty-five years. A physicist loses half of the value of her knowledge in four years. The half-life of knowledge in highly specialized clinical arenas cannot endure a shelf life of more than three years, at which point a clinician can become useless at best and dangerous at worst.

Doctors always have questions on how to proceed. We have them every day. These questions are increasing in frequency and complexity. The frequency of questions that arise in daily practice ranges from one question for every 1.2 patients seen, to a low of one question for every four patients encountered. There's a constant need to refer to colleagues, computers, and colloquia. This is no easy task in the face of financial and professional obligations and an office filled with staff and, oh yes—patients. Often, the amount of time spent seeking answers to medical questions is longer than the time actually devoted to the patient's visit. The reason that 40 percent of physician-generated questions are not pursued is the lack of time. Is that fifteen-minute visit looking more and more generous? It shouldn't.

Offices in lucrative single-specialty practices offer more opportunities to find answers to clinical questions. They have the resources sufficient to send staff off to symposia. They can offer on-site IT training, as well as the hardware and software to put this knowledge to use in a productive, efficient, timely, and care-enhancing fashion. They can also permit a rotating doctor to be a full-time hospital presence. This ensures a continuity and quality of care an emergency room physician can't provide.

Business concerns aren't the only reasons medical groups expand: the proliferation of medical databases has become too challenging, expensive, and specialized to handle in small offices.

3) THE DATA GLUT PER PATIENT
(THE BURDEN OF YOUR COMPANY)

So—a doctor starts a new practice or moves an existing one to a large clinic. He no longer needs to worry about business concerns. He will have a more humane call schedule. The sheer number of his colleagues will protect him from economic winds that could bend and then break a solitary slender reed. He now has at his disposal access to the information technologies and EMR that were previously logistically, financially, and psychologically prohibitive. Eden, you say? Perhaps, except for one feature—the patients (sorry, it's true). *Pari passu,* with all the advantages of a larger practice, patients still arrive in increasing numbers. Schedules groan under the burden as doctors and patients flee to these crowded oases of care in the forever-altered medical landscape.

A physician might be giddy at the thought of being liberated from the quotidian burdens of practice that this larger model provides. He sees that the table has been set and he has been led to his seat. He thinks that the appetite to see the patients that are brought to him in their multitude, once sated, is associated with the possibility of delicately touching his napkin to his lips, masking a discrete belch, and politely pulling slowly away from the table with a "thank you, I'm full." These doctors are not done until someone else tells them they are. This is an "all you can see" buffet. It's a kind of force-feeding regimen in which the doctor is made to see more and more patients, regardless of his inclination or capacity. Is it any wonder that in 2010 one in six general internists quit mid-career?[15]

Even if every possible technique is used to decrease the daily quota of patients doctors must see, by increasing the number of physicians and their extenders, it's still the case that the individual patient requires more time before and after the visit (and much less during it) to be evaluated properly. Patients are living longer, have more complex medical histories, and are treated with more drugs for more conditions than ever before. More patients, more care per patient, and more patient-generated data produce a seismic wave of responsibilities. In 2010 an internal medicine group published data that reflect these pressures.[16] Each physician was on the telephone twenty-four times a day and reviewed over fifty-seven lab and imaging results, e-mail communications, and consultation reports. Office-based time outside of the examination room averaged three hours eight minutes, or 39 percent of the office practice day.[17]

A 2010 research study showed that as a result, doctors become misers, hoarding each second of their day. On a medical search they are willing to spend thirty extra seconds to obtain data that is 99 percent reliable, but won't invest another *two* seconds to assure receipt of information that is 99.9 percent dependable.[18]

Whether you are seeing your family doctor or have been referred to a specialist, whether your visit is an initial evaluation or a follow-up, entering *any* office and being met with a blank stare produced by a blank chart is a waste of your time and a threat to your health. It is a deal breaker.

The avalanche of information that precedes your visit is stunning. These examples are meant to exemplify and quantify, not to edify. Simple cholesterol values are so "'90s." Now doctors look at your apoB/A1 ratio, low-density, high-density, low/high-density ratio, triglyceride, homocysteine and folate levels, and a variety of resultant mathematical constructs.

These results are often accompanied by a page of small-type explanations of every possible permutation that these numbers can produce in different conditions. Extensive marginalia that posit disease likelihoods described as relative risk ratios carry their *own* appended summaries of probability statistics. Even a high "good cholesterol" may not be so good. In December 2008 a "bad, good cholesterol" was discovered.

"We don't need no stinkin' PSAs." Now we analyze free; bound; free/bound ratios; PSA densities; volumes; velocities; and urinary tumor markers. All of this is breathtaking in light of the fact that we don't know if we *should* be getting them, what to do with them once we have them, or how to treat cancer of the prostate if you happen to eventually get it. Whether it should even be treated at all in some population groups is a topic of current debate. There are no normal values for PSAs. They are age-, race-, and weight-specific. Even a high normal PSA in a fifty-year-old may be cause for concern. Gone are the days of casually browsing down dozens of pages with hundreds of lab values while focusing only on the "abnormal" columns. *Normals are the new abnormals.* Also relevant is the fact that trends over time are causing "in range" values to increase but not yet cross into the red zone. This, in turn, requires reviewing not only the current, increasingly voluminous and complex data, but a history of values months or years in the past. The time to intercede is before these values, ratios, numbers, blood levels, and the people who actually possess them spill into the danger zone. Patients with normal lab values and without complaints are no longer just okay—they're just presymptomatic. "Walking time bombs" are the new "healthy population."

Even if you won't be looking for a parking spot at the doctor's office for another two weeks, your chromosomal abnormalities, oncogenes, mutations, aberrations, and deletions have already gone ahead of you via electronic transferals of your records. Doctors are ordering and then forwarding up obscure tumor markers for screening against a variety of cancers. You may be preceded by your alpha-fetoprotein, B2M, beta-hCG, bladder tumor antigen, CEA, CA 15-3, CA 12.29, CA 72-4, CA 125 calcitonin, chromogranin A, and CA 19-9s. (By the way, I am only on the first three letters of the alphabet.)

Your chart is buckling under the weight of markers found in stool, urine, blood, and sputum that detect molecules predictive of various cancers. The spectrum of their specificity and sensitivity will dictate the necessity for action or mandatory observation (entailing more blood work). Welcome to your chart ATC, K-ras, P53, and Tu-M2-PK—who the hell are you? And what about your immunologic, virologic, preinflammatory, and inflammatory markers? There are hundreds of these that relate to scores of the most common, as well as fatal, diseases.

We have not even gotten to the x-rays, ultrasounds, CAT scans, MRIs, and PET scans, and the dozens of their progeny. Most x-ray interpretations are hedging quasi-legal documents that serve to protect the radiologists as much as they do the patients. Thus, "We can't rule out a, b, c and d" sends you on further journeys with the result that more x-ray results, with their higher resolutions, are now replete with "incidental findings." These are the "by the way this may not mean anything but I am going to mention it anyway" findings. They usually are just that—incidental, malpractice-averting comments that don't mean a thing. And radiologists act that way every day with every film. Radiologists' self-estimated risk of malpractice suits are three to four times greater than their actual occurrence.[19] Fears of malpractice actions are not unique to radiologists. A 2010 Health Affairs article cited a "pervasive" fear of malpractice actions. Up to 80 percent of all physicians felt threatened by them. Some live in dread of a lawsuit.[20] Again, as for radiologists, the perceived risks were higher than the actual ones. Regardless, it is important for you to know that almost every doctor during virtually every contact with every patient thinks about her malpractice exposure. This fear is channeled into millions of unnecessary tests and referrals which are seen as a defense against potential negligence suits. Given that my junior partner and I were compared to Nazi war criminals in open court during a malpractice action perhaps you may sympathize, if but for a moment, with our fears.

The advances in bioscience produce a deluge of values that, often, are more anxiety-inducing for your doctor than they are actually threatening to you. Each must be seen, weighed, and discussed. Remember, all it takes are a few checkmarks on a page and you're off and running on an exciting

Homeric medical odyssey. But, often, it's your doctor who needs to lash himself to the mast to avoid the Siren's call for more testing.

According to a physician poll taken in 2010, when the big day comes and you are actually *with* your doctor, the paperwork and data entry alone consume one-third of the few minutes you actually get,[21] so don't expect much eye contact. Despite this it still seems as if some data is missing and more is needed. Additional investigations and referrals ensue.

Under these pressures your care is becoming *non-continuous* with one doctor, *fragmented* in light of the many you must see, and *uncoordinated* when communication between doctors fails. So while business was never the predominant domain for many of us, some clinical duties are becoming as foreign.

The use of physician extenders is one of the many ways doctors avoid clinical duties. Although inelegantly titled (but lately enjoying the better moniker of "mid-level providers") they, when properly deployed, are major assets to your care in the office and at the hospital.

Physician assistants (PA) are college graduates with several years of post-graduate experience. Licensed to practice by state medical boards, they must work under the direct supervision of a physician. Nurse practitioners (NP) are registered nurses with two to four years of graduate education. They are certified by state boards of nursing. In some states they can practice independently or in a partnership with off-site physicians. Most of the time PA and NP job descriptions overlap.

Many clinical duties that doctors perform have become routine. Once mastered, they are routinely avoided. In the middle of a chaotic day and faced with the many obligations that have been mentioned, doctors let these routines go first. Neither elevated through their urgency, nor requiring higher cognitive skills, they become repetitive, box-checking, list-driven chores. Yet, these are the very tasks that are of particular importance in caring for patients with multiple chronic illnesses who require multiple medications and a suite of support services to improve their day-to-day function, comfort, and safety. Properly managed, complications can be averted and resulting hospitalizations avoided. Relative longevity benefits may result.

These important routines are perfectly suited to a physician extender's skills. When there is a need for scheduled surveillance, monitoring, patient education, family counseling, and social interventions it is unlikely that a busy family practitioner or a specialist will make them priorities. Medications' side effects, interactions, dosing changes, compliance issues, and laboratory protocols are best managed by those whose skill sets are most appropriate for these obligations. It is then no surprise that some conditions are better managed by physician extenders than by their supervising physician employers. Family practices that employ nurse practitioners have been shown to provide better diabetic care than those without such support. The nurse practitioner's attention to the time-consuming details involved in the daily management of hepatitis C, HIV-AIDS, chronic obstructive pulmonary disease, inflammatory bowel disease, and rheumatoid arthritis provides benefits that are irrefutable. Because these conditions' medications pose risks, their doses need frequent recalibration in the face of the lab protocols demanded by their use.

The efficacy of physician extender (PE) management of chronic conditions as varied as hypertension, diabetes, congestive heart failure, peripheral vascular disease, dementia, and degenerative arthritis has been demonstrated throughout the medical literature. The fact that these diseases frequently coexist in one patient requires the need for even more intensive surveillance, prevention, and management.

In a 2005 article in the *Annals of Family Medicine*, the authors wrote that "current practice guidelines for only ten chronic diseases requires more time than primary care physicians have available."[22] A physician extender's care allows these otherwise unattainable clinical goals to be achieved.

When properly employed, nurse practitioners and physician assistants will perform clinical screening protocols for your benefit at least as well as their distracted employers. A 2011 article in *JECP* proved this point. Nurse practioners followed screening guidelines for abdominal aortic aneurysms over 98 percent of the time. Under a doctor's care the rate was 15 percent.[23] Nurse practitioners' and physician assistants' clinical histories of patients are often more detailed and nuanced than the narrower, goal-oriented, time-challenged products of clinicians.

A physician extender tends to be more aware of community resources for financial support and available social services. In small and midsize communities they are your neighbors far more often than the more cloistered physicians. Not having an M.D. confers the additional benefit of not having some of the M.D. traits that are so often cited by you as being unpleasant. Arrogance, judgmental attitudes, and paternalism **are**, sadly, *our* domain.

Physician extenders also get to know their charges better and in more subtle ways than doctors. This favorably influences long-term results and patient satisfaction. Physician extenders are less distracted by the burdens particular to physicians. Handling multiple duties—many complex, some novel, occasionally emergent, and seemingly always simultaneous—is *our* domain. We perform these functions better when we know that a physician extender is managing the responsibilities to which he or she is particularly suited. Office schedules become more flexible. Productivity is enhanced.

The year 2011 brings new guests to the best doctors' offices. Coaches and scribes. Welcome them. Medical coaches help make sure your agendas are communicated. After the visit is completed they confirm your understanding and agreement with the treatment plan. Scribes will take your interval medical history. All these activities by the least bad performers allow your doctor to spend those precious few minutes on those things only she is qualified to do.

Hospital-based physician extenders provide a rapid deployment force that provides an initial assessment of your problem. If necessary they will alert their clinician, who might otherwise be hours away from his hospital rounds. As members of a true clinical team, they are familiar faces when you are hospitalized and provide crucial clinical continuity when you are discharged.

"I ONLY WANTED A DOCTOR!" AN ECONOMIC LESSON—HOLD ON TO YOUR HATS

An individual can perform a task in the best possible fashion. Depending on the job, it can also, at a minimum, be performed by a person who does it the least badly. That's why Michael Jordan doesn't cut his lawn. Jordan would, by force of his agility, strength, and resources, be better at this task than most gardeners. Yet Jordan will use someone who will do the job less well than he. And that's okay. It's a zero sum game. The gardener has a job that he does almost as well by dint of having experience. The lawn looks just fine. Michael is better off financially making a commercial for John Deere than riding on one. Some *medical* tasks also don't require that they be done in the best fashion. (This is the "hold-on-to-your-hats part.")

How can this be? How should medical tasks be divided? The doctor must spend more time on tasks that he is better able to perform than the nurse practitioner. The nurse practitioner must concentrate on the tasks that she may perform with only slightly less expertise than the doctor. This is the benefit provided by the "least bad performer." This arrangement provides a less obvious benefit. It prevents the doctor from doing what, in fact, most clinicians do the most badly—listening to patients and maintaining a flexible and realistic schedule.

This "Law of Comparative Advantage," or the advantage of the "least bad performer" was best described by the nineteenth-century economic classicist David Ricardo. It is best summarized by his economic antithesis, Karl Marx: "From each according to his ability; to each according to his need."

How will you know whether physician extenders are being used correctly in your behalf?

Your initial visit must always be with the physician who must be in the office to provide supervision and assistance, regardless of whether he is supervising a nurse practitioner or a physician assistant. You will often see your doctor during the visit. He will either provide a quick hello or appear in your exam room if you, or the nurse practitioner, need advice.

Your care will not be managed exclusively by the physician assistant. Every three to five visits you will rotate into your physician's schedule or your doctor should be present during your scheduled physician assistant appointment. While in the hospital you must see your physician at least once a day regardless of the availability of a nurse practitioner.

Finally, physician extenders are held to a lower standard of care than physicians. The competition for these jobs is less cutthroat and the training is more limited. Whatever their benefits, it is unwise to come to the conclusion that the care provided by them is the same as that provided by physicians. This is unfounded, naïve, and potentially damaging.

FINALLY: CAN IT ALL BE DONE?

Ideally an office, regardless of size, must be akin to a *spira mirabilis,* or miraculous spiral, from the Latin. A *spira mirabilis* is a mathematically defined, but naturally existing, structure that can increase in size while maintaining its shape. It *is* a miracle if a practice can grow, even become a leviathan, without changing the shape and nature which it had at its inception. But it is rare to find a practice that is large yet personal, businesslike yet warm, hectic in routine yet calm in approach, and that has a number of physicians but shared goals. As a practice grows, merges with another, and becomes a clumsy colossus, it can also become institutional and detached. Its doctors, distracted and harried, become disillusioned.

A realistic view was published by the *New England Journal of Medicine* in March 2008. This reality-based assessment noted that 7.4 hours per day are needed to provide preventive care.[24] Offering long-term care for the controlled and uncontrolled conditions in the top ten chronic diseases such as cancer, heart failure, diabetes, and chronic obstructive pulmonary disease (emphysema and asthma) requires 10.6 hours per day. This does not include nonclinical duties, business obligations, and hospital responsibilities. Do the math. That *spira mirabilis* is looking more and more like a *mirabilis,* period.

2

The Hospital

- The 3 *non*clinical duties your doctor must perform, without which your fortunes and futures are in jeopardy.
- Hospitalists—strangers at your bedside. Why they are dangerous to your health.
- How to keep your own doctor when you need him the most.
- How to avoid error while under a hospitalist's care.
- Errors in your care while in hospital are 100 percent guaranteed. There are specific times called transition zones when they are all but predictable. What kinds of errors? Where do they occur and how can you avoid them?
- Going home sicker and quicker. Avoiding readmission—the hospital entrance as a revolving door.

In Book II of John Milton's epic poem, *Paradise Lost*, he describes a place called Pandemonium. Its main characters are Chaos, Confusion, and Discord. Welcome to the twenty-first-century hospital.

> . . . into this wild Abyss
> The womb of Nature, and perhaps her grave,
> Of neither sea, nor shore, nor air, nor fire,
> But all these in their pregnant causes mixed
> Confusedly, and which thus must ever fight,
> . . . Into the this wild Abyss the wary Fiend
> Stood on the brink of Hell and looked a while,
> Pondering his voyage; for no narrow frith
> He had to cross. Nor was his ear less pealed
> With noises loud and ruinous (to compare Great things with small) . . .

The hospital is the place where life starts and ends.

It is a place beyond and above the normal flow of time and the definition of place.

Hospitals treat many on the brink of their own wild abyss.

In spite of narrow frith (windows) for success, it is a place to ponder *your* voyage, while surrounded by noise—loud and ruinous.

Where things Important are confused for the minor and things small for those Great.

Paradise lost? Hospitals are inhabited by people who, having reverted to their natural state by force of disease, are now called patients. Shorn of the accoutrements of civilization, often stripped of their dignity, they struggle on the precipice of the void, helpless and vulnerable. In light of the potential dangers of being in a hospital, it's only prudent and natural that patients should be wary. Others may travel to and from the hospital. You don't travel to a hospital; you reside there, however temporarily. All the best and worst this interregnum provides will be experienced by every patient—yes, every patient.

This voyage has little room for error yet is rife with it. Unfiltered sensations—most unpleasant, some noxious and occasionally calamitous—are the rule and you will find no respite at night. Chaos exists or develops no matter how firm your (momentary) footing. Confusion is a constant. Discord and friction are continual—from every room to every nursing station, from the intensive care unit to administration, from doctor to doctor and between doctor and patient. Discord can be a significant barrier to success; properly and willingly used, it can also be a tool to achieve it.

Hospitals, even the best, are minefields. One moment, you and your doctor are strolling along; in the next moment, you are face-to-face with a crisis—all without an obvious misstep. The most grievously stricken and those on its cusp will suffer these crises in the midst of potential calamity. It's bad enough that you need to go to a hospital, but "Oh, the places you'll go!" I wouldn't be surprised to see Bear Grylls on his Discovery Channel show, *Man versus Wild*, devote an hour to the skills a survivalist needs while in a hospital.

In the face of the dangers and errors hardwired into our system of care, the rate of improvement in our hospitals is an anemic 1.5 percent per year. So common and refractory are the errors, Medicare and other insurers now refuse to pay for "Never events" that have resisted all but the ultimate punishment—non-reimbursement.

The hospital is home to such equivocations as the phrases "I think," "the last time I checked," "as far as I know," and "it's what I was told." Whether they result through apathy or overwork, they circumvent the precision and the persistence your clinician needs in every encounter, and for every posed question. It doesn't matter whether they're said by a doctor, nurse, or lab technician, but if they're granted even a moment of credence, it will auger poorly for your health.

The missing chart not sought after, the neglected pile of lab data, the information vacuum caused by a change in shift, and the frustrations of dedicated staff who are outnumbered, overworked, and outgunned by your needs: all lead, nearly inevitably, to error. The only way to avoid potentially fatal errors is to anticipate the miscommunications, misunderstandings, and misinterpretations that end in injury or tragedy; or the encounters that are typically, even classically, prone to them.

A physician's failure to double-check medication orders, their legibility, their doses, their intervals, their interactions, and their routes of administration will occur with some degree of statistical probability for each variable, for each patient on each medication that a clinician orders. Ill-written and indecipherable notes are subjected to a critical exegesis usually reserved for ancient parchments found on desert floors. As a result, official documents that codify your status, progress, and needs become impressionistic canvases open to creative interpretations.

Errors—historical, procedural, and mnemonic—become engraved on your chart through the failure of their verification and live on through their repetition. No matter how often or how loudly you protest these mistakes, they tend to resist correction because your doctor is being bombarded by "noises loud and ruinous." The perturbations that threaten your physician's equilibrium and accuracy arise from dozens of simultaneous stimuli arriving at his cortex that relate to your care and those of others under his name. Research in 2010 proved this. Each interruption, and there are many, degrades performance and increases error.[1]

THREE NONCLINICAL DUTIES
YOUR DOCTOR *MUST* PERFORM

Empathy

In this crucible that is the hospital there is the need for a unique relationship. It's a partnership in which intimacy can co-exist with detachment and one that is open to honest communication yet occasionally requires close-kept secrets. The goals may be the same, but it is understood that the means to achieve them may be disparate and disputatious.

The ability to arrive at a mutual understanding by putting yourself in another person's place is called "theory of mind." It allows all parties to experience each other's feelings, needs, and motives. Sadly, what should be seen as a basic human endowment is now seen by the medical profession as an accomplishment worthy of praise. This is no surprise when "mind blind" patients, families, and doctors use conscious and unconscious skills to distance themselves emotionally, physically, and empathically from each other. We will explore empathy in depth in part 3, "Choosing Your Doctor."

Validation

You're in the hospital. You haven't shared a room with a stranger since 1968 in a youth hostel in Belgium, much less shared his infection. The food is ungraciously presented, unappealing to behold, much less eat. If you are allowed to eat, the solace food has always offered is yet another frustration.

The humiliation and indignity of being cleaned after bowel movements, the character and frequency of which are often severely altered due to your illness, medications, diet, and surroundings, is beyond description. Even this insult to your sensibilities pales in contrast to the multiple pleas and subsequent delays imposed on you, as you await a bedpan, urinal, or morphine.

Incontinence that leaves you in your own effluvium, and your new role as an unpleasant, distasteful chore, are cause for the deepest despair. Treasure the staff that validate and reassure you during these times.

The inevitable depression, anxiety, and sense of powerlessness brought on by some of these facts of hospital life can affect your outcome as a patient. Depression and anxiety are measurable quantifiable entities. The Hospital Anxiety and Depression scores (HADs) reveals through a few easily posed questions those patients at risk. The score will increase in the face of a doctor's thoughtless offhand comments or deliberate cruelty.

How many times have you heard the phrases, "I wouldn't worry about that" or worse, "I'm not concerned by this," when a doctor's comfort level is confused for yours? Such insensitivity reaches its apotheosis in comments that vitiate your concerns, like "What are you worried about?" or "You're quite a worrier, aren't you?" Such statements deny you the simple acknowledgment of your predicament.

The failure of validation, another nonclinical mandate, may suggest a suite of other human failings that will promote error and complicate your stay. The validation a doctor offers is as important as the tests he orders. The failure to recognize or the denial of the depression and anxiety that patients experience during a hospital stay is the antithesis of empathy. The lack of it can lead to emotional imbalance, which can hinder physical healing. When your feelings are subjected to ridicule, it's time to change your course—even in midstream. If you, as an outpatient, have tolerated your doctor's penchant for trivializing, minimizing, questioning, and making light of your symptoms and concerns, the odds are high you will also be experiencing these traits when they are at their most baneful—as an inpatient.

The affective disorders that arise in the midst of the twenty-four-hour, no-privacy, fluorescent-lit war zone that is your hospital can only be assuaged by a doctor who first recognizes them, then validates your concerns. Your doctor must recognize, if not in detail then at least in its scope, your non-medical discomfort by offering some emotional support. (It need not be a two-handkerchief affair; many studies show that doctors who emote too intensely can cause even more upset.)

Encouraging and acknowledging your strength in the face of pain, embarrassments, humiliations, financial concerns, or simple worries about your eight-year-old daughter's response to your illness will make them easier to bear. Doctors who are worthy of you can predict your worries, and will broach and reflect upon them while at your bedside. There are few times in your life that you want to talk more, ruminate, and even perseverate about what is going than when it seems threatened. The clinician who listens and nods his acknowledgment, rather than ignoring or ridiculing these flights of fancy or fact, is to be expected. This is another scenario when the duties incumbent upon your doctor become endowed with a glow of something special or unique. We will see in chapter 9 why compassion is so often lacking and how patients and doctors can re-establish it.

There are times when you may be too ill or weak to even communicate your feelings. Many doctors use this as an excuse to truncate their visits with you. It is precisely these times when communication that is eye-to-eye and mouth-to-ear provide you with a type of solace that no one else can offer. Gratuitous, even minimal, efforts are not trivial ones. The fact that your doctor ministers to you, in all senses of the word, should be expected.

Advocacy

Twenty-first-century hospitals no longer serve the function of "hosts" from the Latin cognate, *hospes.* They are now "exitoriums," dedicated more to getting you out than greeting you on the way in. The word "discharge" in its original Latin (*discarric re*) means unloading. As a noun, "discharge" connotes something unpleasant that is ejected. Indeed, the rush to get you out leads to the predictably high rate of readmissions. This is a universal indicator that should trigger an inquiry into your hospital's quality of care. Readmission rates within one month of discharge or transfer are up to 20 percent for Medicare recipients. Many such readmissions, if not most, are avoidable.

Why is this? Because you no longer leave the hospital when you are better. Rather, you are discharged when it looks as if you are getting better, when it is felt you are likely to get better, or if it's looking as if you will never get better.

The gravity of illnesses needed to gain admission to hospitals today is far more severe than in the past. Despite this, all the forces you experience after admission are centrifugal ones. You almost have to hold on to your bedpost to avoid being caught in the combined vortices produced by the efforts to expedite your exit. Paradoxically, despite the increasing difficulty in gaining admission, the MASH-like atmosphere in our hospitals means that your visits are getting shorter. Discharges seem more like medevacs. No helicopters, just a cab at the curb.

After being warehoused in this refugee camp setting, you will be relieved that you have survived not only your illness, but the hospital experience as well. The readmission rates, however, should disenthrall many from the notion that they have recovered fully. Physician-initiated advocacy is your only bulwark against a premature discharge and its consequences.

Hospitals teem with functionaries and their factotums whose goals are solely institutional, regardless of their advertisements and highway billboards that portray dedicated staffers delightedly caring for their beaming, thankful patients.

The variants that determine your length of stay are not just your physical state but the fiscal state of your hospital. One example is the prospective payment system, developed to provide arm-twisting incentives through fixed reimbursement schedules tagged to your admission diagnoses. Cost containment drives many decisions, including hospital discharge. Your fate is decided, to a large degree, by algorithmically driven clinical outcome trees empowered by actuarial tables, and probability statistics generated from the historically "similarly afflicted."

These diagnostic categories set the limits of a reimbursed visit. Hospitals receive prospective payments based on your Diagnostic Related Group (DRG). Beyond that you are an income obstacle, which makes your hospital both see red and bleed red on its balance sheets. Medicare and Medicaid both use these formulae. Private insurance companies have chaotic hospital reimbursement policies.

If your doctor is not your advocate you are indeed alone. Both primary care and specialty physicians must serve this unreimbursed, time-consuming, energy-sapping, psychologically bruising, unpopular function.

If the system is corrupt and the demands unreasonable she will lie for you. The forces that delay, dilute, or deny you care will force her to enlist the help of other doctors and your family. She will use her own power and use the weight of her own groups' economic clout to get what you need when you need it and where you need it. Physician-applied pressure to those centrifugal forces is the only way they can be slowed. There must be a willingness to engage in discord in your behalf. However unpleasant to contemplate, it is the "Discord" in the house of "Pandemonium" that stills the "Chaos" in this Miltonian milieu. Discord and conflict lie at the heart of advocacy. An advocate calls, pleads, and argues. No one apart from your doctor performs this function as effectively. She is positioned at the crossroads of decision making and cost containment. She knows the language and the players.

You need a doctor who is an advocate. When the day comes and medical-care rationing is the rule (and that day *will* come) there will be no need for a doctor's passion. The care you receive will be dictated by comparative effectiveness studies that determine the best and most cost-effective therapy. You won't need a doctor who must, if need be, engage in conflict on your behalf. Today you do.

If you are in the intensive care unit, at what point would I allow you to be "bumped" so that another patient can have your bed? At what point would I relent in my requests that another patient be "bumped" from the ICU for your sake? First, there is no current higher organizational level in place to which I would cede authority. That these external agencies may prevail someday in decisions regarding your care is irrelevant in the here and now. Mandated "fair" rules of rationing are too arbitrary to be kowtowed to reflexively. As your doctor, I will keep you in the intensive care unit as long as I feel there's a need for you to be there; or until a "higher-up" comes to your bedside and carts you away against my objections, and without my permission. That's what it would take if I thought you needed any service that the hospital could provide.

But what of another doctor's patient who also needs the bed? I hope these patients have a doctor who also believes in unrestricted advocacy and who bows only to the medical director who sends the transport aids who evict you, thereby ending the discord. These conflicts were anticipated by Sigurd Lauridsen, a medical philosopher at the University of Copenhagen. He wrote that "physicians will become adversaries of each other in the healthcare system. They will mutually compete to allocate resources to their patients. As a result, those physicians who negotiate most persuasively will be able to allocate more resources to their patients."[2]

That's what you want: the physician advocate who negotiates more persuasively than the other guy's doctor. Sometimes a doctor wins, sometimes he doesn't. For patients who find themselves without an advocate willing to fight for them, there are no battles. There will be no individual victories, only societal ones. But until there is a system that demands allocation of scarce resources, it is unlikely I will use you, my patient, as the vanguard in cost containment.

It makes life hard for the medical directors, but that's their problem. You're mine. The only insoluble problem occurs when both of the patients who need the same ICU bed happen to be my own. *Only* in this situation will one of my patients rightly feel that the other patient's needs are greater in my eyes than theirs.

Advocacy: Physician vs. Physician

During your hospital stay you are practically guaranteed a cardiologist, pulmonologist, gastroenterologist, and an infectious disease specialist. Cameo appearances from urologists and nephrologists can be expected.

You will be set upon by interns, residents, and fellows. You won't know their names, who they are, what they do, or if they are integral or peripheral to your care. Nursing professionals and students, social service staff, nurse practitioners, discharge planners, dietitians, rehabilitation and occupational therapists will be daily mystery guests. You will be taken on gurney journeys from CAT scans to catheter labs and stretcher adventures from radiology to rehab. A strong physician leader and advocate will minimize, in the midst of this medical miasma, the errors born of miscommunication, redundancy, needless testing, and wild departures from protocol.

The physician-leader-advocate demands that the specialists he calls in demonstrate competence, comportment, and communication skills.

Too often, a weak primary care doctor is relegated to lower status, thus becoming a third party in your care. Specialists can run roughshod over you unless your primary care physician stipulates that all orders need to be cleared, confirmed, or communicated with him or her before implementation. A surgeon who is either too slow or too eager to operate will be called to task. Respect for a surgeon's judgment and skills does not imply an uncritical obeisance to them. Partners or associates of a designated specialist who give unasked-for advice, or who deviate from the established plan, should be politely dismissed. Your doctor will explain that, barring emergencies, there will be no cross-coverage once a designated specialist is chosen, thereby reducing or eliminating communication gaffes and the errors they can spawn. Once this system is in place, unexpected developments and results, both happy and otherwise, are immediately transmitted to your doctor; and surprises in the chart or embarrassments at the bedside tend not to occur.

Activities in your behalf by doctor-advocates are not reimbursed, visible, or recognized. They go unappreciated by those staff and doctors whose activities must be criticized or redirected. Between-visit care represents 14 to 16 percent of your doctor's day. While, for some, this is the easiest part of the day to pare down, for your doctor it is too important a duty to abandon.

Advocacy: The "Team"

"Medical homes," "teamlets," and "integrated medical groups" are neologisms getting a lot of press in the medical literature.

Teams are necessary given the complexity of care that characterizes contemporary medicine. Patients with acute care needs and those with more chronic problems require precise timing and monitoring of blood work, vital signs, and medication. Overworked hospital staff may not be in a position to provide what is needed.

My PA, nurse, and the consults from various subspecialties I have chosen are directed to the bedside to provide quality assurance, adherence to protocols, support, and familiar faces. This is denied to most hospitalized patients. IV therapies for chemotherapy, congestive heart failure, gastrointestinal bleeding, and intensive nutritional support, as well as respirator and dialysis management and critical vital sign protocols are only a few services that require the timely and expert delivery of care. Scrupulous, exacting, and even finicky monitoring of clinical parameters unique to different conditions often determines their outcomes. The primary care provider monitors your other doctors as carefully as he watches you.

A case in point: You are home feeling nauseated. You lean over and vomit up what seems like a bucket of bright red blood and black clots. Who will be the first person to see you after you have arrived at the emergency room? It better be me or one of my team members. We will be on-site to attend to you almost simultaneous to your arrival or ensure that pre-arrival orders are in place and calls are made to the ER physician in charge.

You will get to the ICU in a timely fashion. Internal bleeding of this severity requires performing a great number of services, many simultaneously. The priorities that I have set for you may not be shared by the hospital staff who must worry about a lot of other patients whose needs may or may not be as important as yours.

The following sequence is not meant to educate, but to demonstrate an emergency's logistical challenges.

I need to know:

1. if you are currently bleeding. If so, I need to know from where—stomach or rectum—how much in milliliters, and what color—red, black, or mahogany—as well as your pulse, blood pressure, and urine output;
2. that there will be updates every half hour;
3. that if your condition changes I will be notified immediately;
4. if the nasal-gastric tube is in place and that its location in the stomach has been verified by x-ray or preferably that the x-ray film is in the patient's room for my review;
5. what is coming out of that tube, how much, and what color;
6. if the urinary catheter has been placed and how much urine has flowed into the bag upon placement;
7. that your blood count, clotting tests, and the "type and cross" for the blood bank have been drawn, sent, received by the lab, performed, and their results obtained and then called to me or a team member (those are six *separate* demands);
8. whether the blood bank has put aside blood, platelets, and fresh frozen plasma, that they are ready for use if needed, and that pre-storage leukoreduction techniques have been employed;
9. that the somatostatin and pantoprazole I ordered are up and running and dose titration orders are being adhered to;

10. that the IV fluids and albumin are up and running and being titrated correctly to your pulse and urine output;
11. that consent is signed for all upcoming procedures that I have previously discussed with you;
12. if the surgeon, who has been personally called by me or a team member and notified as to the emergent nature of the consult, has arrived. Has he given an ETA for his arrival?
13. if I will be called if he is not present within one hour;
14. in the face of continued bleeding, that the blood I ordered has been cross-checked for compatibility and that the acetaminophen has been administered;
15. that the protocols I ordered to monitor for transfusion reactions are being followed (respiratory distress, low blood pressure, shortness of breath, fever, flank pain, and red or brown urine);
16. if resuscitative treatment modalities are in place and ready for administration in the case of a transfusion reaction;
17. if the blood infusion is up from the blood bank, running well and on schedule;
18. if backup transfusion packets are ready and vitamin K and calcium are available;
19. that my follow-up blood orders will be drawn on schedule and I will be informed of their results;
20. that my "call M.D." orders will be honored (e.g., call M.D. for pulse over 120, for systolic blood pressure under 95, for urine output under 300cc per shift, for continued active bleeding of more than 50cc of black or bright red blood, for pulse oximetry levels below 90% saturation, for a blood count under 30% or an INR over 2, a platelet count under 125,000);
21. that the family is at the bedside when I arrive for the endoscopy that will diagnose and then control the bleeding;
22. that the cart that carries the medications and support devices needed during the endoscopy are in the room and inventoried;
23. that the anesthesiologist is aware and available if needed.

All of these steps play out in no more than a two-hour time span. Up to this point we have only stabilized you for the diagnostic and therapeutic intervention. Who will guarantee that my priorities are the staff's priorities? How do I know that I will be called if your status changes or that the orders I left are being followed as written? Who will assure me that everything I need and want is where it must be at a time appropriate for its administration?

There is only one way that I can walk away from your bedside and be sure that you will be under careful observation and that my protocols will be followed. An independent team answerable only to me will share goals, implement long-practiced action sequences, and keep alert to warning signs they have been taught to look for. I, a team member, or an invited consult will be at your bedside every few minutes making sure that all the above steps are being followed in the right sequence and in the proper manner, timing, and skill level. You will know that you are in the epicenter of an emergency but also at the center of the team's concerns.

Most hospitals have staff that will usually be as effective. Some won't. And being "usually" as effective is not nearly good enough.

There is nothing unusual about a gastrointestinal bleed or the activities they demand. There is nothing particularly cognitively challenging in its treatment. There are dozens of clinical scenarios that demand as much and many dozens that demand far more. What *is* unusual is the guarantee that they will be done in a time, fashion, and skill level that leads to a greater likelihood of success. That is what a team does. That's what my team did.

Physician leaders and their specialists, each with their own teams, must be able to hire, train, monitor, and fire each member. Protocols are established. Integration and coordination of resource allocation and clinical activities all flow from the top. The team's culture and goals are never in doubt. Clinical outcomes improve when teams are part of your care. A 2010 *JAMA* article revealed that team members are more likely to challenge each other, use guidelines, employ extensive briefing and postoperative debriefings, recognize warning signs, and use reassessment periods that can prevent transition zone errors (see below).[3]

Team care is not possible while you are hospitalized unless your doctors import them. Hospital-based "teams" often lack the attributes, mentioned above, that contribute to a collective hierarchical approach to your care. They are often overworked, understaffed, variably competent, questionably supervised, unpredictably motivated, and unaccountable to the doctor. Further, the hordes of hospital-created "teams" have not been handpicked by the doctor you have chosen to manage your care.

Any physician who is acting as your representative cannot be coerced into participating in an ersatz team approach. If your clinician bows rather than fights, he becomes a toothless creature, without the power to provide the help you need.

You will be encouraged by your doctor-advocate to provide feedback, to be vocal in your own behalf, and to have at hand the hospital telephone numbers to call when violations occur. There's no such thing as discourtesy when you are fighting for your life or to prevent life-threatening errors. When you can't act in your own behalf, your omnipresent relative, friend, room coach, or proxy will.

If your physician is surrounded with, or you are visited by, his selected representatives, clinical data collectors, nurses, and physician assistants, you are indeed lucky. This type of care is easy to provide but not typically offered.

Advocacy: "Ipsedixitism" and Doctor-Patient Discord

Regardless of whether health care is patient- or physician-centered, at some point decisions must be made. As an outpatient, you will sometimes come to a crossroad in your care. It is often seen from a distance and can be approached slowly and carefully, with mutual planning and deliberative discussions.

By contrast, the hospital is a wild ride. Screeching tires, hairpin turns, and head-jolting accelerations are interspersed with periods of clinical gridlock. Sometimes two pairs of hands cannot be on the wheel. A Yogi Berra trope goes "when you come to a fork in the road, take it." Sometimes that's all you, as the patient, can do when you don't see it coming. Decisions made in the hospital sometimes are subject only to retrospective analyses rather than the luxury of leisurely prospective planning. You and your family are in a state of shock, fear, confusion, and anger. Suffering vertiginous sensory and informational overload, you can't always be a part of the discussion. Typically, the decisions in which you play little to no part are the ones that occur when your welfare and life hang by a thread. Sometimes there is time for only brief explanation. Frequently, this is when there is disagreement: when your desire to gain back a measure of control comes into conflict with the recommendations of the doctor. The tests and therapeutics offered are often met with resistance. It's understandable that you want a measure of control. You want to know what the future holds. It often gives rise to the usually unanswerable questions, "What comes next?" or "What if that doesn't work?" If your doctor tries to lay out a course of action beyond what's likely to happen in the next twenty-four to thirty-six hours he will fail. This failure results in a loss of confidence and, possibly, more aggressive questioning on your part. Years of mutual affection and trust can be lost in the time it takes to hold your breath for a CT scan, the results of which may alter your life in a totally unanticipated way. In fact, I *don't* know what will happen when the results of the next blood draw or x-ray come in. Most often it's the unanticipated that determines the next step. Advocating what we think is in your best interest is always a risky endeavor, especially when you disagree. When it comes to your best interests you are the sole and undisputed expert. Don't give up your hard-earned and closely held views without a fight. Let there be debates and friction before decisions are made.

Advocacy is sometimes unpleasant; it's occasionally tyrannical and always provoking. Informing, explaining, and then proceeding with you in tow are not patient-centered activities. Being your own advocate is fine, but there will be times when it is fruitless. That it is time consuming, frustrating, and divisive is also fine up to a point; arguing and bargaining have their place. So do frustration, skepticism, and disenchantment. Usually it's yours; sometimes it's mine. But it's hard to go on when we *both* feel this way. Is there time for a second opinion, a consult, or a brand-new doctor? Sometimes, but not often. It's impossible to freeze-frame an emergency.

There are times when *"ipse dixit"* (because he said so) prevails. Ipsedixitism is alive and well in many doctors who are confident or arrogant enough to use the "because I said so" argument so familiar to parents. It induces temporary embarrassment for the doctor and anger in their patients and families. Despite this, sometimes it's the right approach. When all else fails it may be time to institute a modern version of the medieval rite, "The Wielding of Authority," a Viking custom many clinicians feel is inappropriate in the twenty-first century.

This in turn leads to another rite initiated by your unhappy families. It too originated in fiercely independent early societies. It's "The Gathering of the Clans," evoking visions of animal skins, horned helmets, rock-strewn tundra, and fire pits surrounded by large, blond, and red-bearded people gathering to talk, argue, and then fight interlopers, brandishing their hatchets and long swords. Both throwbacks are usually fruitless and always unpleasant. It is where today, in waiting rooms, rather than in ancient glacial fields, the apologetic face the apoplectic.

We will engage each other in conversation, not in battle. There are times, however few, when you must relent, back down, and allow the process to unwind with mutual prayers it doesn't unravel. It is always done with the understanding that I am responsible.

What can you do to determine if your doctor is your advocate?

- He will not relegate your care to a hospitalist.
- He will be your doctor and will not relegate your care to other doctors.
- He assumes that you are anxious and probably depressed.
- He asks for, and listens to, your concerns
- He acts on your concerns either through advocacy or validation.
- He provides you with an office hotline to call when you feel that errors are being made, or when stretcher adventures are planned that have never been previously discussed. Be reminded that these telephone numbers are for reassurance, not casual use. Your doctor will see you every day—frequently twice.
- Consults inform you that their orders are pending, until your doctor is called or informed of them.
- Advocates are often mild obsessive-compulsives and frequently unpopular. Hospital nursing staff offer, in pique or praise, "your doctor is a real stickler." "We like him but he scares us a little bit."

- He will help you with insurance problems (lie) if your carrier calls you while in the hospital.
- He will make sure you get a private room, if possible. If not, he will make sure your roommate's problems do not become yours (see chapter 18).
- He intercedes on your behalf—either through action or explanations—when you are dissatisfied with dietary, nursing, or physician services.
- You might see familiar office staff. Nurses, physician assistants, and data assemblers arrive at the bedside. It's nice to see familiar faces. It's important to have a doctor who knows and takes advantage of the superiority of care that comes from true teamwork.
- Finally, when your doctor comes to your bedside, do you feel safe in his hands? A sense of security is not out of place even in dangerous places. A positive reflexive response to this simple question requires faith in his qualities and character. These feelings are not associated with your estimation of his medical skills and judgment. Doctors earn respect and a patient's sense of security by the application of the non-clinical skills I've discussed.

When a doctor displays empathy, validation, and advocacy in her office, you can expect to encounter them again at every point of care. Their absence may not constitute a deal breaker, but something irreplaceable has been lost.

Advocacy: Patient-Initiated Advocacy

Little more than lip service is given to patient advocacy. Often it is misconstrued to mean raising your voice, your eyebrows, or your doctor's malpractice fears. In the hospital self-advocacy means having a constant room companion—a designated sitter (DS), a son, a daughter, a spouse, parents, relatives, friends. Whoever that companion is, he or she should keep a log that records the names of everyone coming into your room, their duties, and the times of their comings and goings. It means distributing gloves and making gentle but firm admonitions to visitors regarding the necessity of hand washing (always!) and protective clothing when needed (see chapter 18).

Rather than seeming rude, this can, in fact, personalize your care and encourage a subtle but discernible layer of accountability. If people don't like this, and there will be some who don't, then too bad. This is important stuff. Apologize to those who take offense and keep writing in your log.

Judging from the media, people seem to be very concerned about the chance of being struck by an errant asteroid. The 1 in 50,000,000 chance is seen, judging by the intensity of public interest, as a more likely event than suffering a preventable medical error. It isn't. Whether an asteroid hits Earth is a question of fate. But you can't leave your hospital care up to fate. It's up to you.

STRANGERS IN A STORM

Emergencies get you into a hospital. *Being* in a hospital itself constitutes a state of emergency. Given the intensity of the experience and the consequences of error, this is no time to experiment with the doctors who call themselves hospitalists.

You chose your doctor carefully in a consumer-driven series of inquiries (see part 3). Perhaps serendipity played a part as well. Either way, these relationships, when successful, are carefully cultivated and maintained. Your confidence in your doctor produces an "endowment effect," in which her skills are deemed irreplaceable. As a result, you don't want to lose her services. It's prudent then to be wary of medical professionals you don't know, because during the storms of illness and hospitalization, it's more likely that lightning will strike twice in one place than that good fortune will. Hospitalists are those strangers. They come to you in those storms.

A medical phenomenon, the hospitalist movement is only eleven years old but is now 30,000 doctors strong. A hospitalist is defined as a physician whose primary duty is the care of hospitalized patients. The hospitalist assumes care of the patient from admission to discharge.

An article in the *Journal of the American Medical Association* demonstrates that your care will likely be in the hands of a stranger. The authors noted that only 40 percent of hospitalized patients in 2006 were cared for by a doctor they had seen in an outpatient setting. Only 32 percent of hospitalized patients who had an identifiable primary care doctor received care from that doctor. All true despite the authors' acknowledgment that "continuity of care is a defining attribute of primary care and a core element of the Institute of Medicine definition of primary care. Continuity is generally recognized to have three dimensions—continuity in information, continuity in management, and continuity in the patient-physician relationship. Relationship continuity is the ongoing interaction of a patient with one physician, which results in increased knowledge of patient preferences, better communication, and improved trust."[4]

Robust growth in the absence of any stimulus that serves to nourish or support it would be a biologic curiosity. It is now a medical phenomenon. The dry clay of cost-saving is the soil in which the hospitalist movement was planted. But even the thin sustenance of "dollars saved" is a doubtful proposition.

Hospitalists do not represent a medical specialty. It is not a body of specialized clinical knowledge, nor is it characterized by unique technical skills. There is no specialty licensure, accrediting or state boards, qualifying examinations, or minimum requirements. There are no core undergraduate courses or residencies. Fellowship programs are few and optional. There are no acknowledged standards for mentorship. There is no consistent data on their comparative effectiveness when compared with your own doctor. Membership in the Society of Hospital Medicine, their professional organization, represents only a fraction of its practitioners.

The heterogeneous patient population in hospitals is ill-matched with hospitalists who do not have the skills appropriate for their care. This mismatch of skills is striking and dangerous. Doctors who specialize in internal medicine comprise most of those who identify themselves as hospitalists (85 percent of the total). They are performing duties in areas they are ill-trained to supervise—geriatrics, orthopedics, neurology, and pre-and postoperative care. According to one source, a third of patients require tasks that hospitalists are unfit to handle.[5] In 2010, it was reported that the number of postoperative patients co-managed by hospitalists increased from under 2 percent to more than 12 percent in ten years. "The growth in care of surgical patients by medicine physicians raises the issue of appropriate training."[6] In 2010 the mismatch issue was raised again and its financial impetus was given voice. The author states, "I would argue that even the economic rationale for comanagement is poor because it really involves shifting work to lower-paid workers (internists), allowing surgeons to spend more time in the operating room, where they get paid more by a dysfunctional reimbursement system that disproportionately rewards procedural care over more cognitive services." Hospitalists become the least bad performers we learned about in chapter one. And it's all about the money. No medical benefit was demonstrated.[7]

Yet, you will find hospitalists in 85 percent of hospitals with 200 or more beds. The acknowledged impetus for the movement and the continued rationale for its existence are monetary—getting you out of the hospital and off its books even faster. Think of your admission and discharge as a fast-moving revolving door. Getting you out even more quickly may require a practical use for time warps and string theory.

The secondary goal of the hospitalist movement bows to your own doctor, who manages and values his schedule more than he does your care. Bluntly, a hospitalist's job is to decrease not only your length of stay in the hospital but the amount of time your own doctor devotes to your care. You are treated as a burden and an obstacle to goals that relate more to their lifestyles than your life. There is no benefit to you. This is the most unacceptable, unethical, and objectionable technique used by your family doctor to rid himself of a cumbersome and inconvenient daily burden. Yes, that's right—you. Again.

Business is a burden, technological updates are time consuming, paperwork is numbing, the telephone is a total pain, off-hour call is a nightmare. All these obligations can be modified. All these unpleasantries can be avoided or minimized. *You,* however, are not a burden. Nor should you be passed off to the hospitalist who is stranger to both you and your doctor.

Read part 3, "Choosing Your Doctor." It's not hard to investigate the variables in order to make a safe choice or confirm the wisdom of your current one. But this, one of your most important life choices, is undermined when you're placed in the care of a hospitalist at a time when chance should play no role in your care. In light of this we will discuss methods to protect you from the errors this system of care typically makes.

Both your doctor and hospitalist are divesting themselves of their obligations to their patients because they don't want to be involved with you any longer than necessary. Your primary doctor doesn't want to provide services while you are in the hospital; the hospitalist avoids providing services after you've left it. We will see that this line of separation is really a chasm—one into which a majority of patients fall and a great number are subsequently damaged.

There is a balletic precision to this. Your primary clinician bows out silently and without flourish downstage right upon your hospitalization. A mysterious stranger, your hospitalist, later makes his entrance upstage left, carried aloft in an arching lift by the triumphant hospital administration corps de ballet. With leaps and bounds, he effects your rapid ejection from the stage, whereupon he makes his bittersweet "Dying Swan" adieu to the wild applause of hospital administrators, accountants, and insurers.

This unhappy *pas de deux* arises from the desire to transfer your care to someone else. Hospitalists are actually primary care doctors who belong in community offices. Instead, the collapsing primary care system, which is now in crisis in part due to their absence, dumps you in the hospital, ironically increasing the perceived need for even more hospitalists. It's a vicious cycle in which hospitals and doctors scramble to avoid the *only* obligation that they should never transfer. Continuity of care is a basic tenet of primary care. Patients who are connected to a particular physician are more likely to have received recommended care than patients who are not. What happens to that connectedness when doctors find continuity of care to be an inconvenience, rather than a basic tenet of medicine? It's lost.

End of life issues make this connectedness particularly important and its loss a poignant fact of life in the hospitalist system of care. In an article in the *Archives of Internal Medicine* (2009), the authors note, "continuity [of care] loss involved the patient physician relationship, distinct from medical expertise. 'I think that it's important that you still have that contact with them even though there isn't anything they can do to make you better,' said one patient, who continued, 'I mean, what are they going to do? There isn't anything they can do. And I realize that, but they can hold my hand, so to speak, to the very end.' A nurse recalled how this abandonment fear surfaced with a sense of 'desperation' over an unplanned hospital admission: '[The patient asked] Will you go with me? Will you come out and see me?'"

The article later points to physicians who understand their roles: "As one physician put it, 'What patients need is to know that you care about them. That you care about their future and that you're there for them.' Another physician said, 'I want patients to know that, when the going gets tough, I don't just bow out.'"[8] Dr. Howard Beckman in 2009 says it best: "After almost 2 decades of admitting to the same hospital, visiting patients there now feels like entering a foreign world. When I agreed to the hospitalist system, I believed that I would be a member of my patients' hospital team. . . . My belief that hospitalist care would result in "abandoning my patients" has largely been validated. As a new system replaced the old, we have lost continuity of care and the core element of effective cross-coverage: skilled explicit transitions of responsibility from one clinician to another."[9]

If you are a patient in a single- or multi-specialty group there should always be a rotating partner, associate, or nurse practitioner on-site and on duty, ready to admit you, with your chart in hand, and a recent discussion with your family doctor in mind. This is one of the reasons you have chosen this doctor and this group. But even if this service is not available, there are alternatives to hospitalists.

The need for hospitalization, whether elective or emergent, will always require subspecialists—cardiologists, oncologists, gastroenterologists, rheumatologists, and others. These "ologists" will provide most of the recommendations for your care. They will be recommending, and occasionally performing, your diagnostic and therapeutic procedures. Hospitalists bring no special skills, cognitive or procedural, to your bedside aside from their purported, but never proven, superior availability and affordability.

The "ologists" are chosen by your primary physician. These specialized medical divos and divas will bow only to the call of a primary care doctor. It's the specialists' mantra: "Never piss off a primary." It's all about referrals and the dollars the primary physicians generate for the specialists.

Private "ologists" should, and typically do, have their own on-site staff by dint of their resources in manpower and money. This assures that the right doctor, in a rapid deployment mode, will appear at your bedside. So there you are—a representative from your doctor's office and/or the specialist you need, all quickly and seamlessly provided.

The fact is your primary physician is the ringleader in this circus. He does not have to have his head in the mouth of the tiger. He runs the show, calls in the acts, makes sure the performances are done well and in the proper sequence—all while keeping an eye on the audience. This is an important and stressful job. But it's not so overwhelming that a doctor should endanger your health by avoiding it.

WHAT DOES THE HOSPITALIST PROVIDE?

Availability?

The purported advantage of a hospitalist's touted availability diminishes when the mise-en-scène is better provided by your primary physician, or his group, and the secondary care groups on-site. The benefits of availability presuppose an ability to perform, upon their speedy arrival, a needed service. Under hospitalists' care this may not be the case. Up to 30 percent of you will, due to mismatching, be met by a person who is ill-trained to do more than say "hello." A hospitalist's presence will not obviate the need for a cardiologist during a heart attack or a surgeon during an abdominal crisis. Indeed, they may retard the process in five ways.

1) The transition as you are "handed off" is prone to the same delays and fumbles as a hand-off in football. The more people who touch you, the greater the chance of a mishap. You are no football.
2) The absolute and inevitable fact is that there will be duplication of tests and the performance of unnecessary ones. Your own physician has immediate access to all your records and prior testing results. He will order only what's necessary, thereby decreasing your risks and delays.
3) Hospitalists first see you, assess you, and then call in the "ologists." Your own ringleader-doctor can, in contrast, make them magically appear with a phone call made an hour *before* you arrive, whether it's an emergency or elective admission. He knows you, knows your history, and knows your health issues. When your primary physician tells a specialist "now," he means "Now!"
4) There may be a delay as you wait to see your internist-hospitalist. If you're lying there with a broken hip, all you really initially need is an orthopedist—not a hospitalist.
5) There is limited evidence supporting the beneficial effects of rapid response teams on clinical outcomes. In 2010 the issue was again studied and yet revealed no evidence that rapid response teams improved outcomes.[10] Hospitals are chock-a-block with medical personnel. Even at night, available emergency department staff will respond to urgent needs. It's best that you and your doctor-advocate lobby hard for the most appropriate setting for your care. When you are in the right place getting the right intensity of care the need for rapid response teams decreases.

Early response teams and paramedics have a quasi-military gung ho SWAT team ethic. These energetic responses to real or perceived emergencies are often the opportunity for high spirits and bad practice. In my training days when an emergency was announced on the hospital P.A. system, the ensuing melee at the bedside looked more like a street mugging than a clinical exercise. I'm sure that's what the patient experienced as well.

When my chief resident arrived at this street brawl, the first words out of his mouth were the roared commands, "Stop what you are doing—NOW. Step back—NOW." Later when I questioned his interruption of an emergency, he told me, "It might mean a delay of four or five seconds. But it's more likely I'm interrupting eight simultaneous errors in judgment and performance."

The more rapidly doctors approach the room of a patient in trouble the more likely it is they will exert their skills inappropriately, incorrectly, and always unhygienically. Emergencies, true or false, can result in a syndrome of treating first and asking questions later. Ready, fire, aim is a deadly combination in well-intentioned mayhem.

Only 50 percent of hospitalists provide care on weekends and off-hours. Most sign off at 5 p.m. I don't know a single, private, primary care physician who can clock out at this hour.

Affordability?

This is an advantage afforded others—not you. Decreasing your length of stay and the resultant health-care costs is the principle benchmark used to justify the hospitalist movement.

Twenty-five years ago, elective hospital admissions for workups carried out at a leisurely pace were common for conditions that now can be safely evaluated in an outpatient setting. Those days are long gone. The cost savings are fully justified. No one today will confuse the hospital room with a hotel suite. The most recent figures available in 2010 show that the average hospital length of stay in the United States decreased from 7.8 days in 1970 to 4.8 days in 2006.[11] So, if a little is good then a lot is better. Right? Wrong. The pendulum has swung to the opposite extreme, which is the current norm.

I've discussed the "ejection seat" mode of patient discharges from the hospital. More common is the furlough of patients who are still in a post-traumatic stupor. Your hospitalist will show you—the stunned, and only recently sensate, patient—to the door, with one eye on your vital signs and the other on his own vital statistics. His statistics represent the utilization figures that are expressed as hours of care delivered to you from the moment you entered the hospital until the second you're history, literally or figuratively. For him, it boils down to the fewer hours, the better. If this is associated with "the absence of harm," it is then viewed as a benefit. *"Not harming you" is the new "helping you."*

Your hospitalist may work with a clear conflict of interest if his salary, bonus, or income withholds are affected by the speed of your discharge.[12] If so, he is disqualified from your care. It would be wise to ask your hospitalist whether this conflict of interest applies. He is ethically under an obligation to tell you. So if you have to ask and he hasn't told you, he is guilty twice.

Don't be afraid to make waves. MAKE TSUNAMIS. It is no exaggeration to say that you are fighting for your life. If you, temperamentally, can't make waves, make sure your room coaches are not afraid to take on anyone who might be blocking your way.

Recently my forty-nine-year-old brother-in-law twice removed (don't ask, it's a twenty-first-century thing) suffered a transient ischemic attack. This is a temporary and reversible neurological deficit that portends future catastrophic strokes. It is usually caused by a clot or embolus that temporarily disrupts blood flow to the brain. Partially paralyzed, he was rushed to the hospital, where he received superb emergency evaluation and timely surgery. The relief of the carotid blockage took four hours. It was an unexpectedly complicated procedure. A leg vein served as a shunt to maintain blood flow to his brain, while the acute thrombosis and clot in his carotid artery were evacuated.

He woke up, post-anesthesia, with two large fresh surgical scars, a lot of pain, and a bag full of new medications. Dazed psychologically and physically from a narrowly averted catastrophe and tissue disruptions of his neck, artery, and leg, he was incapable of processing the changes in his appearance and all the lifestyle modifications that now would be required. It was hard enough to shake away the cobwebs.

It's rare when a patient actually follows through on doctor recommendations to stop smoking, lose weight, or increase exercise. This lifestyle trifecta is rarely achieved when all three are required. It is *never* achieved in the absence of counseling. Yet, sixteen hours from the moment my brother-in-law's eyelids fluttered open, he was home on his couch. His doctors told him that he could return to work in two days, in effect making this horrible event the equivalent of a long weekend.

People can become stricken with life-threatening conditions and injuries in the time that it takes to draw a breath, just as my brother-in-law was. Recovery is always, by contrast, a prolonged affair made up of many cascading events that give lie to the fiction of the "uneventful recovery" so casually, universally, and dismissively predicted by the vast majority of excessively sanguine surgeons. Regaining full consciousness and a recalibration of self—the integration of the old familiar you and the brand-new you that disease or injury has wrought—is not achieved by the classic slap on the face and the "are you awake yet?" rituals of anesthesiologists.

Your wounds must be tenderly explored both emotionally and physically. Adjusting to these realities is not accomplished in the time used to enjoy a July 4th holiday weekend. Nor does it give hospital staff the necessary time to treat you carefully and sympathetically.

Tissues become vital, bones mend, scars heal, purposeful activities return. They do so slowly and painfully, with the need to regain the fluidity of what used to be automatic. That some wounds never heal, and that function returns incompletely to some and to others not at all, is common. Recoveries are roller-coaster rides: stomach-lurching lows are interspersed with dizzying highs, and yet, progress is sometimes too minimal to measure.

The notion of a convalescence, an in-hospital, "in-between" hiatus that occurs soon after improvement and before discharge is now a quaint relic— long abandoned but still desirable. It was ushered out chronologically, if not causally, when hospitalists were invited in. Oliver Sacks, in his book *A Leg to Stand On*,[13] notes a state he calls "patienthood." It is associated with the need to heal but also with necessary surrender to institutional needs as a precondition for recovery. He recognizes a patient's need, albeit brief, for an almost infantile regression resulting from illness that can, through the dependence it fosters, actually improve care. A hospitalist's job description eliminates this brief but necessary interregnum.

And the Results?

You are discharged only eight to twenty hours before your own doctor would have discharged you, had he been caring for you. This tiny "in-between" that allows for an abbreviated "patienthood" and a mini-convalescence is a luxury only in comparison to what is given to you by hospitalists. The monetary advantages range from the modest to the illusory. In a *New England Journal of Medicine* article, the authors state that "Hospitalist care appears to be modestly less expensive than that provided by internists but it offers no statistical savings as compared with the care provided by family practitioners."[14] Their care is characterized by neither superior availability nor greater affordability.

So what *do* they provide?

Quality of Care?

There is no consistent body of evidence demonstrating that hospitalists provide superiority of care over a patient's own physician. In 2010 two studies addressed this question. The authors of the first survey concluded that quality of care measurements for hospitalists showed mixed results. They did note that in some clinical areas care was marginally enhanced.[15] The second study compared hospitalist care with the previous more traditional models of patient supervision. The results: "no statistically significant differences were found in mortality rate, readmission, or length of stay. There was a moderate decrease in adjusted hospital costs after implementation [for hospitalists]."[16]

You are giving up a lot to gain little or nothing. The bar is set very low for hospitalists. "Non-inferiority" is their benchmark. *Yes, "non-inferiority" is the new "better."*

None of these studies address the only important issue: your results as they play out over the time that *follows* your hospitalization. While hospitals, their hospitalists, and insurance companies make even more finely calibrated stopwatches, your success is measured crudely in hours—from your admission to your discharge. But you haven't disappeared just because they've shut their eyes and wished you away.

INTO THE BREACH

In Shakespeare's *Henry V*, the young Prince Hal (future Henry V) exhorts his countrymen into battle with the cry, "Once more into the breach, dear friends, once more." Your family doctor asks you to step into the breach. Twice. Henry's passage unpromisingly concludes, "or close the wall up with our English dead."

While you are in the hospital your care should be seamless. Under hospitalists there are two euphemistically titled "transition zones" that occur on admission to and discharge from the hospital. These are the breaches into which quality of care can come to grief, but they typically aren't taken into account in quality-of-care studies. They occur before you are admitted and continue after you've left the hospital. These black holes in the medical literature are the true indicators of the deficiencies in the system.

The quality of your care decreases and the chance for fatal error increases simultaneously the moment your doctor relinquishes your care to a hospitalist. So many things in our society are nontransferable: hunting licenses, automobile warranties, income tax relief between spouses, invitations and passes to special events, your estate after you die, some computer files, your vote, your identification, and so on. That this transfer from primary care to hospitalist care is so effortless and casual is objectionable on its face. And after the hospitalist is done you are disgorged blithely and usually incompetently back to wherever it was that you came from.

First to the breaches! What happens, why, and finally how to avoid them.

Breach Number One: The Transition from Your Doctor's Care to the Hospitalist's

Inadequate communication is responsible for 50 percent of all medication errors. Most of these occur almost immediately when you step through the hospital doors. An article in the *Journal of Evaluation in Clinical Practice* commented on the prevalence of medication error on admission to the hospital. "Error is a leading cause of avoidable harm suffered by patients, resulting in significantly increased morbidity, prolonged length of stay in hospital and increased mortality. Medication error occurs most commonly at the interfaces of care. At point of hospital admission, variances between the medications patients were taking prior to admission and their prescriptions on admission ranged from 30% to 70% in two recent literature reviews."[17]

Twenty-five percent of these errors are due to an inadequate medical history and the failure to review your prior medical records. These would not occur as frequently if you were under the care of your own doctor. In light of this, you want to minimize your chances of being one of the 770,000 people who die or are injured annually due to a variety of adverse drug events. Your chances of becoming a statistic increase when you fall into the breach in care created by others. It's not just likely, but almost certain, that you will be admitted to the hospital with an incorrect or incomplete name, age, diagnosis, drug allergy history, name of referring physician, and contact telephone numbers for your physician, family, or medical proxy—either separately or in combination.

Breach Number Two: Going Home

The interregnum that occurs between your departure from the hospital and your return to your doctor's office is even more prone to serious error. Now there are all sorts of new things to get wrong. The burden of newly generated data and new medications makes errors more common and, in the aftermath of your hospitalization, these errors have more severe ramifications.

Your reentry to daily life is characterized by as dense a communication blackout as accompanies the space shuttle on its reentry to the earth's atmosphere—only it takes longer. All agree that there is a certain amount of information that is needed when you return home if you are to continue to recover successfully. At minimum, your family doctor will need a discharge summary, your physical findings, the results of your testing, and changes in your medication, as well as the reasons for these alterations. Specific reference must be made to the results of pending labs and testing performed in the few days prior to your discharge. Recommendations for follow-up testing should always be present. Inpatient counseling, condition-specific information, and the opportunity to ask questions should occur before you leave the hospital.

Under a hospitalist's care each of these mandates are prone to error, deficiency, or even omission, separately or, more often, in combination. Errors and lapses in documentation occur in every aspect of your care. Data that is incorrect, incomplete, or obscured from view provides the majority of failures in hospitalist discharges. In this modern clinical fantasy world, 20 to 50 percent of you will experience an adverse event; of that number, 66 to 72 percent will involve medication errors and, of these, up to 75 percent will be preventable.

The results of the tests you endured, took risks in having, and for which you will be unerringly billed are incorrectly listed or missing 29 percent of the time. It was shown in 2010 that in the rush to get you out, you, while dusting yourself off at the curb, will still have 40 percent of your test results pending.[18] Forty-three percent of these will show abnormalities; 10 percent of these will be significant enough to require action; 60 percent of the hospitalists who ordered them are, and will forever be, unaware of them. One to two percent of these abnormalities are so dramatic that they would lead to a change in your diagnosis or therapy. Finally, the fact that fewer than half of the primary doctors were contacted during a patient's hospitalization or informed of a patient's discharge is indicative of the degree to which primary care physicians are ignored, isolated, and marginalized by the hospitalist system. These facts come from a study of 2,644 patients who were discharged from two Boston hospitals.[19] In another survey of over 900 primary care doctors performed in 2009, the investigators noted, "More than half reported not receiving a discharge summary within two weeks, and almost one quarter did not have any knowledge that their patients had been admitted at all."[20]

To hospitalists, you are like Athena—appearing as if from nowhere upon admission. You are also likely to end like Lucky in Samuel Beckett's play *Waiting for Godot*—going nowhere upon discharge. To hospitalists, you exist only while in the hospital. So, yes, you are treated like a Greek goddess and you are "Lucky" indeed. But to state that your risks are no worse with hospitalists while *in* the hospital misses the point entirely.

No surprise then that some studies show that you are 6.2 to 7 times more likely to be re-hospitalized within three months when under a hospitalist's care.[21] This does not include the 23 percent of you who are injured but don't require hospitalization to fix the errors made during your stay.

If that readmission is needed, it's unlikely that your care will be assumed by the same hospitalist. *New* strangers, unaware of critical clinical facts, will appear. Only 48.5 percent of your discharging physicians are made aware of your readmission. Communication between teams occurred only 43.7 percent of the time.[22] There are no strangers; just doctors you haven't met.

There are 100,000 interns, residents, and fellows working in our hospitals. They are the most overworked, inexperienced, sleep-deprived physicians in the country. They may also be the first doctors to see you.

Typically they work at teaching hospitals associated with universities and medical schools. These are the same hospitals that also tend to employ hospitalists. Having two doctors, one a stranger and the other a beginner, is something too awful to even contemplate, much less subject yourself to. Interns and residents who are poorly supervised are prone to errors in judgment and performance. If left completely unsupervised, they increase the chances of error and poor clinical outcomes. A disproportionate percentage of malpractice cases involve them.

Hey, I went through training too. My best memories are of the mentors who shaped the physician I became. My worst flashbacks are of the times I was left alone to improvise.

Welcome these shiny pennies to your bedside. Inform them that you look forward to working with them. Tell them, however, that their orders need to be approved by the attending senior physician, who, you might also inform them, is expected to appear at least once a day at your bedside. They may bridle, but so what? Your health is on the line. Interns and residents should never be the agents who discharge you. Interns are so overworked and anxious to get you out that hospitalists will seem leisurely in comparison.

Even without studies and their statistics, it is intuitively obvious to even the most casual observer that a stranger, no matter how qualified, is no substitute for your own doctor. Only if your primary doctor is a complete dolt might a hospitalist be preferred. That "the devil you don't know is better than the one you do" turns the old adage on its head.

THE ADVICE

In light of this fact you'll need advice on how to avoid the pitfalls while under their supervision.

On Admission

If you must have a hospitalist, make sure you are physically in possession of your personal records. Don't rely on hospital staff to log into a computer in your behalf to obtain your online history. They probably won't. Print it out yourself.

Never go to the hospital, whether electively or in an emergency, without having someone bring your office chart to the stranger who is now taking care of you. Even if your doctor has deserted you, the office shouldn't compound this mistake with the failure to deliver a copy of your entire record. Don't settle for the last note in your chart or a past summary of your care. At the hospital, allow the doctors to review it in your presence or to return it after a specified period of time. If you relinquish it, your records and the protection they offer will be lost forever—guaranteed.

On the day of your admission inform your hospitalist and the discharge planner that you will require, upon the date of your discharge, your entire hospital record. A written discharge summary is unacceptable. Obtain their agreement. Have a check ready for any possible fees that this necessity may require.

Put your hospitalist on notice that upon discharge you will require a follow-up appointment with your primary physician within five days. Obtain his agreement.

A consumer-driven demand for the care you deserve puts everybody on notice without making them defensive. If they resist, ask to speak with the medical director and obtain a copy of the hospital's "Patient Bill of Rights." Okay, now you've raised their defense mechanisms. But remember, better to be rude than to be . . . (you do the rhyming).

If you have been seen as an outpatient by a subspecialist relevant to your admission it is imperative that he be called in immediately. Do not allow strangers to take care of your heart, lungs, eyes, kidneys, or brain if trusted doctors have seen to you in the past. Specialists do not use hospitalists. Specialists can be used instead of them.

When You Leave the Hospital

If you give them a break they'll give you a breach. If the demanded hospital chart or the return appointment to your own doctor is not delivered to you, do not go home. Do not leave your room. Don't even leave your bed. Because if you do, you're likely to be back . . . soon. In 2010 it was shown that those lacking timely follow-up with their primary care doctors were ten times more likely to be readmitted. It's best to be seen in a few days, but longer than a few weeks is unacceptable.[23] Remind personnel that these were required and agreed to on admission. Demand to see the medical director and request again that the hospital's "Patient Bill of Rights" be delivered to you forthwith. Inquire if the hospital administrator on call is available. Accept no assurances that your records will immediately be sent to your doctor by fax, phone, or FedEx—they won't (see chapter 19).

Obtain or prepare a list of all the tests you had in the previous three days. You can compile it by inquiring about each blood draw, each stretcher adventure, and each consult that sees you. Add this information to your log. Now you're officially a self-advocate.

Review your written prescriptions carefully. If any medications taken prior to hospitalization have been stopped, ask, because it is most likely an error of omission. New medications should be accompanied by educational materials. If *you* can't read the name or the dose on the prescription, have it rewritten. The pharmacist probably can decipher them but why should you take that chance? This ensures that any prescriptions will be for the correct condition, and not a product of error. Why treat a condition you don't have while the problems you were hospitalized for go therapeutically ignored?

Yes, it's a lot to do, and yes, you have a lot on your mind. But remember, if you give them an out, they will take it.

What Is Your Primary Care Physician Willing to Do?

First make sure your own doctor knows you're in the hospital. Many of your own doctors who would be able to help might not even know that you are fighting for your life just an elevator ride away. Sixty-two percent of you will never hear from your primary care doctors while in the hospital.[24] Perhaps they don't care you're there. Perhaps they don't know. Let them know and *then* see if they care.

The best doctor is the one who takes care of you both in the office and while you're in the hospital. If your practitioner will not or is unable to attend to you during your personal medical diaspora, will he see you every second day? No? Every third day? Failing this will your doctor make periodic telephone calls to your hospitalist and to the nursing station? Failing this, will he request a daily fax from your hospitalist that includes current chart notes and laboratory data? If not, will he give you the telephone number of a designated staffer within the office who will relay your important concerns and your progress? Will your doctor respond to e-mails?

Failing all of these would disqualify him from providing your care. Given the range of possibilities that he can choose from, agreeing to *none* of them is a deal breaker. When you go home it's necessary to continue your care, however temporary, with the family doctor who has failed you; then start your search for a new one.

What Is Your Hospitalist Willing to Do?

Demand that she send daily faxes to your doctor that include progress and consultative notes and lab results. Demand that all dictated notes and labs be sent to your primary physician. All this requires is a phone call to the lab and the hospital transcription service informing them that your data must have a courtesy copy (cc) sent to your private doctor.

Inform your hospitalist that you look forward to working with her, but make it clear that you are aware of the weaknesses associated with this specialty. "Hey, nothing personal, doc, I don't even know you; but that's the point. Right?" Inform her that you would much prefer your own doctor on-site and that you would expect her to act in your behalf at all times. Inquire if there are any conflicts of interest that might vitiate this request.

Trusting your fate to strangers with fingers crossed is the beginning of a star-crossed course.

3

Medical On-Call

- Why what has previously been viewed as medical abandonment is now considered effective time management.
- Finding your own doctor off-hours is a long shot—why?
- On-call doctors do all they can to avoid you—why?
- Nighttime, on-call "tricks of the trade" are explained by Drs. Justin Case, Willie Soomie, Izzy A. Newcomber, and I. M. Zslypey.
- There are steps to take when you're stricken and stuck at home. What *is* an emergency?
- Establishing your own "do not call" registry is important—when keeping your phone *on* the hook keeps you *off* the hook.
- Why fragmented, uncoordinated, and non-continuous care is now the rule.
- There are no strangers . . . just doctors you haven't met.
- The myth of the telephone as a diagnostic and therapeutic agent.

Being on call (also referred to as "call") is the last duty of a doctor's day. For a doctor, this means a potential thirty-six-hour marathon of work-call-work. Call responsibilities that are too frequent and perilously proximate become unsustainable.

1. Alertness is tested in the face of fatigue.
2. Patience is tested in the face of continuous interruptions.
3. Patient risks are increased in the face of a doctor's sleep deprivation.

All this makes medical on-call an unhappy experience for your doctor and a risky one for you.

This is another instance when our problems quickly become yours, when the burdens of practice are seen as so onerous that doctors will use every possible avenue to minimize or avoid them. Again, it becomes your problem. You could show up at an emergency room today only to find that there are no specialists to assist you with an urgent need. You're increasingly likely to find your erstwhile care provider at his new medical spa rather than his office. More physician/entrepreneurs may be spending their time at these medical-care-cash-registers performing facials and dermabrasions, and offering depilatories and Botox. If your specialist isn't in the emergency room you may instead find him at one of the 2,500 medical laser clinics that are in business nationwide. This is a fivefold increase from just four years ago. These and other medical service models are, essentially, a doctor's "you can't bother me anymore" clinics. These businesses are inexpensive to establish, and reimbursement is by cash only. The examinations are low risk, easy to perform, and highly profitable. These medical careers are now devoid of on-call duties.

Yet, medical on-call duties are now more frequently requested than in the past. There is a demand for mastery in advanced technical skills. Newer exotic-toxic pharmacologics require the presence of an expert. In the not-so-distant past, patients with heart attacks, strokes, and GI bleeding went to their hospital rooms with supportive care only. There were no techniques, procedures, or medications that, the moment they were used, dramatically improved outcomes. Conditions that today would require emergency interventions went undiagnosed in the absence of what current technologies can spot.

Emergency department physicians call for help now, even if they don't need it. The presence of specialists simultaneously decreases their workload and their liability exposure. Both are potent inducements to picking up the phone. Emergency rooms are primary care clinics for millions. As the number of uninsured and underinsured increases, they present themselves to emergency rooms with acute exacerbations of untreated chronic clinical conditions. They arrive in increasing numbers with end-stage diseases of the lungs, kidney, liver, and heart. These duties always require specialized care and are most often requested on nights and weekends.

In light of this, it's time to sit back and reflect a bit about what this means for all of us. A doctor's availability off-hours is no longer assured. *Your* doctor's availability is highly unlikely on any given night or weekend due to larger coverage groups.

If your doctor has been out all night in the open chest of a motor vehicle accident victim, she will be both bleary-eyed and stressed by the time of your 7:00 a.m. coronary artery bypass. How badly will her skills have degraded by the time she performs her third coronary bypass at 3:00 p.m. that afternoon? The answer? According to a 2010 study, sleep deprivation "may result in lowered levels of alertness and an increased risk of errors in people on night duty, such as medical personnel."[1] Your family practitioner, who attended a patient at 2:00 a.m., may offer you less time and detail during your long-awaited appointment. He may be unfocused in his discussion and more abrupt in manner. Your need for new antihypertensives will be less well understood, and your compliance less likely.

If your doctor shares on-call duties with a physician from another group (cross-covering), it's good for him but bad for you. The chances for potential medical error multiply. Sleep deprivation, care under the supervision of a stranger, and now the addition of inevitable communication flaws that occur between groups the following morning, can align in such a way to increase your risk astronomically.

Cross-covering doctors do not have access to your medical records. They will treat you the same way a Volvo dealership might when you bring in your Saab for repairs. Since they have no real interest in the relationship, the rigor and vigor used in your care may become diluted, especially if, in a few hours, the buck can be passed back to your own doctor. When choices need to be made, these variables should not play a role. But they do.

MY LIFE ON CALL

While training in a New York City municipal hospital, I took call every third night. Here's what that means:

Monday: 7 a.m.–7 p.m. (12 hours)
Tuesday: 7 a.m.–7 p.m. (12 hours)
Wednesday: 7 a.m.–7 p.m. Thursday evening (36 hours)
Friday: 7 a.m.–7 p.m. (12 hours)
Saturday: 7 a.m.–7 p.m. (12 hours)
Sunday: 7 a.m.–7 p.m. Monday evening (36 hours)
A 105-hour workweek!

The thirty-six-plus hours of call ran perilously close to each other. A day off occurred once every ten. In the face of the gravity of illnesses that were the stock and trade of any large municipal hospital this was a crushing burden, fraught with stress, depression, anxiety, and unhealthy habits.

Three decades have passed but even in 2010 over-tired trainees are still the subject of discussion and controversy. This is a current cautionary tale. In December 2008, the Institute of Medicine proposed revisions in hospital scheduling to decrease the chances of fatigue-related errors. Even so, there was no serious challenge to the bruising eighty-hour weeks currently allowed. Rather the report urged that trainees work no more than sixteen hours consecutively, at which point a mandatory five-hour sleep break was suggested.

Feel better with this knowledge? I wouldn't.

In 1974, our 110-hour workweeks were compensated for only by a wonderful camaraderie otherwise only found amongst troops in combat. This is what my brothers-in-arms and I were. As much medics in battle as interns on duty, we never left our wounded behind.

I remember a thirty-eight-year-old woman, Irene, who came in one morning with congestive heart failure, in shock due to a massive heart attack. I met her as I entered the hospital because I unwisely used the emergency room entrance. Grabbing her gurney, I took her in the elevator to the coronary care unit. Five days of futile effort left her dead, her large family devastated, and me, her intern, broken up and broken down. I remember visiting her family months later in an unlikely beautiful bungalow perched on the bay under the Throgs Neck Bridge in the Bronx.

Three hours after Irene's admission and in the midst of frantic activity in her behalf, a combative and drunken lady with alcoholic cirrhosis and end-stage liver disease became mine. Yellow with jaundice, abdomen tense with fluid, she was exsanguinating, as well as drowning, in her own vomited blood. Her name was Dorothy. When she awakened she asked me if the Malach ha'Mavet would be coming. When an elderly black woman asks in fluent Yiddish whether the angel of death is coming, she certainly gets your attention. She lived in the Bronx not far from my father's drugstore, and they knew each other well. Her Yiddish came from her long-dead Jewish boyfriend. We were friends until the end—four days later.

After these patients, who I remember with affection and clarity, the shades shut. My memory of the next few patients is not vivid and what made them unique was lost.

Four hours after Dorothy, an eighty-year-old woman in a diabetic coma.

Three hours after that, a young black woman in sickle-cell anemia crisis.

Five hours later, a demented ninety-year-old nursing home patient with a fever of 104.

It was only 10:00 p.m. and the night had just begun. My thirty inpatients, admitted from prior on-call days, still occupied their beds—and my thoughts. They demanded my attention, as did the sixty to seventy patients signed out to me by my fellow interns, now homeward-bound. These unknown patients were time bombs who I prayed would not detonate that night.

My resident and attending physician did their rounds, supervised, and generally kept their distance from me. It took only one look at my "deer in the headlights" eyes that would mercurially turn to a menacing, Travis Bickle–like stare ("You talkin' to me? Then who the hell else are you talkin' to?"). And they silently backed off. Don't for a second be fooled by the doctor/hospital television shows you watch. Doctors then and now have no time for casual conversations, leisurely conferences, and off-site adventures. They did and do have time for the occasional fling.

By seven the next morning I had four more admissions. None had the favored, and much-sought-after, gift of a ROMI diagnosis (Rule Out Myocardial Infarction), which would have meant I could tuck 'em in and wait for the blood work while I got back to more serious affairs.

Emergency room residents who admitted everyone they saw were objects of bitter derision. They were "Sieves." Those who would not even admit their own mothers in agonal throes were our heroes and earned the honorific "Rocks." That night even the "Rocks" crumbled. All my admissions were critical. Denied any sleep, I was, at least, freed from the possibility of new admissions. I went to work filling holes I'd only crudely patched the night before and desperately prayed that the patches would hold until I could get back to them.

An automaton, I walked the hallways of my ward. I used a tool belt that I'd fashioned for myself. It transported empty syringes and those filled with blood from recent draws. Medical specimen containers attached to my belt—empty or filled with urine, cerebral spinal fluid, phlegm, or stool samples—bounced about my hips. Compartments for gloves, masks, tourniquets, chemical reagents, dipsticks, pipettes, microscope slides, capillary tubes, lubricant jelly, and ever longer "to-do" lists had to make room for two packs of Marlboros and a lighter. The lighter did double duty, firing up both Bunsen burners and my Marlboros. In those days, now long gone, doctors performed their own lab tests and smoked incessantly. The two packs of cigarettes wouldn't last the day. It's sad to report that I'd examine, and drain of various body fluids, the occasional 3:00 a.m. comatose patient while a cigarette protruded jauntily from my mouth. Smoke gets in your eyes.

The weight of this tool belt posed no danger of bringing my "whites" down to the levels that might excite comment, if not excitement. I gained twenty-five pounds through compulsive and unhealthy stress-related gorging. My new rounder belly held the belt firmly in place. Now lower on my hips, it too was at a jaunty angle, one side up, the other weighed down by the equipment. I fancied that my belt was a holster and I was a cowboy walking the length of my ward, a place more dangerous than the streets of Laredo. Almost hallucinatory, I'd get home around 7:00 p.m., after thirty-six hours of a sustained high-wire act surrounded by death, and my fears that, during the course of the day, I'd caused it. There were times I was so busy, I wished that those fated to die would just get it over with. My chief resident told me that it was okay to wish them dead; it was not okay to get them dead.

In my fatigue I experienced what I later decided were two cognitive blackouts. On those two occasions, awakening on my recliner at home, I found, spilled over my clothing, an entire meal I didn't remember buying, much less eating. After the last such frightening occasion, I recorded a diary entry I still turn to thirty-five years later: "One day when I am a big deal f-----g specialist this will be remembered only as yesterday's nightmare."

Well, maybe.

When I started my own practice, seven years later, I performed my own on-call duties 95 percent of the time. I worked each day and was on call every weekday night, weekend, and holiday. So much for abandoning the nightmares of yesteryear. There was one other gastroenterologist in town. Our mutual competitiveness kept us in separate orbits. For the first few months, the combination of the novelty of being on call for my own business and its relative unobtrusiveness in my life, enabled by a still patientless office, led to few demands. My frequent calls to my answering service asking "Any calls for me?" were met with laughter and ultimately, impatience. I am sure they had a pool, gambling on when this patient-free doctor would leave town and them alone.

Eighteen months later I was the proud owner of the old "1,000-yard stare" and a fifteen-pound weight gain I thought I'd left behind in the Bronx in 1974. My practice exploded and my personal life imploded. On too many days my family and my patients were subjected to the "new-old me" from my training days. I was once again among the walking wounded. I never had to call my service again. Their calls to me caused physical pain.

Flash forward, twenty-five years later. I was now in the midst of the large group that I'd created and now managed. I had under my supervision seven physicians, four physician extenders, seven nurses, and sixty employees in several office locations. I was on call every eighth weekend and every eighth weekday night. Finally, El Dorado!?

Well . . . in some ways I was still no better off. As my practice expanded and required more doctors, nurses, and offices, the number of patients, hospitals, and inpatients outpaced the meteoric rate of growth of which I was so proud. This conceit turned to ashes in my mouth when I was on call. The collective responsibilities my group shared were no longer divided when I was on call; now the responsibility for the patients of eight doctors and four physician extenders was all mine. I generated my own force field strong enough it seemed to make the hospitals' fluorescents flicker in my wake. My 100 billion neurons, interconnected at 100 trillion synapses, crackled with electricity. My head was a Vandergraff generator.

Almost every on-call experience, especially on weekends, was a guaranteed dawn-to-dawn sprint from one emergency to the next, and a marathon to the far-flung hospitals in our medical kingdom. Phone calls seemed to arrive incessantly, like breaking news alerts from Reuters. Any of the tens of thousands of patients, historically in our care, could call. It seemed to me as if most of them did, no matter how distant their last contact.

It took only a quarter and a question to make the phone ring. I envisioned lines of patients feeding quarters, Vegas-style, into countless slot machines. In this case, the payoff was a sure thing—me! Calls from patients in the throes of crapulence or crises required from me as much guesswork as a contestant on *Let's Make a Deal*. The inevitability of doubts that arose from advice given to patients over the phone, many incoherent with anxiety or pain, inevitably led to a quick response: "Go to the emergency room." I—and later in my career my physician assistant—preferred to see these folks in person rather than tossing about in our beds, waking our spouses, and worrying about them and their lawyers (the "them" and the "their" could refer to my patients, or each of our spouses).

So many easy opportunities for error—so few and difficult are the strategies for success. So many doctors make assumptions rather than confirming readily available facts. "Enter through the narrow gate. For wide is the gate and broad is the way that leads to destruction and there are many who enter through it. But small is the gate and narrow the road that leads to life and only a few find it" (Matthew 7:13).

If your doctor, regardless of her religion, doesn't know this truism, show it to her. There is no injunction in the Hippocratic Oath more important than this one.

My physician assistant, by screening my calls and being the first to the hospital, replaced me as the first soldier over the trench, charging into a medical no-man's-land. During the week and particularly on weekend call, I was open for business to everyone except my family who, like refugees from a natural disaster, took to the exits in a state of mild panic. Calls came from doctors, patients, their relatives, any ward nurse, ward secretary, lab technician, pharmacist, doctor, physician extender, social worker, or discharge planner in any of the three hospitals that made up our little empire. Even people who called us by mistake got unsolicited advice.

Calls from nursing stations were too often blithely passed on—pro forma, buck-passing exercises—to decrease nursing's own liability exposure and that of the hospital. Once it appeared in a patient's chart, the designation "M.D. aware" protected staff from everything but the legal repercussions of a direct, intentional physical assault on my patients.

Overworked and under-informed, the staff met my questions with sighs and almost audible shrugs and eye rolls. "I think so" or "the last time I checked" were the default responses. The "as far as I know" response was my favorite. My retort was, "I don't know how far a road I must travel down to reach the end of what you know. Spare me the trip and call me back in ten minutes with the facts." SLAM. These calls resulted in my own dictation of a précis of the conversation, as I lobbed the ball back onto their court until correct decisions, based on accurate information, could be ensured. I was not a popular doctor. (If your doctor wins the "hospital's most popular doctor" award, I worry about the intensity of his advocacy and his willingness to be ruthless in pursuit of his patients' care.)

Nurses are so woefully overworked, underpaid, unappreciated, and often culturally at odds with their environment that their workplace satisfaction is dismally unlikely. Despite this, "their price is far above rubies" (Proverbs 31), although their pay is far below them.

The hundreds of calls I took in a forty-eight-hour weekend were a descent into the heart of chaos theory. My fate was subject to seismic shifts wrought by but a single call or one abnormal lab result. I heard the flapping of butterfly wings and correctly anticipated tornadoes. The three hospitals, aside from their telephones, also had three intensive care units, three cardiac care units, three emergency rooms, and three recovery rooms, as well as post-ICU step-down units and short-stay units. Hundreds of patients inhabited the general care floors. Drowning in my own success, I would see, on an average weekend, twenty to thirty consults, perform up to a dozen emergency invasive procedures, and be responsible for and perform rounds on the dozens of patients my seven juniors signed out to me. These patients didn't take Saturday and Sunday off. I was not their covering physician. I was their doctor.

Leaving home after hours was routine. Leaving twice in one evening was not unusual. On one occasion, early in my career, I made three separate trips—each a family-awakening, profanity-laden event which brought me to three different hospitals on three different missions, and reduced me to tears—for my sake and for my family's.

By Monday morning I faced another full workweek and geared up for another on-call night. Aware that sooner or later I would hurt myself, or worse, a patient, as well as alienate my family even further, I assembled a true, cohesive medical team comprising my physician assistant, Pat Onate; Barb Reynolds, my nurse of twenty years; followed by Kathy Bullis and me. The unpredicted, but no less tangible, benefits of camaraderie were a welcome bonus. Our on-call nights allowed us the ability to vent our frustrations with, and sometimes on, each other. This spared our families the effects of frayed nerves, overstimulation, and the rants of anger and self-pity.

My family's support, like that of any doctor's family, was like the proverbial faulty faucet. Starting as a mighty torrent, later sputtering with fits of surging gushes alternating with miserly drips, it finally dried up altogether. When there is nothing people can do to help they stop trying.

In the absence of the sympathy I shunned and empathy for an experience that they couldn't fathom, I was happy, temporarily, to be isolated from them and they from me. Members of our small, but potent, team provided each other with mutual support and empathy. We provided our patients timely, seamless care. Our patients came to recognize us as individuals, trusted us, and even looked forward to seeing the three of us in their loneliness and need. *Any* medical group with a minimum of three to five physicians has the resources to use a team model rather than running the hospital gauntlet managing a jerry-rigged team model foisted on them by the hospital.

I miss everything about practice. I have particularly poignant recollections of my patients and staff. I think often about the patients I helped, and those I couldn't. It's been difficult to overcome my sadness at the thought that I will never be able to help someone else medically in a face-to-face setting, and difficult to overcome a sense of melancholy for the failures that are now beyond my future repair. My staff and I enjoyed an intimacy born from the times spent together, shared experiences, affection, and mutual assistance.

I miss being the manager of the group's affairs. The success the group enjoyed was for me a personal journey that none of my partners will ever experience, however brightly the future and their own successes smile on them.

There is one aspect of practice that I do not miss and never will, and you've just read about it. Perhaps some doctors feel less burdened than I did. It's a great solace not to have to embark on an evening or weekend feeling unhappy and anxiety-ridden. The only other aspect of day-to-day care that I was happy to shed was waking up each morning with a knot in my stomach that wouldn't go away until I'd checked the overnight office voice mail that sounded an all clear for those in my care.

On-call duties or services provided to hospitals entail considerable sacrifice, even personal risk. It was an on-call patient who gave me his hepatitis B. My system shrugged it off. Other physician and nursing contacts may not have. Patients have transmitted hepatitis A, B, and C, tuberculosis, and HIV-AIDS to my colleagues; I assisted in the care of these doctors and nurses. The results were never uniformly successful—lives were lost or interrupted and careers ended. This is a fact of life. The sickest patients who spray viral-laden blood and who cough biologically rich respiratory mists in the faces of their caregivers are not inevitably our on-call patients, but they definitely represent a disproportionate number who are.

Most hospitals do not reimburse on-call responsibilities. Even more unappealing is the intensity and breadth of the services that emergency patients require. Uninsured patients tend to let their conditions deteriorate to states that are often end-stage before they come in to the emergency room. The famous 1960s-hippie battle cry, "Suppose they gave a war and nobody came" can be applied here—suppose they gave an emergency and nobody came. It's happening today.

The lifestyles of the minimally invasive: Some doctors retreat to narrow skill sets that are not frequently required during the night. They abandon general orthopedic surgery for the more limited responsibility of hand surgery. Many surgeons restrict their practices to breast surgery, laparoscopic bariatric procedures, and other minimally invasive specialties that also provide minimal invasions to their evenings. The general pool of doctors available for call is shrinking. This is, in part, because of an increasing dissatisfaction with medicine as a career, but there's also a noticeable decrease in the number of doctors on the front lines of on call. The general surgery workforce contracted 25 percent between 1981 and 2005. In the years ahead a 140,000-physician shortfall is projected in the field of primary care. A severe shortage of surgeons is being experienced today in many areas. These losses won't be made up by physician extenders or the legions of internationally trained physicians who will be recruited to fill the gaps. Both early retirement and doctors who switch to allied fields are culling the on-call workforce of its most experienced members at the peak of their skills.

Some physicians and surgeons hire others to perform on-call duties, but per diems fill in no better than round pegs in square holes. They know nothing about the communities and hospitals in which they bivouac. Some groups will hire junior members at night and on weekends. Others may hire trainees to provide a first line of defense.

TRICKS OF THE TRADE

The Great Debaters

Other doctors who are on call, but don't want to respond to an emergency room call, typically engage in debating society tactics over the phone with the emergency department staff. They attack the arguer, and not the argument. They argue from their authority, regardless of the situation's actual merits. They argue that since nothing has been proven, the premise that demands their presence must be false. They pinpoint inconsistencies, ignoring the larger picture. They suggest correlations rather than specialty-specific causations. When all else fails, there is the ever-popular appeal to the emotions.

These doctors win every argument—ask any of their remaining friends. It is here the value of their liberal arts education is most on view.

The Birth of Munificence

Some doctors will do the unthinkable, requesting that a competing same-specialty group be consulted, or magnanimously spread the wealth by recommending that alternative specialty consultants be sought first.

Reverse Cinderellas

Other doctors, rather than leaving home, will leave lists of tests to be performed—some inevitably unnecessary and done simply to run the clock.

When the clock strikes 7:00 a.m., they are nowhere to be seen. These are the "Reverse Cinderellas," When the critical hour strikes their pumpkins turn into Porsches.

The Suddenly Stupid

There are some doctors who suddenly and uncharacteristically demean their own clinical skills as "not up" to the level of care needed when it comes time to perform on-call duties. They suggest that the patient is too ill or too young to be under their care. They insist these unfortunates would be better off at tertiary care centers—pediatric, oncologic, or women's hospitals—than if they submitted to the riskier care of poor country doctors, or hopeless, information-deprived specialists. Thank you for calling.

STRANGERS IN A STRANGE LAND

Okay, you get it. We don't like call. It's a high-risk, uncompensated, family-compromising, unhealthy, psychologically challenging, legally risky lifestyle. And, hey, we can avoid it. But you can't. You will continue to have emergencies and off-hour needs. Here's why you shouldn't like this state of affairs.

The inevitability of strangers is understood in light of the fact that no doctor can cover his practice full-time. It's something to think about before you pick up the phone. We have already addressed strangers in the night, in the hospitalist section.

In the event of a nighttime emergency, you will be dependent on strangers. During a twenty-four-hour day you will not be able to reach your own doctor for 65 percent of the time that the office is closed. It's hard enough to get her even when the office is open. On weekends there is a 100 percent certainty you will not reach your doctor unless she is on call (also unlikely given the increasing numbers of large cross-coverage groups).

In the face of this, I'll go into detail later about what to do when you are stricken and stuck at home.

If you call ahead, the on-call doctor may direct you to the emergency room where he's working. That way, he bundles his patients, travels less, and sees you more expeditiously. If, however, you wind up in an emergency room that is not of your choosing, your own doctor the next morning may find himself in the same predicament when he realizes you're in a hospital where he does not have, or may not want, privileges. *You are now both* strangers in a strange land—a toxic combination.

Before we move on to the errors to which on-call doctors are prone, let's take a shot in the dark, and guess how doctors are likely to behave at two in the morning after their drive in the dark. You are in a state of distress. He is in a state of sleep deprivation and irritation. And both of you are in a state of confusion if neither of you is familiar with the emergency department or its staff.

Unhappy doctors make their patients unhappy very quickly. The unwelcome telephone call, the abrupt interruption of sleep, and the groggy departure into the night often leaves behind a wide-awake and irritated family or partner. This means that you are more likely to meet a sour, dyspeptic, if not dysfunctional, doctor who is terse and tense. He is as worried about his next day (which starts in four hours) as he is about you. So add distracted, disgruntled, dyspeptic, and perhaps dysfunctional to the list. In light of these factors, errors tend to occur far more frequently than when the same services are delivered during the daytime.

What to Do When Stricken and Stuck: So, you're stuck. What can you do? This is, after all, our goal, to help you to understand physician-based issues, which allows you to protect yourself.

If nothing else has been shown in this section, it's that doctors are very skilled in taking care of themselves, their lifestyles, and their incomes—even to the point of leaving you behind, alone or with strangers, to fend for yourself. There are societal issues that need to be addressed, but in the short term they are irrelevant to the problem: what to do when neither your doctor nor his office is open for business. At some point you may find yourself in the hospital, and you will need a blueprint for what to do and how to behave in an environment with so much potential for error and injury.

YOUR PLAN

Developing Your Own "Do Not Call" Registry: The only thing more dangerous than not seeing a doctor? Seeing a doctor. When the doctor who is delivering your care is not your own, the potential for error or injury increases. The vast majority of medical professionals performing on-call duties, though well intentioned, are ignorant of your medical history and have only limited exposure to you. They are apt to do harm, even with the best of intentions. Some, however, are the floaters, drifters, grifters, cameos, and flotsam and jetsam of our profession who leave you prone to their errors during the day, but make you particularly susceptible at night.

Even just one encounter with a doctor who isn't familiar with your history can lead to more errors and injuries than months or years of seeing your own primary care provider. Over time even your own doctor will make errors by virtue of the length of time you've been in his care, the number of times you've seen him, and the weaknesses inborn in any human enterprise. Lesson number one: Doctors make mistakes. This is inevitable. Most mistakes are invisible. Many are innocuous. Through continuity of care and proper communications they will usually be recognized and corrected without sequelae.

By contrast, single contacts with on-call physicians, by phone or in the emergency room, offer more opportunity for errors, but fewer chances for their quick detection and correction. Given these facts, why do you want to maximize needless contacts with physicians? Sometimes you don't have a choice, although these instances are surprisingly few.

Doctors and patients alike share the fantasy of "fix it all, fix it now, fix it fast, fix it completely, and fix it forever." The patient-centered fantasy that all doctors are alike is an equally dangerous fiction.

Don't Call—GO!

If you think that you are having an emergency, get up and go. Whether it's 911, or in your Ol' '55, go as quickly as you can to the emergency department that you have previously chosen.

Although it's beyond the scope of this book, an emergency state is an emergency if you define it as one. This logical tautology is, by necessity, always true because, by virtue of its form, it can never be wrong. When it comes to emergencies, never being wrong means it's never necessary to feel sorry or to find yourself dead.

Symptoms that are new or occur atop chronic complaints that are sudden in onset, and rapid in their progression, will frighten and concern you. This constitutes as inclusive a definition of an emergency as possible and advisable in this forum.

Most people are not Chicken Littles—they are, in fact, the opposite. The problem is not that you don't recognize a symptom that requires immediate attention; the problem is facing up to it when fear, fantasies, and wish-fulfillment paralyze you. Fear is the basic atom in the molecule that is an emergency. A symptom is your body telling your brain that something's wrong—at first your soma speaks softly to your psyche but then, if ignored, it screams! If you turn a deaf ear to both nature's warnings and your own instincts that something is wrong, you are more likely to invite a full-scale crisis. The mantras of "It will probably get better soon," or "I'll tough it out for a while," or "there are people sicker than me who need the care more" are just variants of "I am scared and I don't want to think about it."

Let's return to a transient ischemic attack, which, as previously mentioned, is a major predictor of a catastrophic stroke. A British study found that 56 percent of those having a transient ischemic attack delayed seeking help even when they recognized the symptoms and their implications: only 10 percent went directly to an emergency room.

But if your child has a hint of a problem that worries you, you'll take action far more rapidly than you would in your own behalf. In any emergency your child has no choice—but when it comes to your own care you fantasize that you do. Paradoxically, you resist doing what should be obvious—going straight to the emergency room. You hope instead that a telephone call to a perfect stranger will do the trick.

These calls result in delays, confusion, and errors and lead to advice that was predictable in the first place.

Most on-call doctors will take the safest approach. "Go to the emergency room" will be the most likely advice. No doctor was ever sued for telling a patient to get care. It's also the right advice, and most importantly it allows him to go back to sleep.

It's fine to call the covering doctor when you are preparing to go, or to leave your cell phone number with his service after you've left. It's not only courteous, it gives you the opportunity to demand a call to your receiving emergency room so that a physician-to-physician referral can be made. You also should call the emergency room and let them know that you are on your way. Obtain the name of the staffer you informed. The importance of knowing names cannot be overemphasized. "I called Nurse Smith and told him I was coming. Dr. Jones called the E.R. doctor too." The fact that knowing someone's name imparts greater importance to your statement is as undeniable as it is inexplicable.

When the sun sets, anxieties dawn. Emergencies occurring during the day are frequently ignored in the midst of daily activities, obligations, and rationalizations. This is doubly unfortunate. First, emergencies should always be heeded. Second, the daytime is the *only* time you have access to your doctor and your records. This is when making the call makes all the difference. The office contains both your doctor and your medical records, a combination of inestimable importance. Tell them, "I'm having an emergency. I need help immediately."

This offers the possibility of bypassing the emergency room altogether. Direct admission to the hospital, with your doctor's calls to the on-site "ologists" who can immediately attend you, is of incalculable worth. Thrombolytic therapy for the heart and brain during heart attacks and strokes has only a narrow time window for maximum efficacy. The treatment window for I.V. thrombolysis (clot dissolution) in strokes or impending neurological catastrophes is only three to five hours. During an ischemic cardiac event you should be on thrombolytic therapy within ninety minutes—the window shuts in twenty-four hours. These intervals can prevent impending strokes and heart attacks, and they can limit the damage if they have already occurred.

One in four patients with heart attacks will wait up to fifty minutes in emergency rooms. If you suffer a heart attack, just being in an emergency room is an independent, negative risk factor in your five-day mortality. Bypassing the emergency department is associated with more frequent use of reperfusion techniques. These are called percutaneous coronary interventions (PCI). Angioplasties and stents are PCIs and, although controversial, may, in some patients, provide life-saving therapy. Even if your emergency does not suggest a heart attack or stroke, your doctor's call will still facilitate your care. Direct calls to hospital-based specialists will result in expedited and appropriate interventions.

When I was called by a referring physician, her patients never had to wait. Rather than waiting for me, a team member or I would wait for them. Again this is the embodiment of your goal: "Doctor, your patient will see you now." Your internal bleeding or abdominal crisis won't be played out in the waiting room. My staff would have you and your chart in a therapeutic setting in minutes if needed. A phone call from your doctor has the weight of both her knowledge of you, and her familiarity with the staff. You may even find your doctor herself or her physician assistant at your bedside as soon as you arrive. By making the call to your own doctor you've drawn a crowd!

Don't Call and Don't Go

"I Have a Question"

If you have questions (but no symptoms), or if you have problems that are chronic or minor ailments, well-known to your own doctor and due for routine follow-up anyway, keep yourself off the hook by keeping your phone on it. Don't be an annoying evening telemarketer of your own personal surveys, idle worries, and curiosities.

Questions are fine—it's the answers that will get you every time. Call your own doctor tomorrow. Compile a list of pertinent questions using the databases you worked so hard to amass. By calling your doctor's office the following day the reassurance you need may be offered even without an appointment. Those who know you best are also the ones who advise you best if the need is not urgent.

"I Am Not Getting Better"

If you have seen your primary care physician for a problem that has already been evaluated and treated, which hasn't changed and for which a follow-up appointment pends, but you're still experiencing difficulty—don't call a stranger. Neither you, nor the doctor on call, will find a solution that night over the phone to problems that have been under the supervision of your own doctor for weeks or months. The on-call covering doctor will, at most, confirm that the mentioned variables have been checked off and then inevitably tell you to "call your doctor tomorrow." This is the best advice. There is always a possibility that he will simply tell you to go to the emergency room, where, after a long wait, their staff is sure to tell you the same thing. If your symptoms are changing then don't call—GO! Change in status, as well as fear, is another atom of the molecule that makes an emergency.

"I Am Not Getting Better As Quickly As I Was Told" (or More Likely, "As I Had Hoped")

Getting better, however slowly, for a complaint that was evaluated is a cause for celebration, not dialing. Problems, symptoms, and conditions don't wear wristwatches; nor do they consult yours. People who take their symptoms' temperatures too frequently will never see changes. Make sure you have a follow-up appointment and relax. Call in the morning if you must.

The only reason Dr. Justin Case will send you to the emergency room is to punish you for interfering with his evening and to protect himself from liability, however unlikely in these circumstances. Yes, it happens and yes, it is common. Yes, it's terrible—but you made the call. You pushed the ball.

Renewing a Prescription

Off-hour calls for chronic medications? Shame on you! If you must, do it only for medications that are so crucial that even the loss of a single dose poses a risk. Fortunately, these conditions and their therapies are rare.

More common are the errors that happen when Dr. I. M. Zslypey calls in an emergency prescription that bungles, alone or in some combination, your name, your drug, your dose, its frequency, its mode of administration, or your doctor's name. Wait until morning—it's only a few hours away.

Don't Call—Don't Go

For the want of the following, a visit to the emergency room may be avoided. Sometimes all that is needed is a first aid book, a bulb syringe, adhesive tape, antiseptic ointment, assorted Band-Aids, cold packs, chemical hot packs, gauze and roller gauze, scissors and tweezers, butterfly bandages, cotton balls, or eye patches. Over the counter (OTC) medications to have on hand include antihistamines, calamine lotion, decongestants, antacids, hydrocortisone cream, insect sting swabs, laxatives, sterile eye wash, and an EpiPen, if you have any history of anaphylaxis (although its use still demands a subsequent but healthier emergency room visit). More than 500,000 emergency room visits are just for constipation and millions more are for cuts and bruises.

Chronic Pain Syndromes

More than 25 percent of all Americans are in pain at any given time during the day. If you suffer increasing discomfort from a known and treated chronic pain syndrome, the likelihood of an off-hour phone call or an emergency room visit proving helpful is unlikely. If you are on chronic prescription pain medications, Izzy A. Newcomer, M.D., will not and should not call a pharmacist to increase the dose or change your prescription. Even if such a call were made, the pharmacist would be reluctant to provide a restricted analgesic that is likely already being used at dose levels higher than usually encountered.

Emergency room visits for chronic pain syndromes that are being treated put you on the lowest triage level. You are assured many hours of sitting or lying in pain in the waiting room. Even if you choose to wait, satisfaction is far from likely. Only 39 percent of patients are given any analgesics; 40 percent leave the emergency room still in pain because 25 percent of emergency room doctors simply don't or won't believe them. Most of them will feel that you are engaging in "DSB" (drug-seeking behavior). If we have an acronym for a condition or behavior you can be assured it's common enough to require one. In light of this, the majority of patients feel that they were not treated with dignity or respect.

You Are Hopelessly Unsure

Okay—you truly don't know what to do. The anxiety is scaring you more than the problem. This anxiety may, itself, cause a change in stable symptoms or evoke new ones. In the words of the French essayist Michel de Montaigne, "he who fears suffering is already suffering from what he fears." So go, go already! Always err on the side of safety.

In such cases, consider an urgent care facility rather than an emergency department. Patients who need immediate care for injuries and illness, be it a laceration from broken glass or a severe stomach bug, are increasingly turning to walk-in, urgent care clinics. These facilities aim to fill the gap between the growing shortage of primary care doctors and a shrinking number of already-crowded hospital emergency departments. Appointments aren't necessary and extended evening and weekend hours are available. Urgent care clinics are staffed by physicians, offer wait times as little as a few minutes, and charge $60 to $200 depending on the procedure—a fraction of the typical $1,000-plus emergency department visit. Some offer discounts and payment plans for the uninsured; for those with coverage, co-payments vary by insurance plan but may be less than half the amount of an E.R. visit, which can range from $50 to $200.[2]

Calling a doctor when you can't determine the gravity of your problem at first blush seems like a reasonable thing to do. But this isn't always the case. There are a number of scenarios that can result, and I've listed them from the best result to the worst. Paradoxically, of the scenarios I present, the best possible results are the least likely to occur, while the worst possible results occur more often.

1. Great advice. No need for the emergency room. Peace of mind is yours. What a nice doctor—so smart!
2. Good advice you don't trust—who *is* this guy anyway?
3. Bad advice that you don't trust.
4. Bad advice that you do trust. This last scenario presents the worst possible result and is also the most likely.

So, only one in four of these scenarios will keep you out of the emergency room. Three out of four of these scenarios leave you in doubt or in danger. So go! Relying solely on a telephone call for information doesn't help and is more likely to harm.

Most on-call doctors want to rid themselves of you as quickly and as safely as is possible for them (and you). If they pick up on the earnestness and seriousness with which you describe your dilemma, they will tell you to go to the emergency room. A diagnosis by telephone is as unlikely as the previously mentioned telephonic therapeutics.

Now having divested himself of you, the on-call doctor, Willie Soomie, M.D., will fall into a deep, trouble-free sleep. No nightmares for him about lawyers in three-piece suits or juries horrified by an attorney's vivid depictions of his willful negligence! Willie may awaken only to call in two or three tests that won't necessarily hurt you, but will certainly help run the clock.

It is equally unwise to call the 1-800 number provided by your healthcare carrier. Their opinions, and the opinions of those who work for them, are predictable. Whatever is cheapest, is best. When in doubt they err on the side of frugality. You can't sue *them* if they're wrong. If you must call to assure that the visit will be covered, then make the call. Tell them anything that works. Yes, that's right—lie. I would. I did. Insurance carriers in my experience do not possess institutional ethics so no personal ethics should routinely be afforded to them. Yes, cajole, entreat, implore, and beg if you must. Ultimately the poor people who work for them must toe the line. I worked on an insurance company hotline. I know what the company expected from me. In order to get people where they needed to be, I, too, had to lie to avoid the wrath of my masters.

As you go off to the emergency room your medical day is not over. But before that long night's journey into day, I want to recap what is one of the leitmotifs of this and previous chapters: Doctors are changing the definition of previously inviolate rules of medical responsibility. Some of the newer medical care models keep you at the center of their concerns.

Some don't. What had previously been viewed as medical abandonment is now considered effective time management. Earlier notions of continuous, one-on-one relationships have given way to fragmented, uncoordinated, and non-continuous care. You are now no longer in the ranks of unwary patients. You are less prone to the dangers these new "standards" promise.

The other leitmotif running through this section is that seeing your own doctor is no longer a sure thing. Nowadays expecting a familiar face in your care, whether in the office, at the hospital, or during an emergency, may be as quaint as expecting a house call. We have learned that regardless of the severity of your problem or the time of day, there are no strangers . . . only doctors you have not met.

4

The Emergency Room

- All emergency rooms are not created equal. The average grade is a C-. How to find an A+.
- The five "must have," non-negotiable features for your emergency room.
- Less important attributes that increase your safety and comfort while decreasing your waiting time.
- The emergency rooms you must avoid.
- Triage status—how to maximize your triage level and minimize your wait without drama and exaggerations.
- The waiting room doesn't have to be a long night's journey into day. Two calls you must make if *you're* waiting but your problem *won't*.

The only good time to call the covering doctor off-hours is when you've decided on your own to go to the hospital. Remember, if *you* think it's an emergency, it is one. You may be wrong, but it's better than being the new tenor in the "Invisible Choir."

Bring a downloaded copy of your medical record with you. Always keep a recent up-to-date copy in your safe for such emergencies. In the absence of a detailed past medical history, errors can occur almost as soon as you walk through the door. You shouldn't rely on the hospital's record room to be a trusted repository of your medical history.

You choose your emergency room before you need it in the certainty that someday you will. There are some features of emergency room care that are nonnegotiable; others are highly desirable; and there are some that shouldn't figure prominently in your decision making, however enticing they appear.

Regardless of how much you want a telephone, flat-screen TV, or a fast-food chain providing meals to you in your cubicle, these are neither nonnegotiable assets nor highly desirable ones—and they're not final indicators of the quality of a hospital's health care. The "wow" factors you may value are usually the least important when using strict clinical criteria to choose the proper emergency room. In any case, no choice will be perfect.

EMERGENCY ROOM TAXONOMY

Emergency department services can be divided into a four-tier system: Demanded, Desirable, Disarming, or Deal Breakers.

Tier 1—Demanded

You may find the perfect emergency department: Private rooms, massage therapy, telephones, call-ahead appointment systems, even a pet-care center, all housed in a level I trauma center that is just down the block from your home. But if your doctor doesn't go there, this wonderful facility might as well be on the moon (although you might want to rent it for bar mitzvahs and weddings).

Why doesn't she go to a particular emergency room? Why won't she go to the one of your choice? There are several reasons: she's not familiar with it, its services are not used by her coverage doctors or her medical group, and she may have financial interests in an alternative, for-profit facility. It's best to start with the emergency room she does use and begin your investigation there. If her emergency rooms don't meet the criteria mentioned in this section, then you have a problem. You must realize, too, that bad emergency departments are often housed in bad hospitals. If the emergency department doesn't get you, the hospital might.

It's unlikely you'll have a problem in large cities, where there are dozens of hospitals to choose from. Most doctors have privileges in a few of them.

Small rural communities may only provide the basic services of a micro-hospital. Under these circumstances it's reasonable to assume that you want your emergency and hospital experience to happen elsewhere. A neighboring city may be only fifteen to twenty minutes away. If it's possible to reach it, it's worth the trip. If you find yourself in your town's only solo bed emergency room, perhaps you can use it as a launching pad to a larger facility rather than a landing strip. If you get admitted and your condition permits, you can demand an early transfer to the hospital of your choice. Seventy-one percent of Americans have access to an emergency department of some kind within thirty minutes of their home, and 98 percent can reach one within an hour.[1] Many of these may not provide the technologies you need. The trade-off between the dangers of extended travel times and the quality of the destination-facility's services must be taken into account.

It's easier to say goodbye to stereo headsets and a sushi station than to your doctor, but it's difficult to keep him if his emergency room uses non-accredited staff, or is a specialty, for-profit hospital with few emergency beds but many opportunities for his own profit.

Staffed by Certified E.R. Physicians: Those certified by the American Board of Emergency Medicine must recertify every ten years. Some emergency room doctors specialize in toxicology, pediatric emergencies, and sports medicine. There is certainly a premium placed on the availability of these services compared to facilities that don't staff reliably endorsed clinicians. A hospital that seeks to offer assurances of its staff's training is also likely to offer other advantages. It is always important to remember some doctors do not benefit from degrees earned or lessons learned.

The American Board of Medical Specialties (ABMS) lists its American Board of Emergency Medicine diplomates online. The registration is simple, free, and open to the public. It is one of the "must-have websites" (www.abms.org).

The Services That Are Provided by Its Affiliated Hospital: Hospitals that house emergency rooms don't always provide access to invasive radiological techniques, radiologists who are on-site or on call, cardiac catheterization labs, and crucial surgical care (cardiothoracic, neurosurgical, and vascular surgery). Your emergency department must be able to initiate intravenous fibrinolytic ("clot busting") techniques when indicated and allow rapid access to the more sophisticated therapies that may follow. I've alluded to the narrow time frame needed to access clot busting therapies for heart attacks and strokes. All this takes is a simple intravenous injection that can be given by any of the E.R. staff. Ask your doctor if her emergency room offers this therapy. The availability of this single low-tech intervention may be more important than access to percutaneous coronary interventions (PCIs) like angioplasties, stents, and coronary bypasses, which continue to generate controversy and questions about overuse. (All things being equal, if you are close to a hospital offering PCIs, cardiothoracic, neurosurgical, and vascular surgery, it is an indisputable advantage if their need becomes clear.)

Proximity: Emergencies require some degree of proximity to a receiving facility. A level I trauma center 100 miles away is useless, except as a transfer resource. A level II "regional trauma center" within twenty-five miles is a possibility. A level III "area trauma center" down the block may be your default choice (see below for trauma center designation).

If you locate an emergency department that is attached to a trauma level I hospital status, that's almost all you need to know to make a decision about an emergency room. In 2010 there are 129 trauma level I centers in the United States, most of which have twenty-four-hour, in-house surgery and anesthesiology.[2] About half of them have continuous in-house availability for neurosurgery and orthopedic surgery. Prompt access to radiology and internal medicine specialties are also required to obtain this imprimatur. Not only are these level I centers the best candidates for treating trauma patients in their emergency rooms, they are usually larger, university-affiliated members of the Council of Teaching Hospitals and, therefore, best suited to treat a range of emergency conditions for patients who have multiple comorbidities. They are also attached to hospitals with more acute care beds and larger intensive care units. Neither Pennsylvania nor New York State allows the American College of Surgery to designate its hospitals as accredited. All other states do. That's too bad. A hospital with this accreditation confers benefits too significant to ignore, much less hide from public scrutiny.

Level I trauma centers provide a 20 percent higher survival rate for their patients than do non-trauma centers. Their physicians are better trained and more experienced in emergency care, and there is a greater availability of specialists. A level I trauma center's willingness to be inspected and the high volume of patients it attracts say it all. Even survival rates for a level I trauma center one year *after* the emergency room visit is 25 percent higher for its patients than for their poor cousins. Some hospitals claim that they have "trauma teams" and they may have "trauma directors." This may be better than nothing, but unless they're designated as level I, they are not trauma centers. Level II centers serve just as well in the absence of a level I designee in your area. A level II label reflects only a lack of research or training programs that would have little effect on your care.

Level III centers are for patients who don't need the services of a level I facility. A level III hospital should never be chosen when a higher level is available. When you are lying on the floor at home, unconscious or in pain, or have been injured in a car accident, your future is unpredictable, as are your needs. It is always in your interest to seek out the best, logistically available facility, not the one that is simply the most convenient. No one knows what they're going to need during an illness; maximizing what is available immediately is better than being transferred later. Ask for that transfer when you wind up in a rural level III trauma center. In 2010 it was shown that patients who transferred, even the elderly and seriously ill, enjoyed a survival benefit over those who stayed put.[3]

All states listed on the American College of Surgery website have at least one hospital with a level I or level II rating.

That's it: your doctor's okay, accredited staff, access to cardiothoracic, vascular, and neurosurgical technologies, trauma level I or II designation, and proximity.

Tier 2—Desirable

The second tier of desirable emergency room traits includes: fast track units, short-stay units, designated children's emergency rooms, and the fulfillment of all first tier requirements.

In addition to the essential features in tier 1 facilities, tier 2 facilities have the potential to provide a more pleasant and less emotionally jarring experience. Greater efficiency and less waiting time are also possible. But none of these features are worth tossing your own doctor under the bus to obtain.

Unit Segregation: The separation of the critical from the casual patient has several advantages. First, and most importantly, children, teenagers, and the faint of heart will find them less emotionally disruptive. In contrast to Mark Twain's comment, "I have been through some terrible things in my life, some of which actually happened," *any* emergency room experience will be, by dint of your disease, or the facility's defects, a god-awful one, even to those with flinty dispositions.

Any feature that cushions the blow is welcomed. Neither you, nor your children, would care to witness in full H-D the panorama of assorted bodily fluids, body parts, and unclothed body habitus that typically crowd an emergency room. Any emergency room would be rated X by the Motion Picture Association of America. The only way to get a PG experience is by segregating the unmentionable from the impressionable. This tacitly places you in a lower triage category. But, by separating the dramas from the traumas, your wait may turn out to be briefer.

Patients in the less acute setting have their own staff and the workups are quicker. Although the line may be longer it's likely to move faster.

Fast Track Units: Urgent care centers, treating problems that seem to lend themselves to a less acute setting, offer one big disadvantage. Proceeding to an urgent care facility means that you are doing your *own* triage. If it turns out that you need really, *really* urgent care, then you are in the wrong place, in the wrong line, waiting for the wrong people. If, however, that facility is in a hospital, no matter how distant the emergency room is on the hospital's blueprint, it's still just down the corridor or an elevator ride away. You will be transferred to staff that are close by and waiting for you with all your paperwork in hand. This is in contrast to a lonely, time-consuming excursion across town that finds you having to start all over again.

Short-Stay Units: "Warehousing" occurs when E.R. patients are put off to the side and down some corridor while awaiting test results. This is no euphemism. It's literal. It is also the embodiment of a paradox. The emergency department staff has decided you are ill enough to require several tests that require you to wait before and after they are done. They may even decide that you are ill enough to be admitted. But, despite the acknowledged gravity of your situation, you are then placed on a gurney, shoved against a wall, and deserted in a hallway, out of sight.

This practice, also more benignly called "boarding," was commented upon in a position paper of the American College of Emergency Medicine.

> In 2007, the American College of Emergency Physicians (ACEP) conducted a poll of emergency physicians to measure critical issues facing emergency patients. At that time, nearly 80 percent of the 1,500 emergency physicians responding to the poll said they had significant concerns about the crowded conditions in their emergency departments. Half reported personally encountering a patient who had suffered because of "boarding," and 200 said they knew of patients who had died because of the practice. Further, numerous studies have now linked emergency department crowding and the boarding of patients with compromises in clinical care.[4]

In hospital administrative terms you have become an "input obstacle" to new emergency department arrivals. This is their way of saying an "income obstacle."

It's not unusual for hospitals, on any given day, to run censuses of 110 percent. Competition for beds is as intense as it is for Notre Dame football tickets. Emergency rooms that have short-stay units give you access to dignity, doctors, diagnostics, and the delivery of services that would be denied you in a cold corridor. The short-stay unit may have a separate, dedicated nursing unit, or be in a wing off the emergency department. Either way, you can anticipate privacy and ready access to both a doctor's care and family support. Whether you're in a private or semi-private room or lying around in a space partitioned by curtains, you now have an address on the hospital's computer. Your doctor can find you and specialists can treat you. If short-stay units aren't available, it's not an exaggeration to imagine doctors walking up and down hallways, poking their heads into deserted alcoves, window-shopping for their patients.

Despite the Health Insurance Portability and Accountability Act (HIPAA) that mandates your right to privacy, you will still be reciting your history in front of strangers, if you've been warehoused. Nor will you receive adequate physical examinations if you're in a public space: strangers are meeting, interviewing, and examining other strangers while surrounded by onlooking strangers. Hardly a harbinger for a good outcome.

Presented with these obstacles most doctors will wait, however long, until you have a real home in the hospital before seeing you. If the facility is full, you must wait for a patient upstairs to be discharged or to join "The Invisible Choir" before you can obtain a hospital bed. The only ways to determine if a hospital has short-stay units are to visit it, call hospital information, or look on the hospital's website.

Children's Emergency Rooms: As long as the facility has all tier 1 benefits, this attribute is highly valued. BUT: Children's emergency rooms are housed in children's hospitals. If your child is to be an inpatient, these hospitals have to be reviewed before defaulting to them. This is particularly true if it is a physician-owned, specialty children's hospital.

Everyone has expectations that a child-centered facility offers superior care, fostered by the tender emotions we all have for defenseless tots, toddlers, and yes, even teens. We may view them as we do school buses: vaults on wheels carrying passengers in bubbles that are protected by laws appropriate for the treasures they carry. Is this true for children's hospitals? Sadly not.

As recently as spring 2008, the journal *Pediatrics* published an article demonstrating that drug-related complications in children's hospitals were much more prevalent than previously described.[5] Most were preventable. Many led to harm—usually temporary conditions, such as rashes and fevers. Others were more serious, involving over-sedation and perturbations in glucose and potassium levels.

Tier 3—Disarming

If your community has an emergency department that was recently expanded or renovated, you can't make automatic assumptions about the type of care you'll receive there. These emergency departments may be more modern, more pleasant and consumer friendly, and allow better access to doctors and technology. BUT: If a hospital's money was spent only to attract consumers and profit, be aware that these amenities may be like loss leaders: enticing come-ons behind which may lie a deficient facility. Even if it has tier 1 features, it is still a tier 3 facility.

Private rooms, bedside telephones, palatable food, even wandering minstrels are great, but if that's all it is, it's like getting lots of sizzle but no steak. You're there for the care.

Tier 4—Deal Breakers

Using a specialty, for-profit hospital for elective care has its advocates. But using them in an emergency should not be an option.

Use these four tiers—Demanded; Desirable; Disarming; Deal Breaker—in your search for a proper facility for you and your family. Determine your first choice and an alternate well before you need them. This is a mantra repeated throughout this book. There are no mysteries, there are no walls, and there are no difficulties in obtaining the information you need. This is true regarding the emergency rooms in your area.

TRIAGE

When you arrive you will be triaged. Be aware of the four triage levels that are typically used by the staff: Emergent (waits of fifteen minutes or less), Urgent (waits of fifteen to sixty minutes), Semi-Urgent (waits of one to two hours), and Non-Urgent (from two hours up to the next ice age).

After your triage you can, and should, ask which level you have been assigned to. Contest this decision if you disagree with it. If your predicted wait is longer than you think it should be (in contrast to how long you want it to be), request that the staff note it in your chart. Make a point of it by securing its documentation. Hospital personnel don't like documenting patient-staff disagreements over medical decisions. They may prove, in retrospect, to be embarrassing or medical-legally compromising. They know that sometimes you will be right. Requesting codification of your opinions makes them more important. The fact that you've surrendered your insurance card doesn't mean you have to surrender your right to your opinions at the same time.

Your triage level may determine if you want to stick around, proceed to an urgent care center, or go home. Preparing for a walk-in at your doctor's office in the morning may not be a bad policy if his office hours start at 8:00 a.m. and your wait in the emergency department is expected to last until 10:00 a.m.

It's not wise or proper to play the system by falsifying your reasons for being there. Nor is it wise to minimize them.

Lead with the headline. It decreases the chance that the triage officer will switch off when you start out with, "I'm feeling okay now but you shoulda' seen me . . . " When asked, say instead, "Chest pain." A happy lull in the manifestation of symptoms may be only temporary; it is their stuttering progression that often leads to the worst denouements. Always respond to questions truthfully but use your story to effect correct action.

If your chest and abdomen hurt and you are not sure which is worse, tell them it's your lower chest. It's their job to sort you out, not yours. Try not to engage in self-diagnostics. Try not to engage in soul-searching or second-guessing yourself. Don't indulge in histrionics: veteran E.R. staffers find them entertaining and, as interesting as they are to watch, they serve only to minimize the importance of your complaints. What you say is far more important than how you say it.

Expressing free-floating anxieties with free-flowing streams of consciousness similarly deflects attention away from the importance of your problem. The people who are the most ill speak little or not at all. The most garrulous may get lower triage levels.

Be Aware of "Heads-up Symptoms": If you arrive at an emergency department for a headache, it had better be a doozy. It's only going to get worse when you find that you're facing three hours in the waiting room. If, however, you tell the staff that you've never had a headache before, that this one was sudden in onset, is now getting worse, and involves only one side of your head, you will get care faster. Much faster.

Using your carefully assembled database, educate yourself about emergencies and their symptoms. You can alternatively use a quick, ad hoc computer search to more accurately describe what an emergency team needs to know while waiting for the ambulance.

If you have a cough, common sense, in the absence of self-education, may suffice. Think again about your children. If they had a cough you knew that if it was accompanied by fever, shortness of breath, wheezing, stridor, and colored phlegm, the pediatrician would call you back sooner. If they had abdominal pain you knew to be on the lookout for vomiting, diarrhea, fever, and localized pain.

"You took good care of your children. Now take good care of yourself" is now a television commercial catchphrase. In reality you take good care of your children *by* taking good care of yourself. Use these "heads-up" symptoms to alert the staff why "this night is different from all other nights," lest they pass over you.

You will pay a steep price if you game the system through exaggeration and fabrication. At the least, your reputation for "crying wolf" will haunt you. Doctors do remember and disseminate information on those they've determined to be "problem patients." At the worst, you will get more attention than you want or need. You will certainly receive a lot more tests, many unnecessary, and some too risky, for the real problem at hand. The perceived gravity of your symptoms will lead to more risk taking (yours) to decrease concerns (theirs). Nothing is more frightening to behold than the convergence of doctors and nurses on a patient with an emergency, real or perceived.

Drama and fabrication do nothing to maximize the level of care you receive. It's your knowledge and ability to cogently summarize your symptoms that advance your interests.

1. Request your triage status and contest it, if needed.
2. Don't minimize your complaints.
3. Present your symptoms as they were when at their worst.
4. Don't exaggerate.
5. If your symptoms concern you and you're not sure what to do, err on the side of describing the symptoms that are the most likely to also concern the staff.
6. Do not use histrionics.
7. A spare, even terse, eye-to-eye discussion is best. Amplify your answers when requested.

Ambrose Bierce defined the word "alone" in his *Devil's Dictionary*: "Alone, adj. in bad company."[6] This is particularly true when you are in any medical facility. Never go alone to the emergency room or anywhere on the highways and byways of our medical system. Every floor in a hospital is a bad neighborhood. Street smarts are called for. When you are ill, frightened, forgetful, compromised, and cut off, it will be friends and family who will come to your side. They will stay with you, in shifts if needed, until you are home. If you are admitted to the hospital, a schedule of family or friends who attend you around-the-clock is necessary, even if it is inconvenient. There is no single piece of advice I can give you that is more crucial to your welfare than this. Your ever-alert twenty-four-hour room coach is one of your first defenses against error and injury. Let *no one* deny you or limit the availability of this company. Hospital rules are for hospitals. These rules are for you. This is one of the extremely rare occasions when reaching for your lawyer's business card might be necessary.

One hundred and fifteen million people use emergency departments annually. They will all seem to be there on the same night you are. You need familiar faces. You need their voices.

If you are in the emergency room with a sprain, strain, or bruise, you are in the wrong place. Don't venture into what is surely one of Dante's Nine Circles of Hell with only a boo-boo. First-aid kits or urgent care centers are better options. Review the prior section to help determine whether to call, to go, or to set your alarm clock for an a.m. visit with your doctor.

THE WAITING ROOM

Use the information below while in the ambulance to obtain your proper place in the inevitable line that awaits you.

Prompt attention to medical needs is a universally acknowledged index of high-quality medical care. It is one of the goals of the Institute of Medicine's report, "Crossing the Quality Chasm."

We have said that 1 in 4 patients with a heart attack—and many more who have symptoms that suggest one—can wait up to an hour to be seen. Patients suffering ischemic brain syndromes, which often present atypically, can endure similar delays. Unfortunately, in such cases, a lengthy delay can result in incalculable damage to brain tissue or, worse, death.

Do you ever wonder about the people who deliberately avoid your gaze when they're supposed to be helping you? This talent seems to serve as a prerequisite for their employment; they look through you as if you are cellophane. Restaurant servers, commercial airline attendants, and emergency room desk personnel lead the list. Even if they accidentally look into your eyes, if you listen very carefully, you can hear a switch click off. But it is never an error to approach the desk and get updated on your status. It is never an error to update the E.R. staff on your status if it is changing.

Urban emergency departments act as primary care providers for the uninsured. Because they're almost always teeming with patients, you can expect to wait up to 63 percent longer in a city hospital than in facilities on a city's periphery or in its suburbs. If the emergency room is staffed by trainees your wait will be longer. This may be a mixed blessing because interns' rates of error are greater once you are in their care.

If you are well enough to choose the time of your arrival then you probably don't need an emergency room.

But if you're a white man, in suburbia, with insurance, and a private physician, and you become ill on Super Bowl Sunday, you can forget the need for a magazine. You may not have enough time to take off your pants before you're accosted by Dr. Ben Dover and his staff, carrying stethoscopes, blood pressure cuffs, and lubricated latex gloves.

When you are, or become, acutely ill in the waiting room: People die in waiting rooms. A cross-national survey conducted by the Commonwealth Fund found that America ranks near the bottom among advanced countries in terms of how hard it is to get medical attention on short notice (although Canada was slightly worse), and that America is the worst place in the advanced world if you need care after hours or on a weekend.[7]

It's a sad fact that people die while awaiting care or disposition. A death in an emergency room in Illinois in 2006 was ruled a homicide by a coroner's jury because of the hours the patient waited prior to being found dead in her chair. In February 2008, a paramedics' union in Canada claimed three deaths occurred in an Ontario hospital during a twenty-four-hour period while the patients they'd brought in awaited medical care or were warehoused in the hallways. An account of a janitor who mopped around a patient while she writhed on the floor in abdominal pain was featured in a newspaper. In the summer of 2008 a woman collapsed while being warehoused in an emergency room holding facility in a Brooklyn hospital. Security video cameras captured her death twenty-four hours into her wait for a bed in a psychiatric facility. More shocking was the fact that for one full hour she lay on the floor, first writhing in pain, and then dead. The hospital staff that looked on during this period did nothing.

A quote from the Mental Health Legal Society succinctly sums up the facts: "From the moment a person steps through the doors she is stripped of her freedom and dignity and literally forced to fight for the essentials of life."[8]

If you are in the waiting room, request a caseworker who could advance your cause. If you are suffering an acute illness, regardless of your triage status, a caseworker may intervene. Any ally is especially valuable if your physical symptoms progress while you're waiting.

The modern emergency room is, for the patients, a kind of purgatory. Staff shouldn't underestimate the emotional toll it exacts, and they should make every effort when appropriate to recalculate the estimated time of admission.

But if you're still in institutional limbo, don't hesitate or be afraid to bring an unconscionably long wait to their attention, particularly if your condition is worsening. Walking over to the desk or shouting over the din are fine strategies if you're scared. Demand that this request be placed in your medical record. No one wants to be an annoying troublemaker but dispensation is given for those raising a ruckus in an emergency room waiting area who are sick and becoming sicker.

When all else fails, use an in-house telephone or have a relative call the hospital's main line (thus demonstrating simultaneously the importance of family and cell phones), and ask for the administrator on duty. Alert the operator that you are in their facility, are in distress, are being ignored, and are in fear for your life. Demand that the administrator on duty return your call immediately. Inform him of your status, and of your intention of calling 911 first and the local newspaper second.

If you were given an urgent triage level there is no guarantee your wait will be measured in minutes. Even a semi-urgent triage level can result in a wait so long that, even if your condition is unchanged, it warrants assertive action by you, your family, caseworkers, hospital administrators, or Oliver Twist look-alikes who can plead your case.

The average emergency room waiting time is three hours and forty-two minutes. In Arizona, the weather better be a consolation for the five-hour average wait.

Do not leave the emergency room without a copy of your test results and the emergency room record in hand. Do not leave with assurances that they will be forwarded to your doctor. It won't happen. Ask for a caseworker. Contact the beleaguered administrator on call. Request the hospital's Patients' Bill of Rights. If you don't get your record now, you'll have to employ Herculean efforts to obtain it later. The need for a rapid follow-up at your own doctor's office means that you must have the record.

The more important or recent the data the longer it will take for your doctor to retrieve it. This is the Law of Medical Information Retrieval.

Sir Isaac Newton's Three Laws of Motion were fine during his time but now we observe Kussin's Three Laws of Medical Motion:

1. Any staffer at rest tends to stay at rest. Any staffer in motion tends to seek rest with the same speed and in the same direction as the rest of the staff—unless acted upon by an unbalanced force. The appropriately named unbalanced force is the doctor.

2. The relationship between a staffer's attitudes and incentives in the face of an applied force is in the direction of the path of least resistance.
3. For every action there is an equally valid reason for not acting.

If your condition worsens after you have been released from the E.R. you are now medically alone but you shouldn't feel on your own. Never hesitate to return to the same E.R. Don't be reassured solely by the smiling face of the doctor who discharged you that evening. Inform them that you are on your second go-around. Refuse to wait. No need to be calm now. Demand entry.

Once inside refuse to go home. Being denied proper care twice in one twenty-four-hour period has led to some of the most tragic incidents that I have in my large repertoire of anecdotes. The environment needs you to diminish your carbon footprint. The emergency room shouldn't help you eliminate your biological one. Demand emergency notification of your doctor. The unbelievable clinical stubbornness of some well-intentioned physicians has led to untold horrors when they refused to reconsider earlier diagnoses.

One elderly gentleman, whose family later successfully sued the hospital where he was treated, made several trips to the emergency room and was given the diagnosis of a common but innocent condition—irritable bowel syndrome—three times over a five-night period. On one occasion he left with subtle abnormalities in his lab work, and on another an abnormal CT scan. He returned for his fourth visit, not long after his third, with a perforated stomach ulcer. Acid spilled into his abdominal cavity, causing extensive burns to his internal organs with subsequent infection. He endured six months of pain, multiple hospitalizations, four major abdominal surgeries, dozens of lesser but still risky and painful interventions (catheter placements in the abdominal cavity, bladder, heart, and major blood vessels; tubes placed into lungs, stomach, and rectum, most performed several times; biopsies, spinal taps, intravenous nutritional support and dialysis, etc.), and major infections, complications, and the countless indignities these produce until he succumbed.

It's bad enough when patients must endure ordeals wrought by the severity of their medical conditions. But it is simply appalling when patients who tried to come *in* from the storm then endure a level of suffering brought on by inept, inadequate, or erroneous treatment.

IN CLOSING

In a 2009 position paper, the American College of Emergency Medicine rated our country's emergency rooms. Sadly their findings only confirm the truth of what we've learned in this chapter.

NATIONAL GRADE BY CATEGORY
Access to Emergency Care: D
Quality & Patient Safety Environment: C+
Medical Liability Environment: C
Public Health & Injury Prevention: C
Disaster Preparedness: C-
Overall: C-
(American College of Emergency Physicians 2009)

III

CHOOSING YOUR DOCTOR

5

Choosing Your Doctor: Introduction

- You love us, you hate us—choosing amongst us.
- Dr. Burgher and Dr. Berger—why there's a difference.
- Why word of mouth simply won't cut it.
- Why a medical degree itself does not entitle a doctor to your care.
- Why board certification is a useless benchmark for a doctor's ability.
- The one and *only* physician attribute that is both necessary *and* sufficient. It trumps a doctor's empathy, communication skills, and style.

Doctors: can't live with them; can't live without them. I did a few Google searches. I first keyed in the phrase "I hate doctors." On subsequent searches I entered several very polarizing demographics in lieu of doctors. What I found was instructive. Surprisingly, "I hate doctors" had 30 to 60 percent more hits than the other embarrassingly mean-spirited entries I chose. Only "I hate Jews" came close. This was unsettling for me, a member of that most un-endangered species—Jewish doctors. I then turned the tables and entered "I love doctors" and later, the same alternatives I had previously used and, at last, received a measure of solace. Doctors were the third-most-beloved demographic and Jews the second. Redemption yes, but also confusion. Physicians are both hated and loved. So are Jews—but that's another book. There is a national schizophrenia when it comes to our doctors.

When consumers choose a physician it seems to be a casual affair. Many think that we are all interchangeable. This incalculable error is measured in lives lost. Look-alikes are not always alike. Dolphins and porpoises, crocodiles and alligators, ravens and crows, hamsters and gerbils, Doctor Berger and Doctor Burgher—different species, despite appearances. Why, as a nation of consumers, do we spend more time choosing kitchen appliances than we do doctors? The casual choice of a doctor is, emphatically, not the way to go. Blissful ignorance is not a strategy. Loss aversion for those worth losing is not a plan.

Dr. Berger owns a share in a radiology business/Dr. Burgher has no conflict of interest.

Dr. Berger will enter you into clinical trials/Dr. Burgher will read about their results and then *may* prescribe the medication.

Dr. Berger won't refer you to specialists or offer you second opinions/Dr. Burgher knows when it's time for more input.

Dr. Berger was the first on his block to prescribe for his patients the drugs Rezulin, Lotronex, Propulsid, Pemoline, Dexatrim, Baycol, Vioxx, Zelnorm, and Trasylol—all pulled from the market in the last eight years due to the deaths and debility they caused/Dr. Burgher will, if possible, wait months, even years after FDA approval, anticipating the fallout some new drugs inevitably cause.

Dr. Berger hands you a statin for lowering cholesterol as inevitably as he does your bill/Dr. Burgher won't "statinize" you at will.

Some of us are really bad players and others unforgivable wretches. Some have given up and others are no longer keeping up. Some of us burn incandescent while others just burn out. Being happy with your doctor is, of course, wonderful. Being safe with her is an entirely separate and far more important consideration.[1] Mortal stakes. You might be loving your bad doctor to death.

Like Rorschach tests, doctors are inkblots in white. We absorb and reflect back at you your personality traits, emotional needs, preoccupations, and anxious perseverations. Skilled, ethical clinicians explore, even exploit, your personal expectations to satisfy your clinical needs. Rogues manipulate these expectations to satisfy their fiscal ones: "Yes, you need CT angiography. A lot of people are walking time bombs even when they feel great—remember Tim Russert?"

A skilled, experienced, careful driver has talents that can be measured and quantified. Yet even the drunk driver will *usually* get you home safely. Why would you chance it? Why would you get into his car?

Two surgeons may have admirable personal skills, brim with style, and be smooth conversationalists. Each has a similar number of surgical mortalities over a four-year period. Yet, depending on their respective surgical volumes, putting your life in the hands of one of these surgeons might leave you twice as likely to end in a serious complication. It would be nearly impossible for a layperson (and many referring doctors) to discern the differences between surgeons that have played out over years with hundreds of patients that result in hugely different outcomes for each.

Take bariatric surgery, for example. In 2010, the rates of serious complications are 4 percent for low-volume surgeons at low-volume hospitals but only 2 percent for high-volume surgeons at high-volume hospitals.[2] So Dr. Randam Sutra does high-volume work—250 cases a year. Over four years 1,000 patients were treated. Twenty had serious complications. Dr. Z. B. D. Doudah, a low-volume surgeon, operates on only 100 patients a year and has sixteen complications over the same four years. Dr. Doudah can honestly say he's had fewer complications than Dr. Sutra, even though his complication rate is double. So what's a patient to do? Read this chapter.

Doctors are not impressionistic canvases. We have lines, loci, and limits that can be learned about before the visit rather than regretted later. So let's examine your doctor. Tell him, "Don't worry. It may hurt, but just for a moment."

This section starts with your doctors' colleges and medical schools because when you pick a puppy you know that the first step is checking out its kennel. We proceed to the *only* necessary and sufficient prerequisite for your choice—a doctor's brains. Following this, we explore the necessary but insufficient demands of communication and empathy. Choosing your doctor on the basis of her style is unnecessary and insufficient but, sadly, it's the factor you value the most. We end by discussing the bad news that makes a second opinion a first priority.

6

College and Medical School: Setting the Stage

- You never chose pets without first checking their kennels—let's find out where your doctors came from.
- What's missing in your care?—A process that started after your doctor's high school graduation.
- How prospective doctors are dehumanized.
- Students—getting ahead in aptitudes and getting behind in attitudes.
- Why empathy can't be taught.
- Too little too late. Why liberal arts are missing from pre-med curricula.

In writing this section, I was inspired by Michael Pollan's book, *The Omnivore's Dilemma*. Just as he urges his readers to learn and understand where their dinner starts and how it ends up on their plates, this chapter will examine where our doctors come from, and how so many end up as damaged goods. Unlikely as it sounds, there are parallels between the process of producing doctors and the process of raising beef cows for market. Both pupil and beast are placed in artificial environments and divorced from familiar routines. Students and stock are denied the time and opportunity for natural maturation. From the teats to the streets, the specific and valued traits that are selected tend to develop into unnaturally hypertrophied forms.

For bulls this hypertrophy results in a broad, straight back with thick, heavy, long muscling. Specific emphasis is assigned to bulging musculature in the anatomical regions which contain the highest-priced cuts. Pre-medical and medical students are not prized for their musculature (to be sure), but for behavioral traits. It's not the length of bone but an (as yet) undefined suite of genetic and epigenetic influences, central nervous system circuitry, and a cascade of hormonal triggers that collectively work in a supportive environment to produce a unique product. These are volunteers who put aside many, if not most, of their normal youthful pastimes. They have a blind willingness to devote themselves to countless hours of study.

But success in medical school is not success at the patient's bedside, nor is it defined by success in life. Achievement in medical school, sadly, has never been defined as possessing an ethical framework from which to proceed. Less than 2 percent of the total instructional time in medical school is devoted to bioethics, a field that focuses on morality and philosophy as it pertains to medical decision making, treatments, and technology. Bioethical issues filter down to most patient encounters and percolate up with each diagnostic and therapeutic plan. Hippocrates wrote that, "The patient, though conscious that his condition is perilous, may recover his health simply through his contentment with the goodness of the physician." This was said in a day when goodness was just about all that could be offered.

In college when pre-medical students are exposed to the arts, this exposure is typically offered through core mandatory introductory courses. These are long forgotten when, six years later, they meet their first patients. Poets, authors, and artists-in-residence at medical schools represent a movement still in its infancy.

Alternatively, some medical educators have proposed that empathy is amenable to instruction. In 2010, a call for "neurobiologically informed training" was made to enhance medical student empathy.[1] Being taught that empathy has an address in our brains doesn't make its doors swing open. This is all well-meaning (and fine, go right ahead and teach it in neuroanatomy) but it misses the point. Empathy is not enhanced by tutorials; rather it is systematically and deliberately degraded by the experience of going through medical school. The authors of a 2004 article stated that "seventy-five percent of medical students become more cynical about academic life and the medical profession as they progress through medical school. Processes described as dehumanization and traumatic deidealization characterize the cynical transformation of medical students"[2] (see chapter 9 on empathy).

Recent calls to teach students emotional intelligence may also be futile. "Emotional IQ" has been touted as more important than cognitive IQ as a predictor of future career performance. This is dangerously wrong when choosing candidates for medical school or when selecting doctors for your care. Creative writing, role acting, and other methods have been suggested to imbue this quality. All this is fine, fun, and a worthwhile break from endocrine histopathology. But there is no scientifically proven psychometric standard for "emotional intelligence." Despite the hype, when it comes to cold hard science, it is an unrecognizable, unquantifiable, and ultimately unteachable quality.

A far better argument can be made for tending to medical students' emotions rather than their emotional intelligence. An article in the *Annals of Internal Medicine* in September 2008 detailed a study of more than 4,700 medical students. It noted that almost 50 percent of medical students had suffered burnout in the preceding twelve months and an alarming 11 percent had contemplated suicide. Over the study period, only a small minority fully recovered. I can empathize: my medical school years marked my initiation as a patient—in psychoanalysis. This occurred at a time when my loans were mounting. But financial worries paled in comparison to the anxieties and melancholy that sapped my emotional reserves.

Lessons are best learned in medical school by following the examples and hearing the criticisms from the very, very, (very) few inspirational instructors, doctors, and professors whom students meet along the way. For those coming up, mentors offer the most lasting lessons in a rigid hierarchical system where hero worship of respected seniors is the norm, but thoughtful, ethical exemplars are not.

The laser-like trajectories that our colleges and medical schools have mapped out for students will not be easily deflected by the siren call of "The Arts." A trend to move the already lamentable status quo even farther in the direction of highly specialized databases is being contemplated.

I know that medical students need to compete in and master a demanding body of ever-expanding knowledge and highly technical skills. But I wonder if the more artful pursuits are offered too late in students' maturation process. They become like the proverbial penicillin shot given to a dead man—it can't help, it won't hurt, it's just too late. It may be possible to stimulate intellectual curiosity in the liberal arts in the minds of some medical students. For many, however, the humanities have left only overgrown trails on little-used avenues of inquiry.

Organic Chemistry vs. Organic Medical Education: The skills required in organic chemistry demand prodigious memory that is put to the service of producing, on paper, formulas for industrial solvents starting from basic component molecules. This might serve the needs of a budding chemist but is no basis for medical maturity. Know the formula for a Grignard reagent? I don't. But I did in the fall of 1968 when, for three weeks, the single most important piece of information in my life was the fact that a Grignard reagent has a formula $RMgX$ where X is a halogen, and R is an alkyl or aryl (based on a benzene ring) group. I lived, slept, and dreamt its permutations and myriad reactions with different electrophiles. My future as a doctor, in no small way, rode on the absolute mastery of this knowledge. Its role in medicine was irrelevant. Organic chemistry is not an organic component of the elements that make a good doctor. Selecting students who are more natural products of their environments *is* a more organic process. These aspirants may be a better cut. And perhaps a cut above average too.

Today, medical schools have a lot of students to choose from. There are also a lot of people who, in their post-collegiate years, are actually living their lives: These are the "nontraditional" medical school applicants. The 16,000 each year who become doctors is a number that has been kept artificially low by admission committees. The physician shortage predicted to occur in the next several years may force the net to be cast farther to include these nontraditional students.

When even the finest steak is put into the meat grinder no one should be surprised when they get hamburger. The parboiled residue that's left after twelve to fifteen years in the sealed pressure cookers of colleges, premedical schools, residencies, and fellowships is the field from which you are choosing your doctor. A 2010 study of medical students revealed that 53 percent suffered burnout. Bad for them, but worse for you. Those with burnout were more likely to engage in unprofessional conduct and less likely to hold altruistic views regarding their societal responsibilities.[3] These young people aren't emerging from a petting zoo, but, rather, from a jungle. Doctors become a different type of "folk," with sensibilities and sensitivities that are indicative of a type of humanity still *formes frustes*. Anxious, depressed, resentful, cynical, and deep in debt, they have a highly developed sense of entitlement. For many, finally, "it's time to get out and get ours."

7

Brains

- A medical degree does not guarantee a gifted intellect.
- There are a lot of "very average" smart doctors out there.
- Your doctor's IQ is the *only* entitlement to your care.
- A gifted intellect is the single most important attribute you can never assume is present or dare do without.
- Board games: The myth of physician entitlement based on board certification.
- Physician-rating sites: Save your money.
- If your doctor's from Abu Dhabi . . . : Judging the talents of international medical graduates.
- "Wringing the Bell": Finding *your* doctor on the bell-shaped curve. Learn the fifteen-minute exercise that, more than anything else you can do, pinpoints just how smart your doctor really is.

Published surveys have indicated that when choosing a physician, patients routinely cite convenience, availability, waiting time, talking time, control in decision making, and access to alternative therapies as factors in their decision. Curiously, less than 10 percent mention a doctor's actual abilities. And even this small percentage use faulty inferential reasoning when seeking a doctor who is skilled in his field. It's not uncommon to hear this kind of rationale: "He took over the practice of an extremely competent physician."

Why is this? Could it be that ability doesn't count, or, rather, that it is always assumed to be present? Clearly no one would sacrifice a doctor's skill for any other non-medical attribute. A doctor's ability is believed to be an unvarying, even inviolate constant, beyond which other talents, such as interpersonal skills, availability, and compassion can *then* be commented upon. It is safe then to assume people see most, if not all doctors, as competent. This error accounts for two mutually contradictory but co-existing realities. People trust us, but we routinely harm many and sadly allow tens of thousands to die needlessly each year.

Doctors are still highly trusted because of their perceived abilities and qualities. A 2008 Gallup survey found that doctors' honesty and ethics were cited as "very high or high" by 64 percent of respondents and "high" by 30 percent, placing doctors fourth on the list behind only nurses, pharmacists, and high school teachers, good company for us to be in.[1] The fact is, however, that doctors routinely harm their patients. Not a day goes by without some media reference to physician error and the heartbreak it causes. Whether enumerated in dry statistics or detailed in the vivid reportage of a family crushed under the wheel of a doctor's negligence, the fact that you are not safe with us stands in contrast to the faith you nonetheless feel when in our hands.

This misplaced faith in our ability may, in part, derive from assumptions about the selectivity of medical schools and the rigor of a doctor's training. Yet even the dumbest, slack-jawed, knuckle-dragging student who graduated from the worst medical school in our country (or a few hundred other countries that can send us doctors) is still a doctor. Yours, perhaps?

Lesson one for this section is: *A medical degree alone does not entitle a doctor to your care.*

DEFINITIONS IN YOUR QUEST FOR QUALITY

It is important to define the primary qualities that you are looking for in a doctor, so that lesser or putative attributes you may find attractive can be assigned their proper place. Despite the fact that English has the largest of all lexicons, most of its words have few true synonyms. Parsing the "synonyms" used to describe doctors allows us to define the qualities that you should look for. Once we've done that, we can outline the methods you can use that are most likely to result in locating a doctor who embodies those qualities.

Qualifications and Entitlement

These two words—qualifications and entitlement—are rarely used now when assessing or describing doctors' skills. They are, however, still the chief indicators of a doctor's ability. They are also the most difficult to claim, the hardest to prove, and the most necessary to recognize. Competence, at its core, measures one's ability to perform tasks using intelligence and common sense. It's an error in judgment to assume that just because a doctor has an M.D., he is competent. Medical degrees are granted to people with a variety of talent, skill, and intelligence levels.

In *Synonyms Discriminated*, the nineteenth-century British lexicographer Charles John Smith observed that "Qualification is competency specifically developed . . . powers that are altogether extraneous to the individual and come to him from without or are conferred upon him." Doctors may be competent, but they are not qualified to undertake your care until they've achieved goals far broader than the mere receipt of their degrees. Entitlement is a step higher in the hierarchy, or what Charles Smith called, "an assertive kind of qualification; that is, is applied to cases not only of fitness but of privilege, and denotes the condition to claim with success."[2] Bestowing credentials on a doctor is possible only when the proper qualifications have been earned and the entitlement to be responsible for your care has been assured. Entitlement does not imply arrogance. It is not a mantle or a medal; rather it's an honorific earned and then conferred upon a doctor.

It is here that we come up against conventional wisdom. Credentials and certification in a medical specialty or a subspecialty have always encouraged the assumption of a doctor's qualification and entitlement to treat you. Although certification is necessary, it's not enough. In light of the fact that the vast majority of candidates who take certification boards pass them, it's time to re-evaluate their value and significance.

The American Board of Internal Medicine administers the tests for certification in internal medicine and its subspecialties. Thousands of applicants in hundreds of training programs take "The Boards." The American Board of Medical Specialties boasts that board certification is the "gold standard," by which we judge a physician's "knowledge, experience and skills for providing healthcare within a given specialty."

But if, as is the case, nearly 85 percent of licensed US physicians are board certified by the American Board of Medical Specialties, how can this examination be a "gold standard" for anything? When everyone passes a test, no one passes it. That type of test is not discriminating. When 85 percent pass you are mainly interested in avoiding the 15 percent who didn't, and avoiding placing any special value on those who did. Critics of the board certification system point out that, as an assessment tool, certification is a misleading indicator.

Lake Wobegon Effect

The board certification system reminds me of Lake Wobegon, Garrison Keillor's mythical community where "all the women are strong, all the men are good looking and all the children are above average." Demographic studies have found that people routinely judge themselves as above average in a variety of desirable skills and traits. And you can bet the farm that doctors, a supremely self-satisfied group, are way up there on the scale of self-regard.

It is, of course, statistically impossible for everyone to be above average. When medical specialty boards are passed by the vast majority of those taking them, you're seeing the Lake Wobegon effect in full display, and it essentially renders this distinction meaningless. The board certification credential doesn't reveal any salient truths about the clinical skills of successful candidates. When everyone is wonderful no one is wonderful. "The Boards" *would* be valid discriminators if the doctors' scores and relative rankings were released, but don't hold your breath on that one. What board certification credentials do tell you is to keep a nose-pinching distance from the few who are not board certified, and an even greater distance from the board-eligible physicians. This "title" is just a deceptive way to obscure the fact that they never took the boards, or, more likely, have already failed them, usually more than once.

Some doctors and experts in public policy assign a distinction to those who routinely follow Medicare-endorsed clinical algorithms and specialty generated guidelines. These cookbook checklists, however important they are in standardizing care, are not exercises in cognition; they are exercises in "monkey see, monkey do."

The Peter Principle

When I entered the Albert Einstein College of Medicine, we were all warned on the first day that our admission did not ensure our graduation. We correctly assumed the opposite and were correct: We all became doctors. I was, however, intrigued to note that some of my classmates seemed, well, dim. And I'm sure I was assessed as less than incandescent by those smarter than me, and so it goes.

The Peter Principle recognizes the fact that, sooner or later, some people are promoted to a level at which quite a few will be less competent than the rest, a handful will be barely competent, and an inevitable few will be frankly incompetent at the tasks at hand. The Peter Principle occurs in every hierarchical field and for each stratum within it.

Some of the people on the higher rungs of a hierarchical ladder will always be outmatched by the more complex, cognitive skills their positions call for. At other times people will be advanced to a totally different job for which they are suddenly unqualified. In cognitively demanding, competitive, hierarchical systems, many find themselves perched precariously at the outer edge of their abilities—and some beyond them.

Use your own experience. If you work in an office and have seen bosses come and go, the difference between the best and worst is large. So large, in fact, are the differences that you are unhappy working under the least-qualified supervisor. You might have to carry this character on your own back. Worse, your job performance and productivity may suffer. If that happens, who will be the one to drop the hammer on you? That's right—your bad boss.

The Peter Principle works the same way in medicine. When you're seeking care it's not just the few incompetent clinicians that you should avoid; rather, you should avoid the far greater number of doctors who are treading water as furiously as they can just to keep their heads above the rapidly rising tides of "must know" information. Of even greater concern is the possibility that the more ill you are and the more acute your need for highly specialized care, the less likely you are to get those who are entitled to deliver it. There will be a greater percentage of cardiologists just hanging on compared to general practitioners. Cardiology is on a higher cognitive stratum and, as more aspire to its practice, many will find themselves, finally, outmatched. Those with the éclat of great achievement will, like forces of nature, rise to these levels of accomplishment. Others may appear to float higher on the tides that only a few raise. For the rest, the Peter Principle still holds. In this rarefied atmosphere, more doctors will be practicing on the cusp of their competence although, alarmingly, not their confidence. The higher the wire on which this balancing act occurs, the greater the fall—for you.

It would be unwise to assume that you are safe in a neurosurgeon's office just because he is, after all, a brain surgeon. When you say to your kids, "Follow the directions . . . it's not brain surgery," remember that there are always higher cognitive strata. That means there are brain surgeons who are told, "just remove that brain tumor . . . it's not rocket science."

You don't want someone literally in your brain, heart, or gut who is being carried by his partners' and associates' superior cognitive and motor skills. You don't want to be one of the "easy cases" that are frequently assigned to these under-performers. You want *your* doctor to be invincible to the Peter Principle.

It's universally accepted that there is a link between intelligence and job performance. This association between high IQ and superior abilities is the key to finding a doctor or assessing the ones you have. The problem is finding out just how smart your doctor really is. First let's disavow ourselves of the popular notion that measuring and stratifying intelligence is a bad thing.

People object to the use of IQ tests, in large part, because they result in a single number that, like a doppelganger, can follow individuals for the rest of their lives. It defines too precisely what most see as an abstract, complex, multifaceted range of traits that exist not as dots along a continuum, but as an array of talents unique to every individual. No one doubts the importance of intelligence. It is ranked only second to good health as a quality worth possessing. Intelligence counts so much, in fact, that we object when our children's prospects in life could be determined by an IQ test's single expression of it. We have come to assess and honor a broader spectrum of attributes that are neither quantifiable, nor in some cases easily definable. The very use of the term IQ is shunned. We view our society as a meritocracy that allows us in some way to separate achievement from intelligence. That's not only a futile exercise but a dangerous one. A doctor's gifted intellect is the sole criterion most likely to determine success when your life is on the line.

No one would want to ignore the importance of intelligence when it comes to choosing doctors. Again, raw mental power *is* the only variable we have that serves as the basic denominator for ability. You don't want a merely knowledgeable doctor, you want an exceptional one. You want Dr. Know. This necessitates the stratification of intelligence, which is objectionable to many people. For many it's all about a level playing field.

Intelligence is defined as a comfort with complexity. More complex tasks require more mental manipulation of information: discerning similarities and inconsistencies, drawing inferences, grasping new concepts. How can we measure it? How can we get our hands around your doctor's intelligence, so that we can recognize and then stratify it against others? What are the variables that can be measured that will indicate that your doctor isn't just smart, but nuclear-powered smart?

Who would deny that Tiger Woods is one of the best golf professionals on the scene today? Perhaps he will become one of the greatest in the history of the sport. In a story in the *New York Times* in April 2008, reporter Mark Sweeney noted that despite his prowess, "a look at his statistics showed some pretty average ranking in categories like driving accuracy and sand saves, yet some pretty impressive rankings in categories like greens in regulation, putting and approach proximity . . .Woods was a lowly 152 in driving accuracy in 2007, yet Jose Coceres, who was first, finished 131st in the Official World Golf Ranking."[3]

It is the variables that have the *most impact* on his score that serve to distance him from the crowd.

So, how do we find the best of the best doctors? Where is your Doctor Woods? What are the high-impact variables that make your doctor a champ? A number of variables that can be used to infer a doctor's high intelligence have been suggested. High income, prodigious productivity, a busy waiting room, high rankings in the public and government ratings, fewer malpractice cases, fewer referrals to state disciplinary boards, and, yes, even board certification.

The correlation fails, however, when you rely on only one of these variables. These causal factors must be considered collectively in order to glean valuable information regarding your doctor's intelligence. Most of the data, however, is unavailable to you. It is also difficult for you to weigh the importance of one factor against another. For example, is high income a better predictor of intelligence than the number of malpractice suits? If so, by how much? Where are the high-impact variables that give your Dr. Woods his edge?

I am here to tell you that when choosing a doctor look for the men and women whom you've identified as being intellectually gifted. It is the only truly necessary attribute you want in a doctor, and those doctors that have it are the only ones who are qualified and entitled to care for you. But simple smarts are not enough. Smarts are all over the place. You see smart people screwing up all the time. You are looking for the doctor with the truly gifted mind. This practitioner will excel above his or her colleagues in each and every stratum he or she reaches in the medical specialties.

But how do you recognize those who are the brightest amongst a cohort of bright peers? The gifted medical mind has been perceived as immaterial (Hey, he's a doctor, right? He's gotta be smart.), and it's been perceived as elitist. Is it shrouded behind a wall of privacy? Is it a Freemason-like secret that cannot be revealed?

It turns out you can avoid the woes of the "Lake Wobegon effect" and find those doctors who are invincible to the Peter Principle with relative ease.

Our job is to find, in a group of doctors, those who occupy the stratospheric positions in this stratum of already smart people. It's not enough to seek out the best of the worst or even those who are amongst the best. You want the leaders of the best.

WRINGING THE BELL

Most natural phenomena, including doctors' intelligence, can be arranged on the well-known bell-shaped distribution curve.

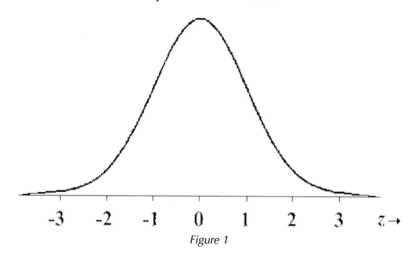

Figure 1

It is a remarkable, and endlessly useful, fact that so many things arrange themselves on this accurate (though approximate) pattern. It also just makes plain sense that extremes are rare while things average are not. Doctors are in a high-IQ profession. As with any bell-shaped curve, it is axiomatic to state that there are *a lot* more doctors with "average" high intelligence than there are those on the extreme positive end of the curve. Sixty-eight percent of doctors are on the hump of the bell curve. This percentage represents one standard deviation above and one standard deviation below the mean, which is the peak of the bell. That's a lot of "average-smart" doctors. A standard deviation is a derived method of measuring standardized distances from the mean. Someone who is +2 standard deviations from the mean is way smarter than someone who is +1 standard deviation from it. A +3 standard deviation is light years from the mean and, for that matter, from a +2 standard deviation. It is here that we find the truly gifted intellects.

It is unnecessary to address what happens to those under the care of doctors who are more than −1 standard deviation from the mean, so horrible may be their fates. Below this level are the garden gnomes and bridge trolls of children's premonitory tales. Thirty-two percent of doctors are poised on each end of the curve. Those on the left are best left alone; those on the right are right for you. We must, by "wringing the bell," extract from it criteria that allow us to identify in a pool of doctors those two to three standard + deviations from the mean. These folks should be your doctors.

Remember that the higher the intelligence, the better the job performance and qualifications. The farther your doctor is from the mean, the more intelligence he has, and the closer the correlation between his intelligence and job performance. Now how do you determine who they are?

All of us who journey through today's education system become sorted out on the bell by application of cognitive stratification. Schools place in our paths the filters that become more selective as we progress onward and upward through their hierarchies. Those who pass through multiple and progressively narrower filters are progressively brighter.

The few and the proud educational citadels strain off from our democracy's "befuddled masses" only the very top students in the population of graduating high school seniors. This collegiate cognitive stratification is given statistical life in Richard Herrstein and Charles Murray's book, *The Bell Curve*. The chance of finding just four graduates from the dozen highest-rated colleges in a random sampling of twelve citizens is less than *one in a billion*. On the 2010–2011 Supreme Court, all nine justices came from Ivy League schools—five from Harvard. Surprised? You shouldn't be.

Those in the top fifty colleges and universities represent a very tight and small circle of extremely bright people. But for aspiring doctors, the filtering is far from complete. The gates narrow when it's time to apply to medical school. Only the best college seniors have a chance of getting into medical school. Those from the elite ivy-covered, ivory-towered colleges are happy to get into *any* medical school. Many fail.

Are we there yet? Nope. To date all these students' work has prepared them for their ultimate careers. All medical school graduates must proceed to postgraduate studies. Most are attracted to the almost transparently thin slice of openings in the most desirable subspecialties in medicine and surgery. Neurosurgery, plastic surgery, cardiothoracic surgery, cardiology, and gastroenterology are a few examples. Dermatology is a handsomely reimbursed specialty with few on-call responsibilities. There were only 320 training positions available in the United States in 2007. Only the best universities amongst the hundreds of others can get to choose between a small rarefied group of applicants that by now would seem to be clones of each other rather than distinctive individuals. Despite this, fewer than 50 percent of the applicants are even interviewed for cardiology and gastroenterology positions. It is suggested that aspirants to these subspecialties apply to thirty or forty programs to improve their chances of admission.

How do you gain entrée to the databases that allow you to recognize these doctors whose offices are just down the street? What number of variables should you investigate on your own? What fees will you incur? How long will you squirm in your chair after having asked your doctor for his board scores, IQ, and income tax statement? What are the high-impact variables that are always and easily available?

All you need to do is look up and see the handwriting on the wall, or in this case, the diplomas in your doctor's office. There are only three certificates that count—the diplomas from college, medical school, and training hospitals that should be proudly framed on their walls. *These are the high-impact variables.* These tell you all you need to know about your doctor's intelligence and hence her job performance. The best institutions take only the best doctors.

A medical educational journey spent at the most elite institutions in the United States and, by inference, the world, pinpoints your doctor's location on the bell curve's tiny tip. Don't see the diplomas? Ask the office for a bio or curriculum vitae. Look for the information on the office's Internet site. Google your doctor. Check with your state medical board. Still no luck? If I went to Harvard and then to Yale and finished up at the Johns Hopkins Hospital for training, believe me, readers, you'd know it. Most doctors with impeccable credentials will do everything but tattoo them on a body part. If you are unable to easily find this information that might be all the information you need.

Bonus Points: In ascending order of importance you may see the college diploma noting its recipient graduated "cum laude," "magna cum laude," or "summa cum laude." More bonus points are given for Phi Beta Kappa. Membership in the medical school equivalent of Phi Beta Kappa, the Alpha

Omega Alpha Society (AOA), is awarded to only 3,100 students out of the 16,000 medical school graduates each year.

After you look up at the office's wall, go home and look up on your computer where each of the institutions you noted on the three diplomas is ranked on the *U.S. News & World Report*. This one site has it all. The comparative rankings of undergraduate colleges, postgraduate medical schools, and postdoctoral hospital training programs are easily available and free. You are looking for the top fifty colleges and universities, the fifty most highly ranked medical schools (in primary care; ignore the research ratings), and the best fifty hospitals. (www.USNews.com/sections/rankings). If your doctor went to these prestigious institutions, he did not get there on his good looks alone.

Free of charge but not of controversy. Yes, the *U.S. News & World Report* ranking may be flawed by aspects in its methodology. Oversimplification, factual errors, and omissions abound. But hey, you're not applying for admission to these places. You shouldn't care about the top five or ten in each stratum. It gets ugly at this level with schools jockeying fiercely for position. This is where the controversy, criticisms, and contumely live. Ignore them. A doctor's educational trajectory through these institutions is the best indicator of his intelligence. This in turn will be strongly predictive of his performance as a clinician. Those three diplomas on the wall embody a "trinity of ability," but they are a transubstantiation of one substance—intelligence. Intelligence counts, and doctors have it. You want the doctors who have it in the greatest supply. The smartest doctors are the best doctors. Period.

Certain patterns that emerge from a doctor's voyage through her education can be as important as her constant presence, across the board, at elite institutions. A doctor who started at a prestigious university but then went to an average medical school and trained in an obscure hospital is the embodiment of the Peter Principle. Perhaps this doctor was a good medical student who erred in choosing surgery as his specialty. Surgery is essentially a new job that requires more than brains and desire. It demands different skills like dexterity and an unusually vivid, three-dimensional visual acuity. Whatever the reason, it augurs poorly for your chances with this surgeon. Conversely, an ascent through the three levels speaks volumes about her intelligence, work ethic, and predicted clinical performance. A hard-earned victory swimming against these filters' unidirectional flow demonstrates that no system is perfect. Pearls, first missed, often emerge later in the processing of students.

The *U.S. News & World Report* includes schools of osteopathy. These doctors, D.O.s, are the equivalent to those with M.D.s—for better or worse, in sickness and in health, and until . . . well you get it.

Many people will ask, "How about experience? Doesn't that count?" The less intelligent but experienced physicians just started the "race to results" earlier. They have had more time but less ability to use that time in practice wisely. An intellectually gifted doctor will typically catch up to an experienced, but less bright doctor, overcoming the distance of time. That doctor's intelligence will usually prevail in any important, desirable clinical endpoint, whether it's the correct diagnosis or treatment or "the ability to save." This ability allows your Dr. Lazarus to save patients who would die in others' hands. Experience plus brains? Priceless!

There are those who can cite their own and others' experiences, both as doctors and as their patients, that run counter to the suggested primacy of elite educational trajectories.

ALTITUDES AND ATTITUDES AND APTITUDES

The group of doctors who have reached these professional heights has been developed to the point of becoming almost taxonomically distinct. They are the foam on a large and deep ocean of physician mediocrity. This tends to affect their attitudes in ways that may not be pleasant. A doctor's professional carriage may suffer in the process of his becoming a doc-star. Severe selection and stratification pressures may further attenuate traits that you value. Character, professionalism, style, communication skills, and empathy increase a doctor's desirability, but not his ability. Intelligence is a label, not a medal. It is the only thing you can never sacrifice.

What happened to physician ratings? Physician report cards and ratings systems would seem like the answer for people trying to evaluate a doctor's reputation and efficacy as a physician. Not only are they unreliable, worse, they can also be deceptive and, therefore, harmful as research tools.

The public correctly has, either through discernment or inertia, ignored the ratings. According to a Harris Interactive poll, only 2 percent of those responding changed their physicians based on a website's doctor ratings or recommendations. Only 1 percent changed their hospital or health plan based on ratings.[4]

Finally, research has demonstrated that when the public uses information found in a health-care report, they tend to value the least reliable information and dismiss the most important data. Patient ratings, anecdotes, and unquantifiable "levels of global satisfaction" ranked first in consumers' esteem when used as quality indicators. The more important discriminators to which the study population had access—disciplinary actions and undesirable clinical indicators—were rated lowest in importance.

State-mandated report cards for heart surgeons have resulted in unexpected consequences. Cardiothoracic surgeons now operate on the low-hanging fruit. Cherry-picking the easy cases allows them to artificially keep their scores elevated. Some surgeons massage their patients' diagnostic codes, making them seem sicker than they are. This can also improve their scores on the state rankings as well as their incomes.

A *New York Times* article in the fall of 2008 reported that "63% of cardiac surgeons acknowledge that because of report cards they were accepting only relatively healthy patients for heart bypass surgery. 59% of cardiologists said it had become harder to find a surgeon to operate on the most seriously ill patients."[5] Deaths were felt to have resulted from this practice.

You shouldn't rely on the anecdotal whimsies of water cooler tips and over-the-fence neighborhood consultations. The Center for Studying Health System Change noted that 20 to 50 percent of us choose our doctors based solely on recommendations made by friends and relatives.[6] Looking up doctors on Angie's List is not the way to make important decisions about your health and the health of your family. Opinions from non-nursing hospital personnel, a rung higher than a Tupperware party, are liable to be too personal and reflect impressions that are limited in scope.

When your doctor refers you to a specialist you might assume he's picking the best one for you. He isn't. Choosing a specialist is a convoluted process involving friendship, loyalty, quids pro quo, a match-up of minimal needs against commensurate skills, and medical politics. Eighteen percent of respondents from a 2002 study in *Medical Economics* said they had referred patients to a physician in their group or managed care network even though they had concerns about that doctor's suitability. Family physicians and general practitioners are most likely to have done so—probably reflecting the fact that they form the core of many closed HMO networks. Similarly, physicians in large multi-specialty groups are more likely than soloists to refer to unsuitable specialists because those consultants are part of their group.[7] A tried-and-true way to find the doctor's doctor is to simply ask "Who do you see when you and your family need a _____ (fill in the blank) doctor?" You may not get an answer or it may be deflected with "Dr. Stew Pydhaso is a great doctor and I trust him completely." This, of course, doesn't answer the question, although by inference it may. If your doctor confirms that your cardiologist-to-be is also his own cardiologist, you know that that heart specialist has a better chance of being a good one.

BUT MY DOCTOR IS FROM ABU DHABI!

International medical graduates (IMGs) represent 25 percent of the physician workforce in the United States. This number will increase in the next several years in the face of an anticipated physician shortage, due to an increase in older and sicker patients, and the 2014 mandate for universal medical coverage that will add tens of millions of long-neglected patients to doctors' appointment calendars. All this is in the face of a shrinking pool of primary care providers. International graduates' life stories, religions, cultures, and odysseys to the West are compelling. Some of these insights were gained as the result of a dinner I hosted with a number of IMGs who are friends and colleagues. These conversations highlighted the process and the pressures of licensure and life in the West. For many it's a Horatio Alger–like journey characterized by risk, sacrifice, competitive victories, hard work, and determination. Strong "in-group" support and the primacy of family ties are the common denominators in this and perhaps many immigrant communities. All this is played out against the backdrop of their belief in, and affection for, their adopted country although their professional standing within medical circles has historically been a tenuous one. In 2010, their struggles and experiences were acknowledged.[8] It starts with the subtle and overt prejudice, bias, and discrimination that they view as pervasive. IMGs feel that they are held to a different standard than US medical school graduates and that advancement to desirable specialties and metropolitan areas is denied them. They rightly view their talents as advanced and, in some areas, unique.

Can these doctors be cognitively stratified in such a way that you can determine which are the elite and which are not? IMGs come from more than a hundred countries and almost 2,000 medical schools worldwide whose graduates can at least contemplate an entry into the process of medical certification that ends with a state's licensure.

There are alternative filters. For many in these countries, a student's access to higher education is not a right. College is, however, the only path to professional and economic success. In India the race to success starts early. Throughout high school, students take up to five tests, the last of which, a national exam, will determine their lifetime trajectories. Technical colleges require students take even more tests for entrance. India has 186 million students; only 12 percent will advance to higher education. The elite schools screen several hundreds of thousands, accepting only a few thousand for admission. Drill schools, extreme expense, and extensive tutoring drain meager family resources. Brutal competition and societal and parental pressures force millions across the world to strain against the rigid and narrow gates through which only the brightest will pass. It's a high-stakes game. In India, students are fifteen or sixteen years old when they commit to medicine. If they wash out, their futures are relegated to careers far less professionally and financially rewarding.

A second alternative filter is the tactical and financial hardships that a candidate endures as part of the process of entering the United States, a process that has no guarantee of success. Byzantine visa requirements demand determination. Thousands of dollars in fees for a series of tests, as well as travel expenses, can amount to more than a year of the salaries earned back home. This culls all but the most ambitious from the herd.

The third filter is provided by our country. All foreign medical students must run the gauntlet of tests administered by the Education Commission for Foreign Medical Graduates (ECFMG). Passing scores for the United States Medical Licensure Exam (USMLE) step one (basic sciences) and the USMLE step two (clinical science) and, since 1998, the Clinical Skills Assessment (CSAs) have allowed for cognitive partitioning of those successful candidates. A 2002 article in the *Journal of the American Medical Association* noted that while the number of IMGs who sought and received certification yearly had decreased, the quality of the applicants seemed to have improved. The percentage of students receiving passing grades on these tests is not so high as to question the tests' rigor. After the test results are in, only 46 percent of aspirants will succeed (2009).[9] Those tests have teeth.

Aspirants also must score "acceptably" on the Test of English as a Foreign Language (the TOEFLs). This test's passing grade is so low that it has permitted many doctors to practice medicine who possess poor English skills. (This issue is explored in the next section.) The cumulative effect of the filters in their native countries, the hurdles they overcome to qualify for examinations, and the testing here in the United States are not without salient results. There is a newfound and well-founded confidence in the equivalence of cognitive medical skills of IMGs to those of American-born doctors. Early candidacy and success in their studies means that they have far greater experience than their Western counterparts when their studies are completed. Dr. Atul Gawande, in his book *Better*, writes "the skills of the average Indian surgeon outstripped the skills of any Western surgeon I know." And there is evidence that he's correct. In 2010, it was found that "patients of doctors who graduated from international medical schools and were not U.S. citizens at the time they entered medical school had significantly lower mortality rates than patients cared for by doctors who graduated from U.S. medical schools or who were U.S. citizens and received their degrees abroad." Patients of non-US-citizen international graduates had the lowest mortality levels, and patients of US citizens trained abroad had the highest.[10] While this is a stunning achievement, significantly, it still does not disclose the rank of doctors who are in the "stratum stratospherics" of their fields.

Although an international medical graduate may obtain subspecialty certification in the United States, it is unlikely, given the competition for these positions, that the training hospital will be amongst the best. If that hospital is, however, high on the *U.S. News & World Report*'s rankings, this individual physician must be considered to be outstanding.

The three diplomas on your doctor's wall tell you all you need to know about his intelligence. But if you don't know where in the world your doctor came from we must begin again. We are back to the basics.

A diploma can't guarantee professionalism. When you can't access training credentials, the first step is to access your state's medical board, which may provide a wealth of information. It's only a Google search away. Go to the disciplinary section for any doctor, homegrown or otherwise. There are many websites where you can link to all fifty state medical boards. Public Citizen offers these links and comparison ratings for the transparency of each state board. It's chaos out there. Whatever else our States are United in, uniform standards of disclosure about medical licensure and doctors' qualifications are not among them.

Highly transparent states like New Jersey will give you access to your doctor's license number, medical school, graduate medical education, board certification, practice information, malpractice actions within the last five years, and the relative significance of any verdict or settlement. Many states include information on disciplinary actions, licensure limitations, out-of-state disciplinary actions, hospital-based privilege restriction, and criminal convictions.

But there are other states that won't allow you to search for anything related to your M.D.'s qualifications—"*e pluribus* anonymous" is more the rule than the exception.

Beyond the state boards and Internet research sites, we are now back to the variables that are individually unreliable but collectively more compelling. These include ratings, report cards, board certification, physician and nursing personnel word-of-mouth, indicators of high income, busy waiting rooms, long delays for appointments, university affiliations, a bibliography of published articles, posted certificates documenting continuing medical education, and Google searches.

Carspotting: I wouldn't suggest arriving early to the office to see what car your doctor drives. But one patient left my care in 1982 because I drove an uninteresting, disintegrating 1974 Audi Fox. He may have had a point.

The next section deals with the traits that, although necessary, are not by themselves sufficient. Can we get everything? In the face of the social pressures on medicine, and doctors' near-universal job dissatisfaction rate, even "the best lack all conviction, while the worst are full of passionate intensity" (Yeats).

8

Communication

- Why the doctor's office is a sensory deprivation chamber, filled with silence or static and statistics.
- Your doctor: as wise as Solomon . . . as silent as a Sphinx.
- It doesn't have to be a brain down the drain.
- Why your doctor and you can't even agree about the purpose and goals of your appointment.
- Setting the agenda—it's your job.
- Why your doctor won't talk with you.
- Suggestions that will get him engaged in your care. How to make "you" matter.
- The doctor-inspired myth that "there's not enough time."
- How to get what you need in fifteen minutes. Meet Dr. Shirley Welby-Tardy and Dr. Seymour Dolittle.
- "Professional patients"—salaried consultants who evaluate and correct doctors' communication skills. Learn their tricks and become a professional too.
- How to give your secrets, worries, and embarrassments a voice.
- Getting around language and other communication barriers—theirs *and* yours.
- Recognizing the friends and relatives who need your help to avoid a "death by benightedness."

Well, you've done it. You've harnessed the high-voltage intellect of a gifted physician. He is comfortable with complexity and he's a master of multitasking. He has the cerebral energy to both analyze and research the questions you have raised, and to investigate your symptoms. He has the mental power to wrestle problems to the canvas and then rise up with reasoned impressions and effective diagnostic and therapeutic strategies that are the most likely to achieve something.

But . . . it's too bad he won't talk to you. He won't be an advocate for his plan; won't seek your participation or opinions; won't bother to make you as confident in him as he is in himself; won't care about you as much as he does about your diagnosis; won't seem to suffer—even a little bit—when the news is bad or savor the results, when it's good.

How can you tap into all that brain matter to get at what matters? A doctor's ability does not confer his desirability. Intellect and interpersonal skills are on distinct and distant cerebral zip codes.

This is all very sad but not really mysterious. In the previous sections, we've warned you about both the blessing and the curse being set before you. Many doctors, especially the bright ones, can become the arid product of selective conditioning, adaptive pressures, and the ultrafiltration that produces cognitive elites. It may come as no surprise that the pleasing, attractive, and necessary qualities of empathy, and the ability to listen and to communicate that should adorn their skills, are shorn in the process of achieving others. But you're not only entitled to proper communication and empathy, you should demand them. Let's find out where they live and see if anyone's home.

Cognitive skills don't necessarily result in the ability to talk clearly and informatively with patients. If your highly rated and expensive wide-screen LCD high-definition television has no audio, it has no value, despite its advanced electronics and circuitry.

When properly used, communication between a doctor and a patient is fluent, rich in metaphor, and concise yet comprehensive. Almost every behavior a doctor displays when she's with you should be seen as a form of communication, good or bad. A doctor's appearance, as well as her movements and posture, reveal something of her inner traits and character. Inappropriate gestures can be judged against more fluid ones that reflect spirituality and a core that's centered.

We judge a clinician's ability to communicate second only to the quality of her mind precisely because that intelligence must be put to use conveying to you issues of great importance. We value intelligence but can't be judged solely on what we know. There is a premium on knowledge that can be communicated. A locked library is not a resource.

You and your doctors are in the Cone of Silence—mutually indecipherable, mutually frustrated. Our first job is to demonstrate the problems patients encounter when communication fails, classify the missteps, and offer solutions.

It was noted in one study that 78 percent of the patients who left the emergency room did not understand what was said and, worse, 80 percent of them didn't even know they didn't understand.[1] With this kind of alarming data, errors in medication and problems in compliance and follow-up are all but guaranteed.

When people are diagnosed with terminal cancer, few of them will know, or be informed of, the difference between palliative and curative care. Even fewer realize that, when offered late in the disease process, palliation can offer either longer lives or more comfortable ones, but often neither, and rarely both. Palliative care focuses on relieving symptoms and reducing suffering when cure is impossible. When offering palliative care many doctors obscure the most important issues by using vague references to a prognosis that promotes both misunderstandings and poor decision making.

"It may buy some time," is a classic example. *May?* (or may not), *some?* (how much?), *buy?* (what price?). Thanks a lot!

In one cancer study, 26 out of 37 consultations failed to offer clear, or in some cases *any*, information on the survival benefit for a suggested therapy.[2] A study in 2010 demonstrated the value of clear discussion of palliative options. Soon after the diagnosis of an incurable cancer, patients who received palliative care not only lived longer but had less pain and depression, more mobility, and a better quality of life.[3] When information is poor, vague, or lacking, some patients may suddenly, in contrast to previously voiced wishes, decline curative therapy. Patients with resectable lung cancer who were denied an adequate discussion often turned down their only chance for cure.[4]

Researchers analyzed audiotaped conversations between orthopedists and their patients who were considering surgical interventions. There is no suite of communication skills that is more important than the discussion of the risk and benefits of surgery. Medical therapy, surgery, or watchful waiting are all options at every intersection on the road to decision making and informed consent.[5] The study reveals that *none* of the surgeons completely assessed the patients' understanding of the proposed surgery or discussed the patients' role in it. These patients weren't placed in the center of the discussion, they weren't even marginalized; it's as if they didn't exist. The surgeons in this study knew they were being audiotaped and are presumed to have been on their very best behavior and "smiling for the camera." One shudders to think what happens when the cameras' shutters are closed.

Research has found that only one-third of physicians studied wrote down instructions for their patients. Only half of them repeated recommendations and few offered more than 10 percent of their complete recommendations the second time around. Very few checked to see whether their patients understood the information they were given. It's rare for a doctor to ask the patient to repeat the information back: the best method for maximizing recall. In light of these poor skills, it was felt that half of the patients were likely to forget what they were told.

In a 2008 article in the *Postgraduate Medical Journal*, John Launer wrote, "The vast majority of doctors in most specialties never once sit down to consider systematically the words and phrases they use when conversing with patients, or the tone and manner in which they deliver them. I suspect that most patients would be astonished to discover this."[6]

I suspect that most patients *do* know that many doctors give little thought to what they say. Clinicians' careless flights of speculative fancy characterize many of your transactions with doctors. Their words can increase anxiety, worsen symptoms, and delay recovery. Your symptom should not provide the opportunity for doctors to view it like a piñata, beating it verbally until all *possible* diagnoses, no matter how unlikely, fall from it like party favors. Idle ruminations over diagnoses are tossed into the wind like so much dross, triggering a Kierkegaardian "fear and trembling," despite the fact that they are, as yet, only possibilities. Cancer, the ultimate "sickness unto death," is more than a word. It is every patient's worst fear for almost any symptom they experience. The utterance of the word "cancer" must await its proof. When a doctor says "cancer," he should rarely be wrong. It should never be casually rattled off because it's sixth on a long list of other possibilities. Despite this, patients leave offices shell-shocked from battles that never needed to be fought. If more doctors knew how to communicate effectively, even difficult conversations would be enlightening, not frightening.

There is often a large gap between your expectations and what the available therapies can offer. A chasm can exist between hope and the sometimes harsh decrees of medicine that deal in the statistical over the spiritual. It's your doctor's job to bridge these divides, helping you to understand the realities of what you now must face. When she won't, you must direct the encounter. Happily, you can.

The ability to limn is the talent to portray, describe, or illustrate, both verbally and visually. A doctor who is unwilling to go out on that metaphorical limn denies to you a critical medical skill. It leaves you frustrated while in the office and at risk for your life while in the hospital. Communication then becomes a matter of life and limn.

You are the indispensable, irrefutable expert on your complaint. You are the definitive authority on the subjective experience that frames a problem no one else can describe. But when you talk, your doctor doesn't listen because he is rushed, distracted, interrupted, unwilling to address your concerns or comment on your research. When he talks you don't get it because of all of the above and because he talks too fast, uses too many technical terms, retreats to uninterpretable statistics, has his own agenda, speaks with an accent, or just doesn't care.

A doctor's "hand on door" habit is worth noting. You know you're off-center when you see the doctor grasping the door handle with a vice-like death grip. You might want to invite him back into the room because when his hand is on the door he's already left.

THE VOCATION OF PATIENTHOOD

We have previously noted that when you are in the office you are the expert on your health and the issues that occasioned your visit. It is time for you to be a professional as well as an expert. There are those who make a living being "patients." They are employed to evaluate doctors' performance. We can learn a lot from their techniques. I will suggest that you become a professional using the tools of a standard patient (SP).

"War is too important to be left to the generals."

—Georges Clemenceau

Medical care may be too important to be left to doctors. A simulated or standard patient is a trained professional who takes on the role of a patient so accurately that the disguise can't be penetrated, even by a skilled clinician. The SP presents an entire picture of what it is to be a person with a problem. The fiction is maintained through the recitation of a history and the use of body language and personality characteristics that make up a three-dimensional patient, replete with the emotional responses to illness, as well as family and job-related stresses. Some SPs judge the entire office experience from the time of the telephone call to the doctor's office to the purgatory of the waiting room. Hey, that's what you do! They just do it for a living. Their evaluations are part of the process toward licensure for IMGs and US graduates.

SPs use templates to assess clinicians' abilities. Marta van Zanten and colleagues introduced a four-tier skill model[7] that works well for our purposes. A physician's communication skills center around four dimensions: skills in interviewing, information gathering, education and counseling, and rapport and personal manners.

You know you're in trouble when the doctor asks rapid-fire close-ended questions. You feel more comfortable when, in contrast, you are given the floor rather than being shown the door.

Must you coax each jargon-infested utterance from your doctor? Or is the information and counseling freely given using language that is clear and colloquial?

You are valued when doctors work to establish rapport. It starts badly if there is no introduction or handshake. If your doctor doesn't pay attention or even look at you, but instead feels free to interrupt, go ahead—judge this character badly. Realize this attitude is what you will be subjected to during your entire clinical relationship. On the other end of the spectrum, you know when you are being treated as an equal. Your doctor is supportive rather than judgmental. He shares your feelings, offers praise when appropriate, and voices his intent to be of help.

There are no skills that SPs bring to an encounter that you can't. You can create the conditions that lead to a successful encounter.

Inspect, interpret, interrupt, inject, and intercede. Inspect your surroundings. Are they conducive to conversation? Can you interpret the suggestions and opinions that are offered? Interrupt when you don't understand what is said. Inject new information when factual errors are heard. Intercede if you don't agree.

Keep, for now, your gifted physician. Her intelligence is the causa sine qua non you used when choosing her. It may be better to have a smart sphinx than a voluble village idiot. Our job is to get your summa cum laude to speak up louder, on and in your behalf.

THE BARRIERS

The barriers to communication are time, unvoiced concerns, language barriers, cultural divides, and health literacy and numeracy.

Tic-Doc, Tic-Doc

Time constraints are perceived as the primary obstacle to proper communication. I will cite two studies that appeared almost simultaneously in autumn 2008. Both point to inexplicably uncaring physician behaviors for which time constraints were blamed. But despicable behaviors are never caused or excused by a lack of time. They are always caused by a lack of organization or, worse, personal inclination. We will debunk the commonly held myth that "there isn't enough time" as an excuse for poor communication.

The first article appeared in the *Archives of Internal Medicine*. The investigation demonstrated that the studied physicians did not respond to the emotional concerns of their patients who were suffering from cancer. Only 10 percent of oncologists produced empathetic responses to the highly angst-ridden, existential, and emotional cris de coeur their patients made.[8] The first reason cited for this heartless lapse was the claim of a limited amount of time available to engage in such activities.

The second study, published three days later in the online *Journal of General Internal Medicine*, also, in part, blamed a lack of time when patients presented with new and severe clinical depression.[9] The depression either went undiagnosed, or the necessary inquiries about the possibility of suicidal feelings were left unasked.

A Pair of Docs' Clocks' Paradox: Dr. Shirley Welby-Tardy is obsessed with time and running late. Because of this she will paradoxically end up spending *more* time with her patients, rather than less, leaving her patients frustrated as she gets further behind on her schedule.

The second practitioner provides the second paradox. Meet Dr. Seymour Dolittle. For Seymour, the poorer the job he did during a visit, the more patient questions he must answer at the end of it, and the more time will need to be spent making it right with the patient because of it. His answers become briefer and more desultory. As his day goes on he leaves in his wake increasingly frustrated patients while his schedule disintegrates.

For Dr. Tardy the explanation for this paradox lies in a "quote of many authors":

- "I didn't have time to make a short letter so I wrote a long one instead."—Mark Twain.
- "I have made this letter longer than usual only because I have not had the time to make it shorter."—Blaise Pascal.
- The final and third attribution is from T. S. Eliot. We can be sure this version took the most time to compose because it's expressed economically and is the most easily understood of the three. "If I had more time, I could have written a shorter letter."

Doctors who spend more time *just once* organizing their resources will have shorter and more informative visits: "If I had spent more time, I could have offered you a shorter visit." Doctors who make this one-time investment don't have to reinvent the wheel every time they enter a room. The proper atmospherics, ambiance, patient flow, scheduling, staffers, and the fostering of informatics will allow the most information to be transferred in the least amount of time. It's all in the medical *mise en place*. Patients' information needs are predictable. Responding to their questions can be effortless if solutions are in place before the patients' concerns are voiced.

"Rapport building may enhance quality of care without taking more time. . . . Physicians trained to fully elicit patient concerns and establish a focus for the visit with patients took no more time and had greater patient satisfaction."[10]

It may be that Dr. Shirley Welby-Tardy should focus on only one topic for a full discussion. Perhaps she should inform her patients that if several topics are raised, their solutions will be discussed on subsequent visits. She should have pre- and post-visit DVDs, videos, and brochures for the common problems she predictably encounters. Informed patients require less time. Clinicians, anxious to inform and satisfy their patients before quickly moving on to the next room, have at their disposal referrals to hospital and community programs that address the common, important problems that require a lot of time to cover well. Diabetes and its management, osteoporosis, cancer screening, nutrition, weight loss, physical activity, smoking cessation, alcohol abuse, and other issues cannot be dealt with in a timely or satisfactory fashion in the office. Yet they cannot be ignored.

Dr. Welby-Tardy should offer office-based seminars to selected groups of invited patients that direct attention to specialized topics of interest relevant to her patients' problems. These conditions often require a lot of time to cover carefully and completely. Doing it well once, in front of many patients, prevents the need for her doing it many times poorly and inefficiently, one patient at a time. Group education can be more effective than the "one on one" hurried and harried exercises you experience today. Privacy issues can be avoided by discussions and agreements before the session.

For busy primary care physicians, the use of specialists should be encouraged. Dr. Shirley doesn't have thirty minutes to discuss constipation; a gastroenterologist does. As we've already discussed, nurse practitioners and physician assistants can be helpful in this regard. The best offices use them as an indispensable resource to monitor, support, and advise those with multiple chronic problems. They have more time to spend with you than Shirley, and are almost always nicer.

In addition to the preparatory work, the doctor also has recourse to a repertoire of metaphors that illuminate rather than obfuscate. Patients who are confused require more time. Explanations need not be longwinded, statistically laden, arcane treatises from the Halls of Medicine. While a doctor is listing an endless stream of pros and cons for every possible action, you're doing your own calculations, figuring out the shortest distance to the fire exit. After all, your kids are waiting.

Any competent and worthwhile doctor should have at her disposal a repertoire of metaphors that allude to daily scenarios, popular culture, and touchstones that patients "get." These have the greatest impact and cover the most salient information in the least amount of time.

The Mysterious Case of Dr. Seymour Dolittle: If Seymour had taken a modicum of time to explain things carefully the first time, he would not be facing the schedule-busting blizzard of questions that come from a frustrated, and now possibly angry patient. These last-minute hand-on-doorknob questions are usually answered in a rushed and impatient fashion, which leads to even more and angrier questions. A better communicator easily anticipates your questions and addresses your concerns in the body of the encounter. This often avoids the needless repetition of information that progressively degrades with each retelling. Don't value the doctor who fields your questions as he leaves; value the doctor who anticipates them on the way in.

This is all very nice, but this book isn't for doctors. So, in light of this fact, let's help make your visit shorter and better.

Tell him:

- "Hey doc, can you skip the biomedical stuff?"
- "Can you give me an everyday example of what you are saying?"
- "Can you clarify or simplify things for me? I am no Ph.D."
- "Give me a few minutes for my monolog now. It will spare lots of time later."
- "Here is what I want to go over today. These are the questions I have for today's visit."
- "Sorry, I'm going to interrupt you here; I want to continue on with my history for a moment."
- "I don't need an exhaustive list of pros and cons. Hit the highlights; I will remember the important stuff better that way."
- "Perhaps there is a hospital seminar that you might direct me to."
- "Please refer me to a gastroenterologist, I have a lot of questions about my heartburn and constipation."
- "I have a lot of questions, perhaps my next visit can be with the nurse practitioner."
- "Before we get further, do you have any DVDs, videos, or brochures on cholesterol therapy? If I have any questions I'll ask them at the next visit."

Studies have revealed that a visit of sixteen minutes, but not less than ten, will suffice on most occasions. Empowered patients are busy people. Many are busier than their doctors. They are happy to be back in their cars seeing the best view of the office—the one in the car's rearview mirror. Sometimes it is you who must set the agenda, change the atmosphere, and be courageous enough to interrupt if necessary. Your doctor is smart, but may be as emotionally awkward as a gangly teen at the prom. Help him out a bit by leading the discussion and directing its flow when things are going astray, away from your agenda.

Tic-Doc, Tic-Doc. The clock's tick should matter to your doc. It should matter to you. Doctors who make better use of their time will allow you to make better use of yours. State your agenda and move it along in the direction that you determine is best. That way, you'll be out more quickly and you'll be better informed.

Unvoiced Concerns and Agendas

How will anything get accomplished when 54 percent of doctors could not determine why their patients appeared for consultation?[11]

How can patients get what they want and what they need when one-third of patients and doctors actually disagreed over the reasons that the appointments were requested?[12] It goes without saying then that, when in the office, much goes without saying. When patients don't say what they want, doctors don't ask. It doesn't stop practitioners from continuing to test and prescribe with predictably poor results.

Many studies based on post-consultation questionnaires completed by patients and doctors reveal what, by now, should come as no surprise. Two people can sit in a room and have the time to talk and to listen; they ostensibly share the same goals; and they possess all the descriptive and analytic tools they need. Nonetheless, each leaves the room with contrasting ideas about each other, the problems at hand, their solutions, and the quality of the encounter. How can the question "What brings you here today?" be so mysterious that its answer becomes equally elusive, and even contentious? The perceived lack of time is the first barrier to open communication. Unvoiced issues are the second.

Patients arrive at their doctors' offices with specific agendas: to discuss symptoms, ask questions, weigh alternatives for diagnostic interventions, review the results of tests previously performed, determine a plan of action if one is needed, or decline therapy if reassurance suffices. Many patients also have goals for the visit: to leave with a renewed prescription, a scheduled routine blood test or x-ray, a return-to-work note, or reassurance about their health.

So, why do your agendas go unrealized? Why do you leave with your goals unmet? Why do you leave the office with things you didn't ask for, don't want, and don't need? Why do you depart more confused than ever?

The mismatch between a patient's and a physician's interpretation of what the goals should be for an office visit leads to needless therapy and overlooks the issues that remain painfully unresolved. Some patients only want diagnosis, reassurance, and follow-up. Many instead get sedatives. Not every antidote comes in prescription form. An example from the literature will serve as the rationale for the recommendations that will follow.

A study in the *British Medical Journal* demonstrated that when patients filled out questionnaires regarding their goals before their appointments, only 4 out of 35 actually voiced them during their time with their doctor. As a result, the outcomes were often poor and characterized by major misunderstandings. Most of the patients had several items on their written agenda, but the questions they actually asked were neutral, logistical, and biomedical in nature. The unvoiced needs were the more personal requirements.[13]

In post-visit surveys, it is the chronic and less intense symptoms that give rise to the most disappointments and disagreements between you and the doctor. You don't talk about them despite their importance to you; and doctors fail to recognize their importance or ask questions because they're old news. In 2011, the military's policy of "Don't Ask, Don't Tell" is dead. In the office it's alive and well. Chronic + nagging = unimportant, in everyone's office math.

Set your agenda. A brief personal note should be prepared for each visit. Inform the receptionist that you want it attached to your chart, so that it is available at the interview during the appointment. The note can be organized around four topics:

1) Your priorities: the expectations and goals you have established for this visit—advice, reassurance, diagnostics, a checkup, information, referral, prescription, a sick note, or a letter to an insurer. Those things you don't expect or want should also be included. That way, there will be no disagreements on priorities or mismatched expectations.
2) Embarrassing topics: folks find it difficult to talk about so many things they perceive as embarrassing. If you write them down you won't stutter, blush, or mumble "Never mind," when facing your doctor.
3) Symptoms: what's new, what's not. Remember that the chronic and annoying problems are the first to slip silently under your doctor's radar.
4) Concerns: how the problems you are presenting with affect job, family, and function.

Mention your theories of causality, as well as any potential diagnoses. List the remedies you've tried and the Internet searches you've used. This is not the venue for soul-searching soliloquies or existential quandaries. This note should be a short, bullet-point exercise. Get your goals and feelings out there in the open. No one seems likely to ask if you don't tell. This précis avoids the "by the way" questions that bedevil doctors as they head out the door. It's been demonstrated that these last-minute issues are the most important ones that you arrive with, but the last ones you address. They will inevitably be treated hastily, if not hostilely.

A note doesn't make you a nudge. It does your doctor the favor of being able to live up to your expectations, rather than having to divine them.

Be yourself. Don't attempt to be a perfect patient. I have always been skeptical, even distrustful, of the self-identified "model patient." Present yourself in the light you wish to be seen, not what you think your doctor expects to see. Bring her into your world. Negotiate with her if she feels that a disease-centered discussion is more important than your concerns about more personal issues. You won't be a difficult patient—just a different one.

Language Barriers

A message to you from Dr. L1, NI, HI (that's me!):
Abbreviations:

EP . . . English proficient
LEP . . . limited English proficiency
NES . . . non-English speaking
L1 . . . English as first language
L2 . . . English as second language
I . . . inflected (accent)
NI . . . uninflected
HS . . . heritage speaker—native-born but speaks another language at home
HI . . . hearing impaired
IMG . . . international medical graduate
TOEFL . . . Test of English as a Foreign Language

Question: What was accomplished when the Hmong-speaking patient went to the Pakistani doctor in Los Angeles? Answer: Nothing.

We have demonstrated that even under optimal conditions the state of doctor/patient communications can be dismal. This is one of the primary reasons that you are dissatisfied with your care. But when you and your doctor can't understand each other due to language barriers you may not even know that you should be dissatisfied. Correcting miscommunications, exchanging ideas, achieving a mutual understanding, and agreeing on shared goals are only possible when there is a common language. But when either party in a medical communion can't fully understand the other, the quality of care inevitably suffers.

Remarkably many medical encounters become exercises in wild gesticulations, pantomime, and the use of medical pidgin. Even more remarkable are the flaws in the use of the only fallback position possible—the use of medical interpreters.

What does the Hmong/Pakistani medical debacle mean to you? Does it even concern you?

Why yes . . . yes it does! Forty seven million people in the United States use a language other than English at home. This represents 18 percent of our population. Fifty-five percent of them state that they speak English "very well." This is certainly an artificially high number, borne from the fact that nonnative speakers overestimate their English skills, as well as the broader truth that everyone overestimates their every ability. Even if it were accurate, speaking English "very well" doesn't confer fluency, much less the skills needed for medical English. Allowing for the unlikely assumption that speaking very well is the equivalent to fluency, then 22 million people in the United States (8.4 percent of the population) have limited English proficiency (LEP).

Medical communication skills are already on life support. We pull the plug when adding the imperfect ability to be understood when talking or to understand while listening.

To some readers the issue of limited English proficiency may seem a distant concern, but it can be problematic for your parents and family. You may think you're immune until you meet your L2, I, HI, IMG MD. As we've noted, the TOEFL bar is set high, allowing the majority of applicants to pass under it on the road to licensure in the United States.

Even when there is proficiency, or fluency, accents and dialects remain. Accents can be beguiling but are more often bewildering. Inflections, word preferences, variations in pitch and tone, different emphases, and syntactical preferences make their comprehension no sure thing. It takes only one to tango when either doctor or patient has limited English proficiency, or a thick accent. The medical environment is now a minefield of potential errors waiting to detonate if a diphthong goes wrong. And finally the unhappy news in 2010 from the *Journal of Experimental Social Psychology*: If your doctor has an accent you are less likely to believe what he says. In medical transactions it is an understatement when the authors conclude, "Such reduction of credibility may have an insidious impact on millions of people who routinely communicate in a language which is not their native tongue."[14]

Even when doctors and patients are native English speakers, dialects can interfere. British, Irish, and American regional dialects are often hard to understand. Vocabulary, grammar, pronunciation, patois, and prosody are all influenced by differences in dialect, and they can affect your communication.

One-quarter of practicing physicians in the United States are IMGs. Most are L2 I, many are L2 I/LEP.

Tens of millions of doctor visits each year present language barriers to patients, their doctors, and often both. So then, for the two or three of you out there who are native speakers, and who have family who are native speakers, and who also have only native-speaking doctors—it's all good.

Posit: There are six types of English speakers: L1/NI; L1/I; L2/EP/I; L2/LEP/I; NES; HS. Any of these six may be a doctor or a doctor's patient. If we placed them on a grid we would see thirty-six potential language interactions. (We are omitting auditory deficiencies but are aware of their frequency.)

In this matrix, interpreters are needed for 20 out of 36 of all potential medical encounters. (Any conversation between two people, one of whom is a NES, or one in which a single party has LEP requires an interpreter.) Deficient communication occurs in 5 out of 36 such encounters.[15] Adequate communication occurs in only 11 out of 36 of these possible conversations.[16] So when we match up 47 million imperfect English speakers with 210,000 doctors who, at the very least, have an accent, we demonstrate that perfect pairings are far from inevitable. As each of us wanders through the medical system, seeing up to a dozen different doctors a year, it is likely that we have had a communication problem based solely on language, accent, or audition, alone or in combination.

Each reader has at one point been confronted with the "Huh?" issue. What about your doctors, who say to themselves when they can't understand you, "Qu'at-il dit?" "Hvad sagde han?" "Ki sa li te di?"

Solutions

Your doctor may need an interpreter when speaking with you and your family. For that matter, so may you when speaking with your doctor if she has an impenetrable accent. Neither scenario is likely to result in an interpreted session. And even if you get an interpreter, their results are often un-interpretable. First, only 6 percent of encounters that require a medical interpreter get one. Second, even when available, most of these services usually provide a poor simulacrum of a regular conversation, let alone a nuanced medical one. When the stakes are mortal, mistakes will be too.

Medical interpreters are generally acknowledged as unaffordable, or logistically unavailable. Sadly and surprisingly, all the interpretation techniques in common use today are unacceptable. Each technique that uses a language intermediary causes problems.

Even when interpreters are available your problems are not over.

A 2008 article in *CHEST* magazine reported on a study in which intensive care patients needing interpreters were audiotaped. Fifty-five percent of the exchanges had errors; more than three-quarters of those errors were judged to have potentially clinically significant consequences.[17]

Many people confuse translators with interpreters. Translators transform one language to another from written text. They can take breaks, research a phrase, or check a cultural nuance, and their work can be checked against the original. Interpreters, on the other hand, work with people in real time and at conversational speed. They must, of necessity, leave much to their own interpretation. There's often no time for a question, let alone a break, nuance, research, or rest. Medical students and postgraduate physicians receive virtually no guidelines or education on supervising an interpreted interview.

The worst technique for interpretation is using the doctor-interpreter.

Doctors, always assured, ever self-confident, and eminently self-satisfied, often allow these character traits to spill over into corners of their non-medical lives. These intrepid individuals often use high school skills, Berlitz courses taken for their trip to Spain, long-forgotten college courses, or "medical" pidgin. They do so to no one's benefit. Some can ask the questions in the patients' language without difficulty. The only problem is they don't understand the answers as they arrive at the doctor's tortured cortex in a blazing flurry of alien syllables, consonants, and syntax. If you or a family member is being interviewed in an ad hoc, invented language, slip out while the doctor is in a self-adulatory reverie.

Ad hoc proximate consecutive interpretations are almost as bad.

ad hoc: For a special purpose at hand;

proximate: Interpreter in the room with doctor and patient;

consecutive: The interpreter listens and speaks only after the primary speaker finishes.

This technique makes up the vast majority of the exchanges between a doctor and a patient of LEP. Each of the three adjectives that characterize this method reveals the fatal flaws of this technique.

1) **ad hoc:** Really means the unanticipated, make-do solutions. It enlists the help of strangers off the street, bystanders in corridors, and patients in the next bed or an adjoining waiting room.
2) **proximate:** *Anyone* in the room other than doctor and patient stunts the conversation.
3) **consecutive:** In medical consecutive communications, one participant often offers too much data for the listener to take in, remember, and then pass on accurately. These efforts are as far from conversation or communication as chalk is from chocolate.

The only presumed benefit for proximate consecutive medical interpretation is the presence of a trained medical interpreter. You may presume the benefit but should not assume it. The high error rates that occur with this technique lead to more than an apologetic "my bad." They can lead to mistakes, poor outcomes, and deaths. Errors in omission, addition, editorialization, substitution, and role changes (when the interpreter offers medical advice) have been documented to contaminate over 50 percent of these exchanges. Their accuracy is akin to a coin toss: heads, your doctor gets it; tails, you're dead.

Errors have been verified in countless studies using spontaneous, scripted, and staged audio- and videotaped interviews. Their content has been deconstructed and analyzed word-by-word. Whether the interviews are between doctor and patient, doctor and family, or doctor and standard patient, the results are chilling. The use of bilingual nursing staff would seem to provide a better chance for accuracy. Surprisingly, nursing errors occurred in one-third of conversations that mediated uncomplicated issues and in two-thirds of complicated ones.

When you find yourself in a medical situation where expert consecutive off-site interpretation is called for, remember Language Line (languageline .com). This is its bailiwick. It's clearly superior to the techniques mentioned above but still unknown to most health-care practitioners. It's not likely you would get this service in states that do not compensate doctors and hospitals for it. Hospitals are financially strapped. This is particularly true in metropolitan areas where the demand for such services is the most acute, and the diseases the most serious. Only 46 percent of emergency departments nationwide currently use *any* interpreters for patients with limited English proficiency. In 2011 the Joint Commission implemented a one-year pilot program. Its goal is to initiate a protocol ensuring recognition of hospitalized patients' communication needs.

What to Do: Avoid the need for interpreters. Find a doctor for you or yours who is a native speaker of your language. Fallback positions: Heritage speakers and "fluent" nonnative speakers. The errors inherent in tête-a-têtes mediated by a medical interpreter are so frequent and potentially harmful it may even be worth a trip to a nearby city to find a doctor who can speak with you, one-on-one. Consult your local or state medical society. Google "medical doctor fluent in _____ in zip code _____." Seek advice from family and friends, and church, hospital, and community groups.

Without a medical interpreter you are lost; with a medical interpreter you are put at risk. In neither case are you benefiting from your doctor's intelligence. *This is the unique scenario where you can prioritize a clinician's communication skills over the indicators of intellectual ones.* Otherwise, at worst, you'll be dealing with a passerby randomly grabbed off a corridor. At best, you get a medical interpreter of unknown skills. A doctor who is a cultural and linguistic partner relieves you from the types of errors that characteristically occur when she is neither.

Every doctor needs to be judged on a continuous basis. Use your own good instincts. Employ techniques found in this and previous sections. Find and use medical shibboleths, and research your own online sources. This helps assure the quality of your doctor. It's a brain down the drain if a gifted genius shares none of your worldviews, traditions, and idioms. These are the touchstones of a good patient and doctor relationship.

Your family members and friends are not ideal choices for interpreters, but it's any port in a storm when your options are contracting. Be sure to discuss the drawbacks of interpretation with the family member or friend who must perform this duty. Do you really want your son to hear about your sexual or urinary complaint? Is it a good idea for your brother-in-law to hear about the survival rate for your cancer? Will your daughter try to spin bad news into good news? Will you neighbor be happy to hear about your psychiatric symptoms? If you have taken every precaution, these mistakes can, through understanding, agreement, and medical necessity, in all likelihood be avoided.

Ask if your doctor will see you on an outpatient basis at the hospital's clinic, where interpretation services are more likely to be in place and the attendant fees are incurred by the hospital. You and your clinician will like this; the hospital will not. *Never* allow strangers off the street, other patients, or housekeeping staff to be recruited to perform these highly specialized and sensitive tasks. These folks might as well diagnose and prescribe for you themselves. It reflects poorly on your doctor if she is willing to use these types of language services in your behalf—it's a deal breaker!

If you must use an interpreter, beware—if it takes 30 to 60 seconds for the doctor to ask his question but 5 to 10 seconds to relay it (or vice versa), something is wrong. If the interpreter's output is a lot longer than the input given to her, beware of editorialization, substitutions, and role changes—when the interpreter fancies herself the doctor.

Recommended phrases patients and accompanying family should expect to hear from their doctor or, if necessary, use themselves during an interpreted session include:

- "I want to introduce you to the medical interpreter. We are using an interpreter because the topics we are discussing are important, and we need to communicate clearly with one another."
- "I depend on you not only to interpret the words but also to be aware of the context for the conversation."
- "If the patient or I say something you don't know how to interpret, please let me know."
- "Do you have any concerns about the family's understanding?"
- "Tell us if we need to slow down."
- "Tell us if you need a break."
- "Tell me or the patients only what is said by us. Do not add, subtract, or editorialize."

When I was young, foolish, and ignorant, I refused to pay a huge interpretation fee that resulted from my first encounter with an NES patient. Within a few weeks I was inundated with a blizzard of federal threats, injunctions, admonitions, and paperwork. Recognizing that I was in the Belly of the Beast, I acted swiftly and firmly. I immediately became a willing, servile toady to the bureaucrat in charge and promised to be a good boy for the rest of my life. I consulted our lawyer and adopted an office policy that minimized our costs as efficiently as possible.

Omigod, I Need an Interpreter!

What happens *when you need a third party interpreter*? Some doctors just talk too fast, or cover their mouths, or turn away; and some suffer speech impediments. Combinations of lalling and lisping, stuttering and stammering, monotones and mumbling, dysarthria and dysprosody will end with the same results, otherwise produced by oceans and far-flung borders. While dodging the salivary explosion of the sibilant plosives or girding your ears from aggressive gutturals, you might miss a lot of important information.

One day, I met a patient who'd been referred to our office. She had no idea why she was there. When I asked her how that could have happened, she told me that she'd had a hard time understanding her doctor. "Even when he introduced himself," she said, "it sounded like he was clearing his throat."

It's not your job to be your doctor's speech therapist. If your doctor won't go to an ESL school (English as a second language) for accent reduction, must you go to an EFL school for accent recognition?

"Dr. Pepper, so misunderstood," is no longer just a soda's commercial slogan; now it's your medical problem. It's not easy to tell your doctor you can't understand her. But you better find a way to do it, or else find a new doctor you do understand. It's acceptable to use face-saving excuses such as "I'm hard of hearing," or to blame the room's acoustics.

Subterfuge that is used to spare the doctor's feelings, or more likely to prevent you from being tagged as a racist xenophobe, won't work anyway. People quickly revert to their normal and unconscious cadences and inflections. Here's what you say when all else fails: "Doctor, I value your expertise and appreciate your efforts. I just don't understand everything you say. I want to be your patient but you're going to have to speak . . ." slower, more clearly, louder, softer, facing me, standing closer, standing farther away . . . in whatever combination is appropriate.

You are going to have to tell her however many times you must that "I still don't get it," or ask her, "Can you write that word (phrase) down?" Being gentle, truthful, and tactful does your doctor a favor, and it keeps you as his patient. Many doctors don't know how thick their inflections are because no one has ever told them. Embarrassment and reluctance to interrupt an authority figure reciting his spiel stop patients cold in their tracks.

Writing things down helps but you can't pass pieces of paper back and forth through the entire exchange—a word or two at most, perhaps. This doctor will need, and you will require, a large repository of personalized instructions that are specific to frequently encountered medical conditions, testing, and therapies unique to his practice.

Has it ever happened that you've taken an overseas trip and searched in vain for a book written in English? Did you never think to go to the foreign language section? That's right. To a nonnative doctor, you're the foreigner with the accent! Let's agree that when there is a language barrier, the problems are mutual.

"If I do my part you will do yours—right?" Do what public speakers are trained to do from a podium. Your exchange doesn't have to be a conversation. Speak in a cadence that seems unnaturally slow—it won't be perceived that way. Raise your voice just a bit. Complement what you say with your body language and paralinguistics. Don't cover your mouth.

Do for your doctor what you wish he would do for you. That's the Golden Rule! Don't ask what your doctor can do for you, ask what you can do for your doctor. That also sounds familiar. These relationships are two-way thoroughfares on bad roads without dividers. Valued doctors are worth a few potholes along the way.

The three things to do if your doctor has limited English proficiency: Find a new doctor, find a new doctor, find a new doctor.

Cultural Divergence

Choose Jews? Chinese, please? A Hindu for you? Is Islamic the tonic? Seek a Sikh? Are WASPs tops? Our new global economics do not necessarily suggest intertwined global philosophies. *Terroir*, a French word with no real English equivalent, points to the qualities of a place: the soil, climate, and exposure to the sun typically used to describe the character of regional wines. There's a lot to learn from it in a more general sense. People, too, are a product of the unique settings of the societies in which they were raised. When thinking about our colleagues from different cultures there is no need for terror when approaching medical care simply because it is delivered by the products of different cultures' terroirs. Many of our advances occur as a result of new perspectives and approaches coming out of countries with rapidly expanding economies and burgeoning middle classes. In these societies, less is taken for granted and the status quo is a moving target. The occasionally maligned Sapir-Whorf hypothesis suggests that different languages uniquely mold and influence their speakers' thoughts. I think it's true. And for doctors, it's largely to your benefit.

In the end, it's not the "who they are," it's the "how they act." How does a doctor talk, listen, and practice; and how do you respond? Choose wisely, carefully, and critically using a consumer's gimlet eye and ear. Find the best doctor using the criteria I've suggested. You may occasionally struggle with a doctor's inflections, but rarely their intentions.

As an aside, my doctor's not Jewish, nor is my accountant, financial advisor, real estate agent, lawyer, or editor. This is a statistical anomaly worthy of its own publication. So much for stereotypes, however shocking these facts were to my parents.

What does it all mean? Aside from the relationship between you and your doctor, one characterized by shared medical goals, there need not be an exact cultural affinity.

Intelligence, Health Literacy, and Numeracy

Not even the brightest clinician can compensate for a patient's cognitive deficiencies. There have to be at least two smart people in the room. This is the fourth, and last, important barrier to proper communication. Half of any population isn't as bright as the other half.

The need for an ever-present room coach or hospital chaperone has been a leitmotif through these chapters. Patients who are alone with their doctors, or isolated in a hospital room, are in environments that are dangerous to their health. This is particularly true for the very young, the very old, those with multiple comorbidities, those with diseases in cognition, those who are sedated, postoperative, or with altered sensoria, and those who have limited English proficiency. We can add to this list those who are somewhat less incandescent than the rest.

Communication, spoken or written, requires understanding. It's a prerequisite for seeking and obtaining appropriate care, utilizing preventive techniques, complying with recommendations, avoiding error through its recognition, and self-managing. Literacy, health literacy, and numeracy are needed in every medical encounter and when sorting through the shameful medical insurance maze that is placed in your path. You need these skills when you care for your children, and, increasingly, your parents. The average American reads at a middle school level. Most medical information, whether written in newspapers and magazines or spoken in the office, is performed at a college level. A federal study in 2010 demonstrated that today's health information is presented in a way that is beyond most Americans. Almost 9 out of 10 adults have difficulty using the health information that is routinely found in our health-care facilities, retail outlets, media, and communities.[18] The frequency of overeducated but under-motivated doctors amongst us often results in conversations laden with arcana, cant, and statistical mumbo-jumbo. These are no substitutes for patient-centered conversations. Anything less will not do.

The 2003 National Assessment of Adult Literacy (NAAL) measured the skills needed to read and understand health-related information used in our daily lives. The Test of Functional Health Literacy in Adults (TOFHLA) is a twenty-two-minute examination that stratifies health literacy. The majority of those studied, 53 percent, had intermediate health literacy, 22 percent had basic literacy, and 14 percent had below basic skills. The smallest segment was the 12 percent of adults who are proficient in health literacy. Source material for those with basic and poor health literacy included television, radio, friends, and coworkers. Almost half of the 30 percent of adults who never finished high school have health skills that are below basic. Those over age sixty-five who have the most need for medical care have the least literacy in it.

Poor numeracy is epidemic. Math anxiety and innumeracy affects the literate and even the literary. You'd never announce in the midst of company, "Hey, guess what, I'm illiterate." You would, however, have no similar hesitation saying "I'm no good at all in math. I can't even balance my checkbook." In fact, being highly numerate is a first-class ticket to geekdom and social ostracism and compartmentalization.

"Fat diabetic needs help in Aisle 10": Obese, diabetic hypertensives must understand calories and carbohydrate counts per serving. Glucose, vitamins, and salt are written as percentages of daily requirements and must be understood for disease control. Yet portion sizes expressed in ounces or in cups are beyond many.

Numeracy is required for dosing adjustments and understanding clinical goals that are numerically expressed. The ability to understand doctors requires basic skills in fractions, percentages, and probabilistic information. Risk stratification and understanding the likelihood of unlikely events is the stock-in-trade of many medical conversations.

Two Cases in Point: "If we treat your cancer your chance of dying from it will be 50 percent less than if we don't." "Wow! That sounds great. Where do I sign?"

But, if the five-year survival rate for your cancer is 95% untreated, and survival is increased 50%, the five-year survival will actually be 97.5%. Not quite the result you were anticipating, was it? Why are you disappointed? Because 50% carries with it the idea that something is being halved. This, the *relative* risk reduction of death of 50%, offers only an *absolute* risk reduction of death of 2.7%. When the risks of therapy, including death, expense, inconvenience, and forced alteration in lifestyle are taken into account, the benefits of treatment become less certain. Now the response becomes, "Let me think about it," not "Let's go for it."

Almost everywhere in medicine, risk reduction is expressed in relative—not absolute—terms. You now know the difference. Most never will; almost none are ever told.

The second case in point was a woman I met while I was in medical school. She had the misfortune of being diagnosed with breast cancer and was given a five-year survival rate of 30%. Three months later she was diagnosed with advanced colon cancer. This carried a five-year survival rate of 20%. When I asked her how she was doing in light of this, she was in good spirits. "With the breast cancer and now the colon cancer I have a 50% five-year survival," she informed me. This neoplastic Anschluss led her to add her survival rates, coming up with good news, rather than bad.

Numbers count. Do the math (http://www.medpagetoday.com/Medpage-Guide-to-Biostatistics.pdf provides a valuable primer on medical biostatistics). Also see the bibliography for *Know Your Chances, Understanding Health Statistics,* by health numeracy gurus Woloshin, Schwartz, and Welch. See, too, the list of best sites for other online tutorials.

The three questions that follow comprise an adapted Woloshin Schwartz numeracy test that was given to a sample of medical students.[19] 1) Imagine that we flip a coin 1,000 times. What is your best guess about how many times the coin would come up heads? 2) In the lottery, the chance of winning a prize is 1 percent. What is your best guess about how many people would win a prize if 1,000 people each buy a single ticket to the lottery? 3) In the publishing sweepstakes, the chance of winning a car is 1 in 1,000. What percentage of tickets to the publishing sweepstakes win a car?

Ninety-four percent of the medical students thought that they were good with numbers. Only 77 percent answered all three numeracy questions correctly. Eighteen percent answered two questions correctly, and 5 percent answered one or no questions correctly. From a sample of healthy female veterans,[20] 16 percent answered all three questions correctly. Twenty-six percent got two right, while 28 percent were able to answer only one. Thirty percent could not correctly answer any question. Full disclosure: I missed one, and so did my son, Efrem. (I promised to use his name in this book though I doubt he'll appreciate its context.) Answers: 500, 10, and 0.1%, respectively.

Low cognition and lapses in health literacy and numeracy are predictive of increased rates of death and debility. Being less than average in "medical intelligence" carries a price—in longevity. In a studied population, 40 percent of individuals with inadequate health literacy died during the follow-up period; 28 percent with marginal health literacy died; and only 19 percent with adequate health literacy joined the Invisible Choir. Those with dim lights or those getting their health information solely by the television's dim lights did not fare well.[21] Television viewing is bad for your health for a lot of reasons. In 2011 it was shown that watching more than two hours a day more than doubled the risk of cardiovascular events over the four year study.[22]

If your dad can't pass a TOFHLA and his doctor barely made it through his TOEFL, disaster will follow. It's a case of a low TOFHLA + low TOEFLs = TOE TAGS. Your input becomes mandatory. Ideally, it should be routine to accompany every patient who visits any doctor and, if they are hospitalized, to be their designated sitters or advocates. Not every medical encounter may need a chaperone, but all medical encounters will be improved by them. It's always better to proceed proactively than to rue, retroactively.

It's not your job to administer a TOFHLA or IQ test to your friends and relatives. It *is* your job to know when to accompany them or to seek help for yourself when you feel you need it.

Several years ago, in a medical malpractice case, I served as a defense expert for a doctor who had been accused of negligence. The defendant-physician, a gastroenterologist, was called in by a primary care doctor to comment on an eighty-five-year-old man's abdominal pain. The gastroenterologist ordered a CT scan to learn more about his patient's discomfort. The plaintiff's lawyer argued that the doctor ignored his patient's history of severe kidney disease by sending him for an IV-enhanced CT scan. Patients with poor kidney function should not get CT exams with intravenous dye. The dye predictably produces further renal failure. For this man the dye did what dye does; it induced kidney failure and, not long after that, his death. The plaintiff's lawyer's principal obstacle was that the patient never provided the doctor with his full medical history, including the fact of his kidney disease. He even denied having kidney disease when asked by the consulting gastroenterologist during his ill-fated visit.

This eighty-five-year-old man did not have dementia. What he did have was a wife, children, and adult grandchildren. Despite this, all alone, he wandered into the storm. The family was all aware of his history. The patient himself was documented to be aware of his kidney problem. After each visit to his primary physician the doctor's nurse called him at home. She documented in his chart that he understood his problems, including the kidney disease. Over the years his awareness of this problem was noted dozens of times in his medical chart. So why hadn't the now-deceased gentleman offered the accurate medical history he was acknowledged to be aware of?

Maybe being "aware" is not being knowledgeable. Maybe the doctor used the phrase "renal disease" or "urinary problem" instead of kidney disease. Maybe the patient felt he had a "condition" or "problem," rather than a disease. Maybe he incorrectly felt it was irrelevant to his abdominal problem. Maybe this, maybe that. Either by the force of cognitive or literacy problems, he was now "Toit indeed and toit in drerd." (This is Yinglish—a Yiddish-English amalgam—and is translated, "dead indeed and dead in the ground.")

The doctor was doubly innocent. It was the radiologist's duty to determine this man's risk for IV dye infusion. It was the radiologist's responsibility to refuse to perform any test if he felt the risk was excessive. It was his job to obtain a history of renal disease. Despite these extenuating circumstances the verdict was guilty. My guy should have gotten the records from the primary care doctor. It is an unwise physician who trusts his patients' stories.

If this nice family had had any one of its members accompany the patient to the defendant doctor and the radiologist he would not have died this way. (When I'm eighty-five, I'm not going to the movies alone!) This man did not die from renal failure; he became collaterally damaged as a result of the cognitive defect of forgetfulness, health literacy issues, and the family's false assumption that the doctors would be cognizant of all the pertinent information.

So, how do you know when to go? C'mon, you know! Assume that you should always accompany your family member. Remember, ideally, no one should go alone into the bad neighborhoods in our medical world. The medical system often plays with patients as cats do with captive mice. Sorry, it's true. It's not cruel (neither is the cat), it's just the way it is. If, however, a patient is going to be questioned by a doctor, there are scenarios in which their answers are going to be frequently wrong as a result of age, multiple chronic diseases, a lifetime in front of the television, avoidance of reading materials whether through illiteracy or the more common aliteracy (can read, but won't), living alone, the kind of stoicism that says, "I'm fine," and those enfeebled and made meeker by age. I also worry about people who no longer get jokes or understand simple wordplay. If Mom and Pop carry notebooks to write down instructions, can't balance checkbooks or make change, or turn to each other when either must answer a question, they will need a hand. Finally, it may be hard for you to acknowledge it, and impossible for you to impart it, but some people you love just aren't that bright or are, in fact, recognizably and dangerously obtuse. Being dim means they won't likely know it. Anyone brighter than they are will. Paid or unpaid, friend or family, neighbor or parishioner, private or state agent, there must always be someone for everyone. There *is* always someone for everyone. Everyone needing it should be in a "witless protection program."

Your Role: Sending those least able to deal with the system is not the same thing as human sacrifice—sometimes it just looks that way. The presence of a third party in the room prevents a loved one from becoming a statistic. Everyone is put on notice by your presence. Active participation by a third party prevents the manipulation of a patient who is unable to understand what is being communicated.

No, the "I'm with Stupid" T-shirt won't work. It is best, whenever possible, that patients speak for themselves. Prepping them for the visit is wise. Patients can readily admit to their weaknesses without confessing to them.

Team up with the patient. "Doc, neither of us is an Einstein." "I'm not sure we understand that, doctor." "Neither of us is much on numbers." "Sorry, but we don't understand a word of what you are saying. You really have to make this clear."

Your subsequent questions and comments will show that you are a force to be reckoned with without hurting the feelings of those in your charge. Make sure that the visit doesn't end without a request for a summary of its content. The patient should be able to repeat it back, and if he can't, go over the information again.

Sometimes you must be the "go-to" party.

"My mom says it is okay for you to call me instead of her with results and information. Here's my cell number. If you give me the telephone number you use to call patients, I will put it on my caller ID and will always answer right away. I won't waste your time playing phone tag, and I won't use the number for any other purposes." (Good luck on that one, but give five stars to the doctor who agrees.)

So, there's plenty of time, you've prepared carefully and you have voiced all your concerns. There is no need for an interpreter and you are proficient in health literacy. You can take charge of the agenda and speak frankly with any doctor. It's all going to be fine . . . right? Well, maybe.

Some clinicians simply won't talk to you, however little time it requires. They do not care a whit about your priorities. They will not value your medical insights and opinions. They will, in fact, summarily dismiss them. Despite what you can bring to the table by preparing for the visit and the synergy possible during it, this doctor never had the intention of speaking with you. These people are politely referred to as miserable wretches and you know perfectly well that they are not rare. Maybe this Sphinx is pleasant and engaging at home. At parties, maybe he'll be the one who puts the lamp shade on his head to resulting appreciative hilarity. Perhaps when this Doctor Jekyll gets to his office he transforms into the evil Edward Hyde—a mysterious case indeed.

Just as likely, he is a dour misanthrope despite his material and social standing. Perhaps he is a mildly sociopathic, Asperger-like product of his genes, brains, training, and entitlement. Maybe he's just a jerk. Who cares! Dump him.

9

Empathy

- Your doctor: Smarter than Bill Gates, chattier than Oprah, but as cold as Darth Vader.
- The definition and origins of medical empathy: Why your doctor *shouldn't* feel your pain.
- Why compassion is in short supply, where it went, and how to get it back.
- Fake empathy: When your doctor cares enough to send the *second-best*.
- The value of schmoozing your doctors: Becoming your doctor's behavioral therapist.
- *Your* use of fake empathy: Paraphrasing, mimicry, and charm to enhance mutual identification.

Your doctor is as smart as a whip, as communicative as cable news, but cold as a block of ice. Two out of three! Not bad, right? Well, no. Empathy is the last feature that completes the Trinity of Traits all patients should expect from their care. As with communication, empathy is necessary but not sufficient in itself. The hand-holding, handkerchief-wielding, hand-wringing pinhead will not advance your agenda.

You want your doctor to care about you, while caring for you. This establishes trust, which is perhaps the most valued sentiment in effective doctor-patient relationships. You are correct in assuming that a doctor should acknowledge your emotional concerns. And if he does this, it will enhance the care you receive, your compliance with medical orders, and your long-term welfare. Just because medical therapy is determined to be unnecessary or deemed futile doesn't mean you have no further needs. You will not be abandoned by a doctor with whom there exists reciprocity of feelings. A working alliance will remain in place that supports and validates you in the event of non-medical issues that still leave you symptomatic.

What is empathy? Why does it seem in such short supply? How do you recognize it? How do you get it?

There are as many definitions of empathy as there are researchers who study it and scholarly articles that describe it. The three qualities of understanding that are used when approaching others in times of difficulty or distress are pity, sympathy, and empathy. The definitions of these words are demonstrably confused when each is cited as a synonym for the other and each is used in the dictionary's definition for the other.

Perhaps we can clear up any confusion, for our purposes, by making note of the preposition that often follows each when used in speech and writing: Pity *on*, sympathy *for*, and empathy *with*.

Pity separates the observer from the sufferer. No one wants to be pitiable. It is an emotion that is placed *on* its victims. It can be considered, at worst, a type of contempt. It identifies its target as pathetic. At best it is an understanding of another person based on the observation that "there but for the Grace of God go I."

Sympathy *for* a sufferer suggests an association but not an identification with the stricken party. You have observed someone else's distress, and you demonstrate sorrow or concern for that person. This is a shared experience but not a mutual one. There is no resonance, a key concept when differentiating sympathy from empathy. Resonance in physics refers to the property of an object that, vibrating vigorously, produces a similar but less intense vibration in other related proximate objects. The expression of sympathy does not produce an emotional resonance in the observer that shares what is experienced by the sufferer. It finds its best example in the act of consolation, when an uninvolved party shows support for someone in mourning or distress.

Empathy *with* is a quality that is shared. It has the subtle connotation of an exchange that is made after a cognitive and emotionally based evaluation is completed. Empathy doesn't simply understand another's emotions. It *shares* the feelings, if not their intensity. Sympathy understands others' emotions; empathy resonates with them. It's not the experience of "being in someone else's shoes," as is commonly cited. It is more usefully thought of as "being in someone else's head." It's an understanding of someone else's situation, combined with an emotional arousal that is brought about by an identification with them. It is a cognitively advanced, yet an affectively primitive, response.

We prize those things that are in short supply. Empathy now joins brains and communication skills as traits you must seek out in a doctor rather than expect as a matter of course. Study after study in the medical literature bemoans the loss of what would seem a prerequisite for medical practice—an empathic response to your voiced and unvoiced concerns.

There is no pursuit more demanding of a doctor's empathy than oncology. What other field is more characterized by patients suffering illness and pain, who dread the possibility, and frequently the certainty, of death? What terrible emptiness must inhabit these patients' thoughts? What other field of medicine attracts those clinicians who are able, even desiring, to enter into discussions that demand understanding, validation, and support?

Despite this, three articles that were published in a span of less than three months, based on hundreds of audiotaped discussions between oncologists and their patients, suggest that an oncology office is a "compassion-free zone."[1, 2, 3] Hundreds of expressions of negative emotion, fears, worries, and existential concerns regarding morbidity and mortality were identified. In these studies the oncologists responded with empathy only 10 percent, 27 percent, and 35 percent of the time when there was an opportunity to do so. Rather than picking up on emotional cues, vague statements, and out-right repeated entreaties, oncologists dodged, diverted, or summarily ended the discussions without empathic acknowledgment. Even tasteless humor was employed as a distancing technique. This state of affairs was summed up in 2009: "Emotional support from physicians was most consistently associated with patient trust. Addressing patient emotions, however, remains an infrequently conducted task in oncology."[4]

These results are not unusual, nor are they limited to oncologists. In surgery and general medicine,[5] doctors missed opportunities to respond to patient clues 62 percent and 79 percent of the time, respectively. When ignored, some patients had to repeat their concerns two or three times. Some physicians denied patient emotional issues and others were cited for the use of inappropriate humor.

On the other hand, doctors don't need to "feel your pain." It's not helpful, possible, desirable, or honest to hope that they can or should. Over-identification with patients is not necessary, nor is it empathic. That said, physicians run from the opportunities to provide needed acknowledgment as if the emotions were contagious. A contextual cognitive appraisal and a show of appropriate emotional resonance is a minimum requirement, and sometimes all that is needed.

Empathy isn't gone—it's just hiding. Empathy is always present. We are all "empaths" from birth. It's our job to learn why you don't see it when you are with your doctors.

Why do you have a heartless cardiologist? The short answer is: he does have a heart—he just checked it at the hospital door.

To learn why, we return to a passage quoted in chapter 6, "Seventy-five percent of medical students become more cynical about academic life and the medical profession as they progress through medical school. Processes described as dehumanization and traumatic de-idealization characterize the cynical transformation of medical students."[6] Dehumanization and traumatic de-idealization? Why, it sounds like boot camp!

Medical school *is* like boot camp for the same reasons, and with the same goals. This article's title should not be "The Decline of Empathy . . ." but rather "The Modulation of Empathy." In the military de-idealization and dehumanization are directed toward the enemy. For doctors this process is directed toward you.

How do we hurt you—let us count the ways. People stricken by illness often experience sensations so lamentable and threats so dire that most people who witness it would, in shock, be paralyzed with horror. We, the doctors, see and react, but neither suffer, nor suffer hesitation. You may be writhing in the pain of multiple trauma, struggling for your next breath or bleeding uncontrollably, but if you attempt to clutch our hands or catch our gaze you will fail. Sorry, too busy.

Our knives cut, needles pierce, catheters invade, cauteries and lasers burn, and our medications poison. Complications inevitably require us to perform all these medical tortures again, fixing what went awry. The ubiquity of preventable error forces us—we who tried to help you—to now do far, far more to correct the suffering our poor judgment has left in its wake.

Every doctor has had the experience of confronting those patients they have damaged, often beyond repair. What allows us to continue in the face of a horror you now face? How do we look into your eyes when, so briefly before, you were denied entry into ours?

How do we deliver the news of the disease that will affect every subsequent day of your child's life in ways too horrible to contemplate, much less witness? We often inform you of the manner and timing of your death—and then attend you during it.

We see, and often don't register, the terror, medical indignities, and painful daily declines even your family cannot witness. When these duties fall to recent medical school graduates they shock by their novelty. By contrast, weathered veterans do not bend under the cumulative weight of the thousands of similar tragic scenarios they have witnessed over the years. Your pain is, after all, our stock-in-trade.

For doctors there *should* be no pain more easily experienced than yours. We are nonetheless reminded to employ models of practice that include "the Four Habits": (Invest in the Beginning, Elicit the Patient's Perspective, Demonstrate Empathy, Invest in the End); "the Four E's": (Engage, Empathize, Educate, and Enlist) model; and the "PEARLS" paradigm: (Partnership, Empathy, Apology, Respect, Legitimization, Support). Do all *that* 300 times a week! It's just not going to happen. The empathy that is so routinely called for in our routines will interfere with them and your care.

The talented intellects that have endured the psychological conditioning dished out by medical school have produced the strongest top-down, cognitively powered modulators of empathy. So despite the uniform chorus of calls for tutoring doctors in empathy, our medical education and our careers actively promote its suppression.

This shouldn't shock any of us. How many children, alone and in pain, would you walk past until you had assured yourself of your own child's safety? We all modulate our displays of compassion. Doctors use all the common modulators, and the one that seems uniquely ours—the "expert" modulator.

This concept was introduced in 2007 in an article in the journal *Current Biology*. A group of doctors experienced in acupuncture was compared with a control, non-physician population. The two groups were scanned with functional MRI while watching videos that depicted needles being inserted into various body parts, including the mouth, hands, and feet. The object of the study was to determine the pattern of brain activity these stimuli produced, and then to determine if there were differences between the doctors and civilians. It turns out that doctors do not activate their anterior insula or the anterior cingulate cortex. These areas are empathy's P.O. boxes in our brains. In the non-physician group these zones lit up like Christmas trees. The areas that ignited in doctor-brains were those regions associated with emotional regulation, cognitive control, and the self-distinction that separates us from others and from you. The doctors also reported that the images were less unpleasant and painful than did the controls.

The conclusion was that doctors "know that . . . situations can be painful for their patients and have learned throughout their training to inhibit their empathy-pain response. It is important for them to regulate their feelings of unpleasantness generated by the perception of pain in others and is, therefore, necessary for successful professional practice."[7]

We don't need to be taught things that we already possess, and that can be identified right down to the cellular level. It's impossible to teach what cannot be defined, quantified, or tested for. Finally, we don't need it when we are in practice. There are substitutes for empathy that will reassure our patients but not paralyze us. Too much empathy results in poor care, psychological distress, emotional hardening, and physician burnout. "The heart must first pump blood to itself."[8]

Will Dr. Sy Berg be a cyborg? In the aptly titled *The Fragility of Goodness*, Martha Nussbaum writes about Hecuba in Euripides' Greek tragedy. She could just as well be writing, however, about a grieving or stricken patient's reflection in her doctor's eyes. "The pupil is where the image of the looker is reflected in the eyes of the person seen. It is an image of the reality of the connection between me and you, of knowledge and its mutuality. I make my appearance inside your eyes."

Nonetheless too many of you stare into doctors' eyes that are about as reflective as bottle caps. When doctors are afraid that others' emotions will become contagious, they will limit and constrain their expressions of empathy. They may, in fact, appear to be cyborgs to their patients. Even in the face of this, it is critical that the doctor offer you something, some essence of humanity. Yousef Karsh, the photographer, caught such moments in the millisecond it took for his camera's strobe to flash. He referred to it as "a brief moment when all there is in a man's mind and soul and spirit is reflected through his eyes, his hands, his attitudes. This is the moment to record."[9]

Why would a doctor deny to you his gaze, followed by a meaningful downcast glance to the floor; his hands, with an offered touch; or his understanding attitude, with an accompanying sigh? What is the price of a touch, with the half-smile and furrowed brow that transmits, wordlessly, an understanding of your problem?

If you long for an emotional connection with your doctor you may be asking the impossible, although there may be some doctors who can both maintain a necessary distance and evince true empathy. The rest of us must realize *that all of our patients expect and demand something*. But where will it come from?

Doctors strain against the biological leashes that demand empathy. Doctors are well aware of the normative, in-group expectations that patients require emotional support; and they know that this support is therapeutic. With all of these pressures, the glance, touch, smile, and sigh can easily come from us, even if it's not within us. How? By acting! Yes, faking it. This is genuine artifice.

This is medicine's dirty little secret? Are we lying? No. If this is lying, then so is the routine prescription of placebos, which are universally acknowledged as beneficial. Placebos are the ultimate and literal expression of "trick or treat." Think of genuine artifice as a form, or more likely a *forme fruste*, of caring. It's when you *don't* care enough that you send the second best. Not exactly a Hallmark moment. But doctors bow to their understanding of the need for empathy when they fake it.

Genuine artifice is no oxymoron. It is an active, voluntary process that calls in other areas of our brain's circuitry. Its sincere demonstration softens what otherwise would be the harsh blast of our profession's form of medical autism. Its use improves our impoverished relationships and communication skills. It is the fulfillment of your expectations based on doctors' emotional intelligence. It is a calculated, rather than inculcated, craft that is made possible by a doctor's will to learn it and then use it in your behalf. The use of this form of sincerity is not only acceptable, it's admirable given how helpful it is, how easily it can be provided, and how rarely it is used.

In Paul Eckman's book, *Telling Lies*, Erving Goffman, a sociologist well-known for his analyses of human interaction, says, "When the situation seems to be exactly what it appears to be, the closest likely alternative is that this situation has been completely faked; when fakery seems extremely evident, the next most probable possibility is that nothing fake is present."

That's how the fake can be real, and the real can be faked.

Another less cynical way to look at it is to remind yourself that courtly etiquette, although also a veneer, acknowledges your status by providing the kind of good manners that are often lacking in your exchanges with doctors. Call it style or bedside manner, we will discuss a doctor's carriage and expand on the concept of etiquette-based medicine in the "Style" chapter that follows.

Schmooze 'em or lose 'em. Stressing any similarities between you and your care providers reinforces native empathy. It builds social capital. It sustains long-term relationships. Social capital allows you to establish some measure of mutual feeling and familiarity. These are the ties that bind, and they often awaken *true* empathetic feelings in your doctor that improve care and provide greater mutual satisfaction while it is ongoing. The tools that are used to promote your in-group status are based on shared experiences, physical similarities, social closeness, shared views, and similar socioeconomic status. It is time to use *your* ability to display genuine artifice to achieve this mutual regard.

It's not enough to be your doctor's patient. You want to assess your doctor's personality and manipulate it for mutual benefit. Patients seem to judge their doctors' behavior as if it had nothing to do with their own. If you expect bad behavior, poor communication, and a failure to see the world through your eyes, you will likely get it. Your behavior affects their behavior. By playing up similarities between you and your doctor, it may be possible to arrive at a point where the physician *recognizes herself in you*.

The techniques for doing this are neither new nor mysterious. They are used by therapists, salesmen, managers, and those in advertising to create a need and promote rapport when it might otherwise be absent. Before your visit, learn something about your doctor so that you can use it to demonstrate shared interests, hobbies, community service, or acquaintances. If you undertake a web search, review the doctor's C.V., or talk to her other patients and allied health-care personnel, the chances are better that you won't encounter a blank slate when the doctor first walks through the door. Pick up on any clues your clinician offers about her life. When she asks you about your interests, ask questions back. Medical appointments will never be conversations but they may become, however briefly, more meaningful than just the exchange of data.

Of course, there are time constraints that make it more difficult to establish a rapport, and stake out your identity. When you're sick, there are also psychological disconnects between the provider and the patient, the healthy and the ill. You can help to narrow these gaps and establish an identity with a doctor through the use of humor, a confident bearing, and strong attitudes and opinions.

Be a personality that stands out. Be interesting. Be memorable. Anatole Broyard, author of *Intoxicated by My Illness*, wrote: "A critical illness is like a great permission, an authorization or absolving. It's all right for a threatened man to be romantic, even crazy, if he feels like it. All your life you think you have to hold back your craziness, but when you're sick you can let it go in all its garish colors."[10]

In your doctor's eyes you can become a one-dimensional cutout—quickly assessed, categorized, and filed away. Fight it. Promote your personality and interests. The family picture you show your doctor demonstrates that your life is also peopled with parents, children, and friends. Carry a book into the room and ask if she has read it. Recommend it and offer a brief comment. You just came back from a movie—ask if she saw it. Make a recommendation to her. It's your style too—flaunt it.

You are being judged as much as you are judging. Your clothing, presentation, and facial and verbal acrobatics are all part of your self-expression. When called for, demonstrate your own cognitive calisthenics. So be the first to smile and offer a handshake. Put on that nice jewelry or wristwatch you have in the drawer; it demonstrates social and financial parity and projects power—that's why good doctors do the same thing. You are a person, not a supplicant. You are not a sufferer but someone confident, seeking a health-care confidant. Your dress and manner go a long way toward bridging any psychological and socioeconomic gaps. Your humor and individuality will separate you from the pack.

There are concrete things you can do during an interview or consultation with a doctor that will help promote your own interests and encourage the doctor to place you within her circle of empathic concern, usually devoid of her other patients.

Paraphrasing what your doctor says both compliments her and complements what was said. It sets up conditions conducive to a merging of interests. Paraphrasing uses your words to acknowledge and interpret her ideas, attitudes, and point of view. The paraphrasing of her words puts you in her frame of reference. It acknowledges that you have heard her ideas without necessarily agreeing with them. Your interpretation of what she is saying may spur her to correct errors or to amplify her thoughts. This, in turn, provides the opportunity for further discussion and stimulates reciprocity and identity. Paraphrasing is easy. Take the lead in statements like "What I hear you saying is . . .", "In other words . . .", "So basically how you felt was . . .", and "I hear you saying . . ."

While you shouldn't parrot the doctor, it's okay to mimic her syntax, particularly if she regularly uses a particular word or phrase. This may help the doctor to feel a closer rapport with you.

Mimicry is a form of paraphrasis. The synchronization of your mood, body language, speech rate, and breathing pattern works subtly to establish common ground. Mimicry can be mocking if it is used simultaneously, artlessly, or excessively. It may be unconscious or learned as an acquired talent. Mimicry extends to facial expressions. You use it to mirror the doctor's expressions, but most critically to allow her to mimic yours. For example, smile for a while—your mood will lift. Others around you may smile too. As contagious as a yawn, your mood invites others to share in it. Facial muscles are linked to the brain's emotional centers. Observing emotion in others evokes emotion in us. It changes behaviors and attitudes and shrinks the distance between two people.

Preparation, paraphrasing, and mimicry are invaluable tools, but there is one final, critical ingredient—charm. Camus wrote that "charm is a way of getting the answer 'yes' without asking a clear question." Because it's a rare commodity, it makes you stand out when you use it, and, not coincidentally, its appeal helps you to further your own agenda. Its effects linger long after its expression is gone.

Whether you inquire after your doctor's health, remember her family landmarks like birthdays or graduations, or send a holiday card, a thank you note, or a box of homemade cookies, these courtesies will make your doctors actually more deserving of them. How they treat you is likely to change. Yes, gifts are controversial when taken from pharmaceutical companies, but not when they come from you.

I know two doctors who benefited from the magnificent largesse of their patients. One received a car (and a nice one at that) and the other acreage on Martha's Vineyard. A birthday card and a cheap tie will do.

Summing Up: Do all you can to promote a doctor's identification with you. This requires preparation; the use of paraphrasing, mimicry, charm; and establishing physical and socioeconomic identity. Consciously promote personality traits that make you the memorable and interesting person you are. All of this allows your doctor to see at least a partial image of herself in you.

What a doctor says is indicative of someone who either seeks to enter into your world or does not care to. The few examples below demonstrate how words can reflect the presence of a patient-centered empathy. Listen for them to develop perfect pitch in detection of compassion.

Inquiries: "How do you feel when that happens?" "What effect does this have on your life?" "Can you tell me more about this?" "What worries do these symptoms cause?" "How would your life be different without these symptoms?"

Clarification: "Let me see if I understand what you said," "Tell me more about . . . ," "I'll summarize what you told me," "Correct me if I'm wrong, but . . ."

Responsiveness: "Sounds like you are . . . ," "I imagine that must be . . . ," "I can understand that," "I am worried about how you feel."

Praise: "You are doing a great job," "You've done a great job at keeping things in perspective," "I admire your ability to . . ."

Reassurance: "We'll get to the bottom of this," "I and my staff will help you all we can," "Call if you need to," "I am, and will always be, your doctor."

Support: "This must be a difficult time for you," "Is there anything else I can do that would make this easier?" "When people have this diagnosis they often want a second opinion or specialist."

10

Style

- Dr. Frank—a parable about a patrician physician.
- Why patients value a physician's style above all else.
- Style's dangers:
  - How it mimics a doctor's brains, communication skills, and empathy.
  - Why Dr. Bland is a better choice than Dr. P. Zazz.
- Style's minimum requirements.
- Etiquette-based medicine—Old World charm.
- When are you being dissed? What to do about it.

Say hello to Dr. Frank, the Patrician Physician . . . a parable on style. Dr. Frank is tall and spare in physique. His eyes, periwinkle blue, sparkle behind filigreed, gold-rimmed spectacles. His hair is as white as this morning's snow. Except for slight laugh lines, his face is smooth, bathed in bay rum. He is encased in a tattersall vest from which an antique pocket watch fob dangles elegantly. A polka-dot bow tie, self-tied, that is slightly, but rakishly, askew sets off the collar of his button-down broadcloth white shirt. He sports a crisp, starched, double-breasted white lab coat with woven buttons. A large black Montblanc fountain pen peeps out of the pocket of his professorial gown. His shoes, old cordovan wing tips with tassels, have been shined to a reflective gleam. His voice is mellow, with a slight midwestern accent. He projects Jimmy Stewart's "Aw Shucks" modesty, Gary Cooper's moral fortitude, and Clark Gable's beguiling charm. Besotted by his manner, you sign the consent form for your coronary artery bypass.

What style! But . . . if *just one more* of his patients suffers a postoperative complication, Dr. Frank will be remanded into custody and extradited to

172

face trial at the International Court at the Hague for crimes against humanity. That is what style can do. It can blind you from what counts most. A doctor's brainpower is the only necessary and sufficient criterion for choosing a clinician. Communication skills and empathy are necessary but are not, in themselves, sufficient. Remember the voluble village idiot? Recall the hand-wringing, hand-holding, handkerchief-wielding pinhead?

Style is "the outward show that deceives the world with ornament."[1] It's neither necessary nor sufficient for your care. Think of it as a meal enjoyed in an elegant setting served with an unexpected spice: the spice alone won't transform the insipid into the inspired; and it adds no nutritional value. Similarly, a doctor's style won't magically transform bad advice to good, and it adds no medical value to his opinions. Whether you are in a café or the clinic, the proof of pudding is always in the eating.

Ideally, it is only *after* you've see the diplomas, judged the communication skills, and felt the compassion that you can then place a value on his personal style. Style's dazzling display is incandescent, blinding patients to the primary, and far more important traits. It's more tangible and immediate than a doctor's IQ. Style's verbal flourishes are often confused with communication skills, and its drama with empathy. We all conflate comportment with a sense of an individual's moral and social character. A person's appearance and appurtenances appeal to the part of our nature that makes quick judgments of an individual's worth and skills. It can falsely elevate the mediocre while hiding the lights of the gifted but insipid amongst us.

External trappings are just that—traps. They take advantage of what Malcolm Gladwell calls the "thin slicing" that allows us to use a narrow spectrum of input to produce a broad spectrum of impressions. There are many simple, efficient ways to evaluate your doctor: The displayed diplomas, the use of "standard patient" templates, and the techniques for the rapid recognition of empathy.

Despite this, when a performance of great éclat dazzles, it's hard to separate stylistic frills from medical skills. It's been demonstrated that patients obtaining excellent care often don't recognize it because of problems with the style with which it is delivered. Investigators observed that "clinical care delivery and the patient's experience of it represent distinct activities . . . patients using such data to select a primary care physician may need to make trade-offs between technical performance and interpersonal performance."[2]

However unhappy you may be in the midst of a monochromatic medical experience, it is preferable to the legerdemain of a lightweight. Personalities expansive and surroundings expensive may prompt you to forgive or, worse, fail to recognize error. A contemporary of Johannes Brahms expressed this contradiction when he said of the composer's performance style, "Brahms did not play the right notes but he played them like a man who knew what the right notes were." Fine at the concert, fatal at the clinic.

Despite this, there *is* a minimum standard of behavior you should expect. Your doctor may not be in medicine's *Who's Who*, but you don't want him to be on a "What's That!?" list either. There is undeniable comfort in an appropriate behavioral display. Once you feel secure that your doctor has the requisite talent and skill, go ahead and value whatever style he or she brings to the job.

Style, for some, is a veneer so thin it inevitably warps, allowing a peek beneath to what might be a beast within. For others, style is part of their woof and warp. It can be either a reflection of how its owner wants the world to view him, or a reflection of his own worldview. Style for some provides credibility. For others it exploits credulity.

A clinician's flair is undeniably appealing when he remembers your child's name or asks after a recent marriage or similar milestone. Smart doctors have these morsels tucked away in your charts, update them frequently, and dispense them regularly.

There are baseline stylistic requirements that acknowledge that a doctor's first job is to put a patient at ease. There are certain non-medical criteria that doctors need to meet in order to be effective. They must present themselves in a way that demonstrates respect. The absence of these minimum standards, even in talented, talkative, and tenderhearted doctors, is problematic.

The public expects a white lab coat with the doctor's name affixed or embroidered. While ties and suits are now optional, cleanliness is not. If you see stains on lab coats, bloody scrubs or surgical clogs, sandals exposing bare feet or a distressed and disheveled appearance, you aren't being taken seriously. Such displays send as ominous a signal as the dead plants in their offices.

All of us have seen and experienced deficiencies in attire and even hygiene. When I was injured in a car accident I met one of the attending physicians, a minor player in my care. I was impressed by his starched white coat and commented on his handsome necktie. Each subsequent time I saw him he wore the same coat and tie. After four visits in as many days in which he wore the same outfit, I became alarmed at his increasingly disheveled appearance. There is a risk that overly casual and sloppy attire can reflect overly casual and sloppy care. Disinterest in personal appearance can reflect more global problems. Personality and emotional disorders may show themselves in the loss of self-esteem, which often becomes apparent first in people's attire, later in their bearing, eventually in their attitudes, and finally in their skills.

The minimums of attire, comportment, and hygiene follow only one rule: "Offer no offense." Some doctors take pride in their independence and laid-back attitudes by flaunting stylistic idiosyncrasies. As long as they obey the Hippocratic medical imperative "first, do no harm" and then the stylistic injunction "second, do not alarm," that's enough.

Arrogant or abusive doctors are one extreme of the spectrum. They can be aloof, louche, or indifferent. This nonchalance begins by addressing you by your first name or its diminutive without asking permission, and without the possibility of reciprocity. Using your first name doesn't bring you closer. The doctor isn't your pal. It's a technique meant to distance and separate, and it is the acknowledged first step toward exerting authority, however false. It's also frequently used by police and IRS agents.

So, unless you're Madonna or Beyoncé the use of your first name is insulting and demeaning. Tell the offender, "I'm fine with being Wally. Your first name is Bobby—right?" The paternalistic physician-centered era is as dead as the attitudes that propped it up.

Deportment is a word that refers to the use and movement of the body. This, too, has its standards. No doctor should sit on your hospital bed or exam room table without permission. The doctor who leans against the wall at the maximum distance possible from you, while working at that pesky scalp rash on his bald pate, is delivering as severe a slap to your dignity as one physically administered.

The thoughtful stroking of beards (one's own) is, of course, allowed. I grew my beard in college but since have consciously cultivated this affectation that suggests, or can substitute for, deep thoughts. My beard, now gray, implies an Old Testament–like wisdom. (I hope.) If I thought I could get away with it and it served to establish trust, I would fake a British accent, wear a pince-nez, and use a quill pen to make my chart notes.

No doctor can get away with being a buffoon. Patch Adams, who is both a physician and a clown, is unique, but he's not a role model. Oliver Sacks, who is a role model, has it just right. In his book *A Leg to Stand On*, his own doctor "smiled, but not widely; he shook my hand, but not formally; he was cordial, but not amiable." While it's true that style alone shouldn't excite you, the absence of the minimum standards may incite you.

Michael Kahn, in a 2008 issue of the *New England Journal of Medicine*, originated the concept of etiquette-based medicine, which he based on his own experience.

> During my own recent hospitalization, I found the Old World manners of my European-born surgeon—and my reaction to them—revealing. . . . Whatever he might actually have been feeling, his behavior—dress, manners, body language, eye contact—was impeccable. I wasn't left thinking, "What compassion." Instead, I found myself thinking, "What a professional," and even (unexpectedly), "What a gentleman." The impression he made was remarkably calming, and it helped to confirm my suspicion that patients may care less about whether their doctors are reflective and empathic than whether they are respectful and attentive.[3]

Good manners are the centerpiece of Kahn's short, yet influential treatise. The use of simple courtesies seems intuitive, yet it's strangely revelatory, even quaint, to the contemporary medical reader. Kahn recognizes that the style in which a service is delivered should be no different for doctors than it is for other tradespeople who have a product to sell. Consumers expect that good manners and common courtesies will be at the heart of medical service. Sadly, we have learned that most doctors are unable to naturally show empathy; they must learn to simulate it. But all doctors need to acknowledge the importance of manners. They help reassure the patient that she is in good hands.

You hear a knock on the door of your exam or hospital room. Once you've given your permission, the doctor enters and greets you, and if you have been kept waiting, apologizes with a brief explanation, and then introduces herself. She smiles as she washes her hands. After the symbolic hand christening comes the now-hygienic handshake. A generic statement should be made that acknowledges your discomfiture as the "person in paper pajamas."

"I hope I can be of help to you today," she says. The doctor then discusses her role in your care, which is particularly important if she is just one of a team of doctors involved in your case. Once this is done, then you both can proceed to the business at hand. Sound familiar? Probably not. But what a wonderful way it would be to begin, or continue, your association with this clinician. Being courtly is the distillation of style and is just as refreshing and reassuring in medicine's New World as it was in the Old.

11

Second Opinions

- In medical care the right therapy is not always the best therapy.
- When is second opinion desirable? When is it mandatory?
- How do you ask for one?
- Where do you go?
- What do you get for your trouble?
- How often will the second opinion change or modify your diagnosis or treatment?
- Avoid asking a barber if you need a haircut. Learn how to get unbiased opinions.
- What cancer centers offer that you can't find *anywhere* else.
- Which cancer centers to avoid and which are worthy of your trust.

Think you're done? Not quite. Even if you have chosen your doctors carefully, sometimes you will need a second doctor for another opinion. (From the English language's phonetic habit of dropping and blurring word endings comes "secondopinions" and from that arises "secondopes," referring to those that offer them. That's why these doctors privately refer to themselves as the "second dopes.")

First, it is important to distinguish the need for a second opinion from the acute or chronic unhappiness you may have with the doctor who offered you the first one. When you are dissatisfied or disenchanted with your doctor *all* his opinions will be cause for distress and uncertainty. You don't need another opinion, you need another doctor.

When do you need a second opinion? When do you need a specialist? The need for both may overlap. You may return to your doctor after the second opinion. A specialist may become a full-time partner in your care or make periodic cameo appearances.

There are many reasons that 19 percent of us seek second opinions. First, because of the certainty that little is certain in medicine. While doctors claim "science," you see almost daily flip-flops in opinion that turn today's tenets into tomorrow's taboos and yesterday's prohibitions into today's panaceas. The battlefields of medicine are lined with the cemeteries of its bad ideas.

You are also aware that health care is a business with something to sell. The lies will follow. Consumers have logically concluded that it's not wise to rely on any one opinion when pharmaceutical giants, insurance companies, and hospitals and the doctors who work for them increasingly seem to operate with clear conflicts of interest. You are correct to conclude that it is not wise to rely on any one opinion, particularly if that recommendation turns your head and can turn a dollar. Patients might well worry if they knew that 94 percent of physicians (yes, you read that right) have "a relationship" with the pharmaceutical and medical device industries, according to a survey of physicians published two years ago in the *New England Journal of Medicine*.[1]

There is a rising tide of generic distrust of once inviolate institutions. Medical practitioners now join congressmen, bankers, and car salesmen. Newspapers frequently publish public health pieces and medical stories, recurring series, op-eds, and blogs. Television provides a.m. warnings to moms, midafternoon misty-eyed patient narratives, and, at dusk, the primetime national news medical correspondent picks up the baton in advance of primetime specials. All focus their imperfect lenses on a variety of health-related issues. Most of this boils down to flogging new techniques while simultaneously flaying those who purvey or use them. "Revolutionary new scanning device offers earlier diagnosis of cancer!!" is juxtaposed, with no sense of contradiction, alongside "Increasing use of scans reaps windfall profit for doctors while increasing cancer rates!!"

We are now living in the dawn of a new era—patient-centered care. It turns out it really *is* all about you! You expect doctors to act like it when you want something—even if it's a new opinion. Patients control their own health-care decisions. You have, and are exercising, the option of obtaining health services from whomever you wish. Later we will discuss, in detail, how you can ask for an opinion without the need for self-mortification or penance. Some of us still haven't gotten the memo that it is now all about you.

Those are the "whys": you want second opinions even from those you trust. Public and private doubts are borne from scrutiny of the health-care industry's scruples and of medicine's science, which seems ever more similar to a palm reader's séance.

Even when you are happy with your care and trust your doctor, there are times when you will want to get a second opinion or consult a specialist.

When your routine care becomes anything but, it's time to reflect. Your doctor's advice may not be wrong, but it *always* reflects an individual philosophy that may not be shared by others. Each physician has unique practice perimeters beyond which he or she will not venture. When a doctor is presented with a patient with a variety of symptoms and has at his disposal the ability to perform a variety of clinical activities, some will move, while others will wait.

I have called these "perimeters and parameters." These are the boundaries within which doctors function, and the toolbox they use within those boundaries. Each doctor has a unique set of perimeters and parameters dictated by training, habit, continuing education, and personal philosophy. It's what a doctor will do, and how far he or she will go for any given presentation. Dr. Goldy may do too little too late. Dr. Locke, too much too early. Where is Dr. Goldilocks who will get things "just right?"

A diagnosis that requires long-term medication and follow-up should be confirmed by others. If you fail to improve with that diagnosis, a second opinion would then be mandatory. Many doctors, as we have noted, are very comfortable with your pain. The "Hey, doin' great!" is an opinion *you* should offer, not receive. This disconnect suggests the need for another helping hand.

You should seek a second dope or specialist when your trusted medical databases are at odds with your doctor's recommendations. When all your sources are singing one tune but your doctor another, it's time to get an additional opinion. When in the course of medical events, it becomes self-evident that your doctor is in doubt, you'll be able to tell. Your symptoms lead to evaluations that lurch from one possible diagnosis to the next. Treatment trials fail. There is no diagnosis on the horizon. Some confusion is occasionally inevitable. But there'll be a point in time when you'll feel better if another clinician confirms your current course, or finds that the solutions to your problems are not so elusive after all.

It may be that your doctor is not confused, but that you are. If the burden of illness is compounded by doubt, it is time to seek alternatives.

A treatment may be recommended that carries risk, expense, and inconvenience. This unhappy trifecta requires an independent confirmation regardless of your confidence in your doctor. The general public-access online resources referenced in part 1 of this book offer lists and tips. The medical journals and proprietary websites that have been recommended primarily exist to inform their physician readership. Now it's *your* turn to discover that a medical problem you suffer should have prompted an immediate specialty referral. If your doctor doesn't heed the calls from his own literature, you may have to.

No one with diabetes, inflammatory conditions of the bowel, deforming arthritis, chest pain, shortness of breath, periodic debility wrought by headaches, or local pain syndromes should be going it alone with just the family doctor. These are only a few examples. If your problem has a name, look it up. Your reference material will tell you when it's time for a more specialized opinion. However brief, however pro forma, there are times you should be seen in consultation. Dangerous diagnoses, delays in recovery, doubts, and conflicting databases demand corroboration.

Sadly there may come a time when too much will be at stake to assume *any* doctor is doing what's best. The key is the realization that there is a difference between getting the right therapy and getting the best therapy. The answer to the question "Is there better care out there?" is always "Yes." There are diagnoses, therapies, and surgeries so grave that they trump trust, even in a cherished family doctor. In these situations, you can't afford to be complacent.

When you care enough to get the very best, it's not a "Hallmark moment"; it's a "fire up the Buick moment." Personal and local resources may bias your doctor. He may not know about, or have at his disposal, all the tools that are needed. We have learned from prior chapters that some doctors are smarter than others, that some work for themselves rather than for you, and that it is a high-tech world out there. That's when you go elsewhere, however briefly, not just to shore up your confidence, but to save your life, extend it, or make it more bearable. The troika of unnecessary procedures, profit motives, and inevitable errors, alone or in combination, sometimes means you have to press the reset button.

Any condition that will last a lifetime or shortens your life span will demand a lifeline. Don't ask the audience or phone a friend. Your doctor won't give you a 50/50, eliminating two of your options. Who wants to be a millionaire, if the money comes as a result of your death and a subsequent malpractice suit filed by your survivors? You need more input. Even when you are willing to accept the diagnoses, doubts, and dithering of your own doctor, at no time should a diagnosis of cancer or recommendation of elective surgery be accepted at face value or go forward without a second opinion.

Cancer almost always requires some combination of surgery, chemotherapy, and radiation. You should never rely on one doctor's opinion. Even if your cancer is indolent and you are told you don't need therapy—get another opinion.

First research your AAA map, then your disease. You are going to travel and you are going to travel smart. You are going to a cancer center. If you have not seen your local oncologist first—you should. You need to judge her on all the previously suggested criteria. You better be happy because it is likely that you will return to her after your second opinion. If, in your opinion, she is not qualified, communicative, or compassionate, you may choose to return to the cancer center for therapy, however logistically challenging it may be.

Ideally, your local pros are in the best position to make a referral to the nearest national cancer center. The local oncologist is best suited to refer you to the physician qualified to serve your needs. But it's not smart to go to a national cancer center, no matter how renowned, unless the doctor who practices there is renowned as well. The quality of these institutions in large part redounds upon their doctors' abilities, not vice versa. The name and address of a world-famous hospital on a doctor's letterhead can confer false confidence in those who don't deserve it. Just look at Congress. All oncologists have clinical contacts in the largest, nearest, and most prestigious cancer centers. They routinely work with them on the myriad therapeutic protocols that cancer diagnoses spawn. Your local oncologist will expedite the appointment. (See part 4, "Choosing Your Hospital," for advice about "going it alone" when seeking the best doctor in the best hospital.)

Never ever go to a doctor for a second opinion without handling your own medical records. Don't rely on a referring office's promise to mail, fax, forward, or FedEx your files. You must have in your own possession copies (never originals) of your records, x-rays, and, most crucially, slides of your microscopic pathology specimens. Summaries of your data, or local interpretations of your x-rays or pathology material, are unacceptable. Only the films and slides, please. Don't bias the second opinion with local interpretations. Otherwise why make the trip?

The specialist is looking for an error or misinterpretation that, at best, may change the diagnosis, or at least alter the opinions on the best treatment. So many doctors will, without a shred of reliable information, act on nothing more than your faulty histories, vague memories, and wish-fulfillment fantasies.

Remember the defendant in the malpractice case I discussed? The man with the kidney disease who came to the office without a clue or his crew? That's why I would suggest that you hand-carry copies of your records with you anyway, even if you think the doctor's office has received your medical records. The promises and good intentions of others are too unreliable, and the data too vital, to assume that other people's interest or competence, much less both, will be in play.

Large cancer centers have multidisciplinary boards, extensive support services, laboratories, and technologies for diagnosis and therapy, many of which are cancer-specific. Multidisciplinary boards are peopled by specialists in radiation, and medical and surgical oncology, as well as pathologists and radiologists specializing in cancer diagnosis and therapy.

Invisible Second Opinions: There are doctors—radiologists and pathologists—whom you will never meet. They play a crucial role in your care. Never seen, these invisible second dopes sometimes offer the most important input when you are at a cancer center.

A large review of second opinions in cancer patients summarized the literature in 2008.[2] In one study the authors cited, of 715 cases referred for a second opinion, a lack of important clinical information was found in 5 percent and a major disagreement in 6 percent. The latter included a change in diagnosis from benign to malignant, or malignant to benign, and identification of a different neoplasm or a significant change in the tumor's staging, all of which dramatically alters your care. In another study the routine performance of second opinions in 194 patients among liver and gastroenterology pathologists reported missing information in up to 26 percent of cases and incorrect diagnoses in up to 9 percent. In 6.7 percent of cases the second opinion had a major clinical consequence. In five series published between 1991 and 2004 on second opinions in pathology, the overall rates of disagreement between the two opinions ranged from 7 percent to 19.3 percent, depending on the body system in question; for gastrointestinal pathology the rate was 12.4 percent. There are many other studies that confirm the wisdom of seeking a second opinion that *really might* be a second, and better, one.[3, 4]

Errors in the pathologic diagnosis for rare tumors can be as high as 60 percent.[5] The pathologists in a major cancer center will stage a tumor's aggressiveness more accurately, and offer both more precise determination of its cell type and the markers that predict its future—and yours—than will local pathologists. They are crucial guides to surgical decision making.

Radiologists in cancer centers have access to the most sophisticated imaging technologies and know how to use them. These physicians also offer invisible second opinions that change diagnoses and serve as guides for therapeutic recommendations. In neuroradiology alone specialists find major discrepancies of up to 13 percent between their readings and those of local radiologists.[6]

It all boils down to the simple observation that things not seen often, are often not seen. But the unusual and rare are frequently encountered and expected at cancer centers. When I trained at Memorial Sloan-Kettering Cancer Center in New York City, I saw, in volume, patients with diseases I never saw again in thirty years of practice. These centers can't routinely disregard the possibility of zebras.

Surgery performed at the time of the diagnosis is a major predictor of a patient's survival rate. The right initial surgery can prevent the need for the second and third operations that are so common in cancer patients. Even with the common cancers of rectum and colon doctors can use surgical methods and specialized techniques that are associated with improved survival.

Controversy continues in the fields of breast and prostate cancer surgery. Surgeons tend to recommend the techniques they do best. Local technologies and support services can limit their repertoires or inhibit any incentive to expand them. Surgeons also choose the surgery that reimburses them the most favorably. The surgical treatment of breast cancer is an example. Mastectomies are performed with the expectation that a reconstruction phase will occur at the end of the procedure. A restored breast also restores the woman who owns it.

Employing the proper technique to make a patient whole again is a priority that cannot be overemphasized. Usually the reconstruction phase has involved the placement of a saline implant. These are quick to do, technically easy, and profitable. Newer technologies are more complex and time consuming but, sadly, reimburse no better than implants. Surgeons unschooled in the newer techniques rarely mention this reconstructive vascular, microsurgical procedure, called "DIEP free flaps," despite the fact that it promises a more natural look and feel to the breast. These more advanced techniques also may obviate the 30 percent rate of additional surgeries that result with older implant techniques. You should at least hear about these newer reconstructive techniques.

Most surgical procedures are elective, and most are necessary. Elective surgery can be defined as an intervention that is not urgent. They can be either suggested by a doctor or requested by a patient. Some may be required (repair of a heart valve), others are optional (cosmetic surgery).Cataract or hernia surgeries, tonsillectomies, tubal ligations or vasectomies, hip and knee replacements, and even most cancer surgeries are elective. According to the latest data fifteen million operations were performed in 2007. Only 20 percent of the patients who went to the operating room (OR) were in the category of those with the highest degree of disease severity. OR patients were in fact *healthier* than non-OR patients. This means that when you are contemplating having elective surgery, there's usually plenty of time. Plenty of time to think, study, and inquire, because hundreds of thousands of these procedures are not needed.[7]

Cesarean sections, hysterectomies, pacemaker implants, coronary angiographies with or without stents, and, most recently, coronary bypass surgery for stable angina have been cited as the most overused and unnecessary procedures in the United States. Seven of the fifteen most frequently performed surgeries have come under scrutiny. Both the increasing volume of these operations and the lax, non-evidenced based indications used to rationalize their performance have been questioned. Almost all cosmetic surgeries are elective, and most are not necessary.

The pervasiveness of unnecessary surgery is the acknowledged reason many hospitals and insurers now either suggest or demand a second opinion before elective surgery. Medicare pays 80 percent of the Medicare-approved amount for a second opinion. Many of the interventions that now require a second opinion have, as a result, seen precipitous declines in their frequency.

Does this suggest that most doctors are lying profiteers who subject you to unnecessary risk, death, and debility? No, not most. Most doctors offer opinions they feel are sincere and correct. It would be naïve to deny that some physicians deliberately send people for unnecessary surgery, but it's more likely that many doctors are influenced by their own honest biases, by exposure to faulty, dishonest, and conflicting data, and by the public's demand, spurred on by the media, for a "quick fix." For doctors it is as true as it is hoary that if your only tool is a hammer, every problem looks like a nail. Need a cleanup of those clogged coronary arteries? Cardiovascular surgeons will operate, cardiologists will catheterize, and medical doctors will prescribe. Who's right? They are all right. You ask then, "How can they *all* be right?" Well, you're right too. Such is the state of the science. There are always alternatives. Doing nothing is an under-utilized strategy.

The most important lesson to impart regarding elective surgery is: if only a little can be endured, a lot can be avoided. Give time a chance. That said, all medical studies accept that the majority of the millions of annual elective surgeries are necessary and some lifesaving. But even a small percentage of a huge number is itself a large number. There are hundreds of thousands, perhaps millions, of unnecessary tests, invasive therapies, and surgeries each year.

What about *your* recommended elective surgery? Is it reasonable, is it necessary, is it being done by a talented, experienced surgeon?

Seeing another surgeon for a second opinion, or any opinion, raises the "never ask a barber if you need a haircut" dilemma. When it comes to performing your surgery, the second doctor may want to become your first choice for it. There is incentive for that surgeon to strongly encourage the surgery, but to belittle the local surgeon who recommended it.

What do you do in this situation? Inform the second surgeon that no matter what his opinion is, you love, love, love your first surgeon and want to return home for the procedure if there's agreement it's needed. This may not be true but it takes the salesman out of the surgeon, and you may get a better opinion as a result. Judge both doctors using the criteria we've suggested, and your own sources. Study. A subscription to the *Archives of Surgery*, for example, is inexpensive and inexpressively important in researching your options. It can be searched for free on the Internet, and many of its full-length articles are available at no charge. The best option? See part 4 for information on UpToDate.com's $20 one-week access to its incomparable resources.

You can obtain an opinion from a non-surgeon. A neurologist can opine on back or cervical spinal surgery. A gastroenterologist should be well-qualified to offer opinions regarding gallbladder, pancreatic, esophageal, and intestinal surgery. A rheumatologist would be in a good position to make recommendations regarding orthopedic procedures. It's a good idea to visit a dermatologist before making an appointment with a hair transplant surgeon or a plastic surgeon if you have questions about facial cosmetic surgery. By subtracting profit motive you enhance the value of the opinions given.

Cosmetic surgery is by definition unnecessary. This does not include reconstructive surgeries that are important, or restorative interventions that correct the disfigurements wrought by trauma, burns, operations, and genetic defects.

People suffering from body dysmorphic disorder obsess over exaggerated or even imaginary physical defects. In our society this form of obsessive compulsive disorder ranks only second to what I call the Ponce De Leon Syndrome: the perpetual search for the Fountain of Youth. According to the American Society for Aesthetic Plastic Surgery, over one and a half million cosmetic surgeries were performed in 2009 to either fix what was never broken or force the clock backward from its inexorable circuit. Not included in this number are the countless Botox injections, body art enhancements of tattoos, tribal piercings, scarifications, brandings, and scalpellings.

As a rule of thumb I would suggest that despite the "benefits" and in light of the risks, those who are contemplating these procedures note the following: The cosmetic surgery never treats the underlying psychological disorder. Cognitive behavioral therapy and the use of some pharmacological agents do, and they are a better substitute for surgery. Finally, if you think that plumped-up lips, age- and gravity-defying breasts, buttocks and thighs filled with stem cells, silicone and collagen implants, or transplanted body fat will look good when you are in your golden years, go ahead; but consider this: Gentlemen, those buttock implants *will* cause you to slip from your cabana chairs, golf carts, and wheelchairs. Ladies, the lovely and fetching butterfly tattoos on your breasts will, with Newtonian certainty, flutter down to your navels. When the rest of your body ages gracefully and naturally, those gravity-defying body parts will look stranger then, than your current fantasies about how they look today. Think twice when you consider the horrors of the countless cosmetic surgeries gone wrong. Think twice before you subject yourself to clubhouse chatter or nursing home staff finger-pointing. I can and will face the future bravely, despite my shortcomings, as long as my dignity is preserved.

If you choose not to inform your doctor that you want a second opinion, you are making a mistake. You're denying yourself the benefit of this doctor's advice. He knows your problem and is the best and the most suitable colleague to offer criticism or corroboration. We love second opinions. They are a layer of protection against malpractice suits. And they add another layer of trust that will be needed in the trying times ahead.

If you go it alone, without your primary care physician, you'll find that access to your medical records is delayed rather than expedited. Remember that you must have your records in hand for the second opinion. You will feel the full G-force of office inertia when you plunge into the freefall of self-referral. The second dope will not communicate as readily or rapidly with your own doctor. While ties between physicians who are too close can skew results, some association can be beneficial when doctors need to consult with each other.

Leaving your doctor behind will lead to otherwise preventable bad feelings. Most doctors want to be in the decision-making loop. Short-circuiting it clearly suggests a lack of trust, making it that much more difficult to return to the first physician and his wounded psyche. You are then treated as being "on your own," so, "good luck and have a nice life." Even if you have your own second dope picked out through careful research, let the provider of the first opinion know. No, you don't need permission. You do need a way back if that becomes necessary. Good manners, honesty, and patient professionalism provide this route. It's Patienthood 101.

How do you ask? Yes, it's difficult. Yes, you need to phrase it all carefully. Yes, there is a risk of bruised emotions. No, there is no need for Far Eastern rituals of humility and prostration. So go ahead and ask your O-Doctor-San for her opinion about a second opinion. Here is a template that sets the right tone. If it results in bad feelings, it's best to learn about her brittle ego early on.

"I appreciate your advice and trust it. I am aware of your excellent reputation. But this is a very difficult choice during a very difficult time. I am going to need more input. I would like your recommendation for a second opinion and your help in obtaining it. I have every intention of coming back to you if I decide to go through with the recommendations you have made. All my doctors and family are here in town and I will not let anyone else interfere. Perhaps there is someone at a local academic university center you occasionally use or send patients to when *you* need more input. I know that you understand that this sudden turn of events finds me unprepared to act right now. I am grateful for your help and will tell my referring physician how happy I am with your care."

This type of statement will make it more likely that you will return to open arms rather than closed doors. If you can't bring yourself to say it, write it down or have a partner or family member do the deed.

In our next section we will discuss the key question you need to ask both your hospital and doctor prior to any service. The response to this *single* inquiry may provide the only information you need to know.

Try not to rely on for-profit cancer centers. These are the ones that advertise on television. They may be okay but the words "may" and "okay" do not belong in the same sentence when you are deciding about your cancer care. The National Cancer Institute accredits thirty-nine comprehensive cancer centers in the United States.[8] The National Comprehensive Cancer Network recognizes twenty-one.[9] If you are near a member hospital complete with a doctor you trust, either through referral and/or your own research, that's your best option. However, twenty-five states don't have a designated cancer center. Only one, Montana, doesn't have a contiguous state offering this advantage. There may be a trade-off between convenience and your clinical outcome.

Good luck. Be fearless. Be brave.

IV

CHOOSING YOUR HOSPITAL

12

Choosing Your Hospital: Introduction

- Not all hospitals are created equal.
- Why we pick our appliances with greater care than our hospitals.
- The two factors you value *most* in a hospital have the *least* predictive value for your survival—how to set priorities.
- You listen to your *health insurance company* for a hospital recommendation?!!
- Kamikaze hospital loyalty. Why people would sooner die than change hospitals—and do!

The casual attitude people demonstrate when choosing doctors incurs a steep price. Let's direct our attention to your consumer powers when choosing a hospital.

The imperative "caveat emptor" (let the buyer beware) carries the most consequence when you purchase health care. When it comes to hiring a hospital's services, it's more caveat empty than caveat emptor.

It's time to impart the same lessons for hospitals as we did for doctors. All hospitals are not the same. Each is its own unique brand. We, a nation of shoppers, are obsessed with brand names that tout their distinctiveness. In reality, most consumer products in any given category are all but indistinguishable from each other. We think we can see the smallest pixel a human brain can process on a video display. We taste the figs and peaches in a $9 bottle of wine. We claim the sensory hyperacuity possessed by dogs, dolphins, and nocturnal predators.

Few use these consummate consumer skills when choosing a brand of hospital. "Aren't they all the same?" Imagine the consequences if 1 in 500 of you died as the result of using HD-DVD over Blu-ray players. Rather than the three-year war for your loyalty, HD-DVD would have suffered an extinction event within seconds. Yet, 1 in 100 of you *will* die or be damaged by preventable medical error when you lie in hospital beds that were so casually chosen. For many surgical procedures there is up to a 3-fold greater chance of dying at "your" hospital than at a carefully researched facility that may be only a few minutes or hours away. The choice between Sony and Samsung is a minor one. Not so for St. Sony or Samsung General. Let's show you how to choose the right hospital in the certainty that you will, one day, need one.

Yes, it is confusing out there. Hospitals are variably touted for their safety, high-volume, elevated-rankings, report cards, or placement on some publication's list.

Some "top" hospitals are not on the list of "safe" hospitals. Aggressive clinics are not all high-volume institutions. *US News & World Report* (*USNWR*) hails hospitals that HealthGrades (HGs) and the Leapfrog Group (LFG) ignore. You would think that all of Forbes' largest and safest top ten hospitals would find a home *somewhere* on *USNWR*'s 170 "Best Hospital List." Only half did in 2008.

As for *USNWR*, an article in *Circulation* noted that "13 hospitals not in the *US News & World Report* cohort did better in providing . . . evidence-based aspects of heart care than did any of the 41 top *US News & World Report* organizations, and 313 nonranked hospitals did better than half of those ranked on the *US News & World Report*.[1]

In 2011 LFG's "Top Hospital of the Decade" can't be found on either *USNWR*'s or HGs' top hospital lists. It's not even listed amongst their second tier hospitals. What does this all mean?

And how about that familiar old pile down the street? That's right, your local hospital, St. Wutsisz. It's on no one's honor roll. It's not a designated "Hospital of Distinction" or a "Center of Excellence." It missed the cut of *USNWR*, HGs, LFG, Reuters, and *Consumer Reports* by a country mile.

Maybe you tried investigating hospitals but surrendered, stymied by the bewildering varieties and numbers of hospitals vying for your business. Perhaps your nascent consumerism was nipped in the bud by skeptical media reports shrilling over the flaws and frauds associated with the hospital rating systems.

In light of all this, very few of you go shopping for a hospital. In 2008, fewer than 15 percent of the population referred to hospital ratings or report cards. Most people have never seen one. Seventy percent don't know they exist and a mere 1 percent actually use them when making health-care decisions.[2]

The features the public do value most, cost and convenience, have the least predictive value for survival when you are hospitalized.

The public remains passive recipients of their health care, relying on friends, family, familiar doctors, and, alarmingly, their medical insurance companies' websites. Nobel Laureate Paul Krugman sums it up best when he offers two pieces of advice about health insurers:

1) Don't trust the insurance industry.
2) Don't trust the insurance industry.[3]

People follow the path of least resistance, staying with familiar hospitals that are close to home regardless of the problems they or their hospitals suffer. It is astounding that many would sooner die (and do) than leave their neighborhood for better care when it's needed.

In a study published in 1999, patients were asked to imagine that they had a resectable pancreatic cancer. They were given the option to choose between local or regional care—a four-hour car ride from home. If the risk of operative death were doubled at the local hospital compared to the regional institution, 45 percent of the study population preferred to stay close to home. If the local risk were quadrupled, 25 percent would still stand pat. How about six times the risk compared to a regional center? Eighteen percent of local die-hards (or more accurately die-easys) wouldn't pack a lunch and gas up the Buick. As the odds of death increased, there remained a significant number of stalwarts who remained stalled at home. Finally, under the promise of certain death, a 100 percent local operative mortality (compared with a 3 percent regional hospital death rate), 10 percent accepted their fates and would march off to their hospital *qua abattoir* without complaint.[4]

Attention Darwin Award Committee! So stunningly counterintuitive are these results they might be thought of as a poorly designed outlier with aberrant statistical anomalies gleaned from an unrepresentative patient population. Nope. A clinical survey in 2000 by the Kaiser Family Foundation and The Agency for Healthcare Research and Quality (AHRQ) concluded that "Personal recommendations and familiarity are so important that they often outweigh more formal indications of quality . . . people are more likely to choose a hospital that is familiar (62 percent) over one that is rated higher (32 percent)."[5]

In the past, choosing a hospital was unnecessary. You were lead in tow to the hospital where your family doctor practiced. There was no choice. "It's the doctor, stupid." With the rise of the hospitalist movement your doctor may not work in *any* hospital. The "where" becomes your choice. Let's work out a simple, but rigorous, plan. One plan for routine hospital care and another for emergency regional backup, and a strategy to find a national center when all else has failed and you are told nothing else can be done.

13

Staying Local

- Whither the community hospital.
- There *is* no place like home: the case for your local hospital. Why it might be better, safer, and cheaper than its downtown big brothers.
- When size *doesn't* matter: why small hospitals rule and why a technology delayed can be a technology avoided.
- Which is better, a great doctor in a "so-so" hospital or a bad doctor in a great one?
- The ratings game—the good, the bad, and the ugly.
  - Understanding and getting the most from hospital rating sites.
  - And the winner is . . . the "you never heard of it," hands-down, thumbs-up best site when seeking local care.
  - A case in point.

Everyone should have in place a carefully chosen community hospital. Yes, ignored by the ratings, and perhaps a bit threadbare in atmosphere, it's a destination hospital for no one but its town's inhabitants. When you need hospitalization it should be your first step if not your last stop.

Most problems will lend themselves to your old pal—your community hospital and your own doctor in it. Emergencies demand them. Even though the answer to the question "Is there a better care out there?" is always "yes" regardless of your location, let's start at home. First let's make the case for local hospitals. After this, we'll demonstrate the method to find the best one, whether it's down the block or across town.

We are not looking for a hospital located at the end of a path of least resistance. We do not prioritize convenience. You should choose your community hospital carefully, elevating one above all others. There's nothing wrong or dangerous about local loyalty—though not the seppuku variety demonstrated in the previously cited studies.

Small, local health-care facilities have traditionally been objects of derision and scorn. In doctor argot, these "pus pockets" still exist but have been increasingly overshadowed and supplanted by institutions that are characterized by their cultures of safety and, in many cases, that have become hotbeds of innovation. Many provide sophisticated technology, electronic medical records, and computerized physician order entry systems. Many are case studies in excellence, following the benchmarks prescribed by private and public groups dedicated to greater patient safety—the Institute of Medicine, the Commonwealth Fund, the federal government, and the Leapfrog Group. Small community neighborhood hospitals stack up well against larger urban centers. In many cases they are superior to their downtown or neighboring city's university hospital. "A Harvard University researcher found that community hospitals did just as good a job treating most common illnesses as academic medical centers, but provided that care far more cheaply."[1]

A hospital's wealth can no longer be transmuted into a promise of health. Not only is there a lack of association between quality and spending, some hospitals that spend more give you less favorable outcomes. *Health Affairs* in 2009 comments, "For all of the quality indicators studied, the association with spending is either nil or negative. The absence of positive correlations suggests that some institutions achieve exemplary performance on quality measures in settings that feature lower intensity of care."[2]

Hospital size and urban location no longer serve as proxies for quality. A hospital survey on patient safety generated by the US Department of Health and Human Services in 2009 found that smaller hospitals (forty-nine beds or fewer) had the highest average percent positive response from their surveyed employees on all twelve patient safety culture composites. Large hospitals scored lowest on the percentage of respondents who gave their workplaces a safety grade of "Excellent" or "Very Good."[3] The medical behemoth twenty exits and six Denny franchises down the highway is no longer your default medical destination hospital. *Health Affairs*, in 2008, commented, "Despite concerns about the availability of high-quality health care services in rural communities, we found only a modest relationship between hospitals' geographic remoteness and hospital-specific mortality . . . despite the challenges faced by hospitals in remote small rural areas, many perform as well as or better than hospitals in urban areas."[4]

Large urban hospitals are also 15 percent more likely to offer you an infection while you pay up to 30 percent more for its services. Patients in smaller hospitals are more often cared for by their primary care physician rather than a hospitalist. Small hospitals routinely excel in the performance of less intensive duties that require careful and thoughtful on-time administration of drugs or other therapies. They follow care-based algorithms more methodically. This is why patients with pneumonia fare better at smaller, community-based facilities. The timely administration of antibiotics, oxygen, and respiratory therapy relies on institutional personalities that are characteristic of local hospital centers.

As community hospitals continue to thrive, academic centers are more frequently establishing alliances with them. Two-way conduits allow "big-time docs" a small town experience and small town patients a rapid egress to big-brother hospitals if the occasion demands.

If a small community hospital is judged side-by-side with the largest and most aggressive academic teaching center, there may be fewer highly sophisticated services available. Some of these technologies, and the doctors who use them, are deemed indispensable in certain emergencies. This availability of "man and machine" is considered lifesaving and, by inference, mandatory. Multiple studies between 2007 and 2009 have questioned this assumption. Dr. John Wennberg is renowned for his studies on regional patterns and costs of medical care that suggest we suffer an epidemic of unnecessary interventions. In 2009, he and his colleagues noted that "patients hospitalized in regions with greater inpatient care intensity tend to rate their hospitals unfavorably and are more dissatisfied with their hospital experiences for tangible reasons—dirty rooms, noisy nighttime, poor pain control, and shortfalls in communication with doctors and nurses . . . illness- and severity-adjusted mortality is higher in regions with greater use of acute care hospitals. . . ."[5]

For the benefit of a relative few who need such care, the several hours of acute care, stabilization, and discussion may not have an unduly negative affect on their outcomes. It has been shown that patients with mild heart attacks can delay intervention up to twenty-one hours.[6] Only 25 percent of acute care hospitals offer invasive revascularization techniques (PCI or operative bypass). For those with severe heart attacks who actually need these procedures, there is still a six-hour window of interhospital transfer (assuming the use of fibrinolytic therapy) without unduly affecting their results.[7] Many are mindlessly rushed headlong into the maw of these invasive strategies. Starting your journey at a hospital without these technologies might save some from the resulting mortality, morbidity, long-term disability, and psychological trauma when "*doing something*" is not needed. It may be the absence of these types of services serves as a relative advantage.

How many *well* patients must suffer so that one *sick* patient benefits? In medicine, many must take the risks of a given technology they ultimately don't need in order to extend or save the life of the occasional person who does. Known as "needed to treat" (NTT), it's the number of innocents who must endure our technologies, tests, and invasions so that a much smaller number will benefit. Take statins as an example. The number NTT for using a statin is 100:1 over three years of use. One hundred people who never needed it must take it so that one very happy patient is spared one very unhappy event—a (usually nonfatal) heart attack. It works because everyone who takes statins must think that they will be the lucky one who will be spared a terrible event. I think that in community hospitals your NTT numbers are lower when all aren't, lemming-like, marched off technology's cliff to cushion the fall of the few who need it. Dr. Nortin Handler in his book *Worried Sick* might agree. For invasive cardiac interventions the needed-to-treat ratio is also sky high. One hundred patients with coronary artery disease must be put at considerable risk to extend the lives of three who do need it. Many patients can be treated medically for their coronary artery disease. Those who need intervention have a several-hour window to be transferred to it. So whether you "opt for the top" or feel "less is best" the chances are good that, properly chosen, a community hospital is a good bet to be worthy of your care.

In less than a generation, my community of 100,000 people has gone from a medical backwater to a sophisticated teaching center. Medical services then unimaginable or requiring distant referrals are now routine. Newer and younger physicians, imbued with the philosophy of evidence-based medicine, are arriving fresh from training. Over the past several years our community has gained the bragging rights for six MRIs, two CT/PET scanners, and three cardiac electrophysiologists that assure no waiting, much less lines. The most sophisticated CT scanners churn out ionizing radiation like our now defunct mills once spewed out chemical pollutants.

The psychological benefits of local care are critical. A hospital that's close to home anchors you to your life. Familiar newspapers, television, and radio channels, and the landscape viewed through your window, keep your mind engaged in familiar routines and happier thoughts and allow you a more sanguine contemplation of the future. Family and friends at the bedside protect you from isolation's progressive erosion of your norms, prevents alienation, depression, and withdrawal. The ever present company of friends, enabled by your hospital's proximity, reminds you of your role in their lives and the roles they play in yours. They also bring food! Familiar surroundings while being surrounded by family are conducive to your welfare and recovery. I think that there is a logarithmic drop-off in the number of people able to visit and attend you for each fifty miles you travel from home.

The medical benefits of local care? It's where your doctors are! It always boils down to the doctor. I have previously noted that going to a top hospital means nothing if you are about to be cared for by that name-brand hospital's village idiot. Every village has one. Every hospital has quite a few. They are the most dangerous when they have the imprimatur of a "top hospital" to prop them up. They may be a full professor of this or a clinical director of that. It all means nothing. Yes, there is a correlation between the quality of the hospital and the doctors who practice there. The degree that a hospital's attributes correlate with its doctors' abilities is too weak to count on when the chips are down and it's the last roll of the dice.

Which is best? Your own great doctor working in, for the sake of argument, an average hospital, or a bad doctor in a great hospital? That bad doctor is like a child playing with a loaded gun. A bad player with all the tools and technologies available will use them indiscriminately. Your carefully chosen doctor, using his clinical and nonclinical skills of advocacy, validation, and empathy, will rise above what might be his hospital's relative weaknesses, making it a better place for your care. The local doctor, properly chosen, has the benefit of your trust. You have benefited from this trust in the past and count on it in the future. You found him by asking the right questions, listening for the right words, and recognizing the right attitudes. You made the right decision. If the time comes to evacuate to a larger, more prestigious center your own doctor will know it—often before you.

Later (see chapter 14, "Abandon Ship!"), I'll show you how to find your own backup doctor and hospital that's only a short hop away if things go awry in your local hospital. So for now let's keep your trusted local family doctor and the specialists you have seen in the past. There is no doubt it's hard to keep your doctor in the age of the hospitalists. If you risk losing your own doctor to a hospitalist, use the three phrases that may turn the tide: "I trust you," "I need you," and "I thought I could rely on you." Hit those guilt buttons. As noted earlier, at least bargain for your doctor's periodic inpatient visits or ask that your care be supervised by a specialist you've seen in the past.

This section's leitmotif is that no two hospitals are the same. The quality of community hospitals lies along a distribution curve. Knowing about bell curves, you are aware that some of your local hospitals are great, most aren't, and a few are god-awful terrible. Most communities have several hospitals to choose from. Some cities offer dozens. How to choose? It's time to enter the brambly thicket provided by the hospital rating systems.

Hospitals are rated and ranked by the federal government, the states, for-profit rating companies, nonprofit foundations, proprietary and nonproprietary websites, and the media. Some rating systems share common databases. Others use unique points of reference. Source material for the sites come from patient charts, and hospital billing records, diagnostic codes, health insurance sources, and Medicare and Medicaid public access sites. Data is available from hospitals' departments, particularly from pathology, which registers diagnoses. All of the information is assembled and sent for statistical analysis to a number of independent contractors who use a variety of software programs to tweak, massage, and torture the data. The results are published, sold, or made available on Internet sites to the public, insurance companies, and hospitals. *USNWR* and HGs review virtually every US hospital. The Leapfrog Group (LFG) invites 2,000 hospitals to respond to a medical questionnaire generated by a panel of experts who confirm hospitals' safety, quality, efficiency, and improvement methodologies. In 2009, 1,206 hospitals completed the survey. In the 2010 survey, only one of the fifteen hospitals that are within fifty miles of my city responded to the LFG questionnaire. Forbes tweaks HGs' data to come up with unique (and weird) categories like "Safest Top Hospitals" and 'Top Destination Hospitals" and "Top Luxury Hospitals."

When released, the results bring on howls of righteous indignation or chest-thumping self-promotion. Unfavorable reports produce board room profanity and finger-pointing, semi-convincing counterarguments, publicists' spin, and the contrasting opinions from hired gun statisticians. Favorably rated hospitals call news conferences and ramp up advertising and fundraising campaigns that spread the word and the wealth.

The innocent are fired, the guilty promoted. It sounds like hospitals are big businesses. They are. It's a $2.5 trillion a year industry that represents one-sixth of our entire economy. Hospitals take in the largest share. You can bet that for some there will be blood; for others there will be buzz.

In light of the chasmal differences between hospitals and your fate while in them, everyone should want to know and be able to measure a hospital's quality.

The competition, high stakes, and honest desires of public health experts have confused physicians and alienated the public. The weaknesses, methodological flaws, and outright frauds have caused a measurement nihilism. Ratings are approached with cynicism and distrust. As a result, many of you may be tempted to ignore good information and go off in search of the bad—hearsay, anecdotes, and advertisements.

First, you can trust many of these sites. Second, to benefit from them you need to know how to use them, and, third, to put things in context, flaws are inevitable in this type of quest. Most sites lean heavily on a hospital's mortality rate. Death is an irrefutable end point for a hospital and even more so for its patients. Yet, since 1863, when Florence Nightingale published mortality rates for a London hospital, debates have raged.

Hospital mortality rates, a seemingly straightforward statistic, can be radically altered by the manner in which they are calculated. Some procedures are so safe there *are* no mortality rates. Low-volume, low-mortality diagnoses and procedures like pediatric cardiologic surgery require a huge volume of cases, often thousands, before small, 5 percent differences between institutions can be seen. Mortality rates are not able to comment on errors, poor medical practice, or lax standards, nor do they shed light on other factors such as long-term disability and other more subtle end points.[8] Many rating systems use a hospital's case volume as a proxy for quality. Is it the total volume of cases by the hospital or the volume generated by the hospital's individual surgeons? This represents a large potential difference in your results when you face a low-volume surgeon who works in a high-volume hospital. HGs charges hospitals a licensing fee to use its data in marketing campaigns. Does it have an incentive to make more hospitals happy? Some hospitals are like schools that "teach to the test." The school is terrible, the teachers inept, and its students deprived. But wow, don't they do well on standardized exams! Hospitals too may concentrate on Medicare's 2010 thirty-four quality indicators and ignore the performance of other equally important clinical services.

We will use the rating systems. We will use each in areas where they are the most helpful and reliable. Some are best when choosing between hospitals. Others are better when you're looking for a destination medical center. Others allow national rather than regional searches. One rating system stands alone when you've narrowed your search to two or three hospitals and now need crucial information about your own condition—not the hospital's. Don't confuse your status with your hospital's. You won't be sporting a bumper sticker that reports "My Husband Was an Honor Patient at St. Zachary's ICU."

Let's rate the raters: There are a lot of them out of there. So far we have mentioned only a few. The federal government, the state governments, HGs, Thompson Reuters, *USNWR*, LFG, Forbes, and more are all vying for your attention.

For our current purposes we need a rating site that allows a single screen display that gives us a hospital-to-hospital comparison that goes beyond the confines of a zip code or state. We want to compare local choices, "almost local" regional choices (see chapter 14), and those hospitals that require all but a passport to visit (see chapter 15).

And the winner is . . .

Whynotthebest.org (WNTB). Why not the HUH . . . ? Yes, the "you never heard of it" Commonwealth Fund's whynotthebest.org is the absolute, number-one, hands-down, thumbs-up favorite. This site has it all. It uses rigorous methodology and current statistics, and it offers on-screen comparison for an unlimited number of hospitals regardless of location. Just keep picking hospitals, adding them to "my hospitals" on your "my profile" section. Cross zip codes, go regional, or compare hospitals nationally if you wish. After choosing the hospitals you wish to size up, it's time to select "choose benchmarks," which allows you to compare your choices to local and national benchmarks. Then just click "choose" and all your hospital choices will be listed and ranked against your benchmarks and for any chosen features, including mortality rates, care of heart attacks, pneumonia, heart failure, or surgical care improvement. Compare your hospital to others for patient satisfaction, as well as readmission and hospital-acquired infection rates.

You can register for free and save or e-mail your searches. This is perfect for vacations. Why be a stranger in a strange land when you travel? Before setting off, choose and compare all the hospitals in the city, region, or hamlet you are visiting. If stricken, you will know more about that area's hospitals than the locals. You'll know *a lot more* than the night clerk at your Super-8 motel. Registering is simple, fast, free, and has many other advantages.

This is a superb effort from the Commonwealth fund—a private foundation dedicated to improving health care through research and education. Get on this site, register, and start to learn it. It's almost fun! Cranking up your computer while waiting for the ambulance's wail is not the way to obtain its benefits.

With the information available on WNTB let's return to our premise "stay local" and prove it. Rome, New York, is my town's sister city. Rome Memorial Hospital is its sole health-care facility. Some Romans and all those passing through it might think they would be safer traveling thirty-seven miles to Syracuse and its University Hospital. Many who would need a routine hospitalization might go to Syracuse or travel 200 miles to Manhattan's New York University or New York Presbyterian Hospital. Others might journey 670 miles to North Carolina's Duke. On WNTB's "overall quality—all topic composite score," Rome Memorial Hospital topped University Hospital in Syracuse in all but one category. Rome Memorial Hospital outdistanced Duke, Presbyterian, and Syracuse for pneumonia care. For heart failure it was surpassed only by Duke and NYU. For mortality rates Rome was comparable to Duke and way better than Syracuse. Yet on the ten patient satisfaction metrics Rome didn't do as well as in 2009. It was outscored by the others on the levels of highest patient satisfaction. But in the 7 or 8 out of 10 metric it was the equal to them all. And being close to home . . . priceless.

Now, I am not suggesting that if you live on Duke's campus you should hop on a plane to Rome, New York, for your medical experience. I'm sure you'll find a distant hospital that beats Rome Memorial Hospital and your own carefully chosen health-care facility. For certain treatments I wouldn't dream of setting foot in Rome Memorial Hospital. But for routine hospitalization for common problems and treatments a local patient would otherwise travel far and lose all his hometown doctors, local support systems, friends and family, and familiar surroundings. So, when in Rome do as the Romans do—stay local. Jay Neugeboren gets it right in a *New York Times* piece when he writes, "To get diagnoses and treatment plans right, we need doctors who know us over time, and who have the time to know us."[9] Why bother consulting a map unless the trip is mandatory (see chapters 14 and 15)?

WNTB allows you to narrow down your local choices. If there is a photo finish between two or three hospitals you may need more information before bringing your choice to your doctor. Enter HealthGrades (Health-grades.com). HGs is a serious industry. It uses millions of data points, studies thousands of hospitals, employs hundreds of consultants, and adopts dozens of quality, safety, and clinical end points from federal agencies and independent foundations. Log on to HealthGrades.com. Its 2010 site asks you to choose your state and city. This takes you to a page that lists over thirty conditions and diagnoses. Link to one that is relevant to your search. The local hospitals appear with their quality ratings for your problem. Click on the hospital with the best ratings. HealthGrades brings you to their web-page for that hospital. The page contains more information on the hospital demographics, its benchmarks against national averages for a variety of procedures. You can see comparative data on costs and lengths of stay. Then it's time to link to the hospital's "Quality Ratings by Procedure or Conditions." There you can choose among dozens of diagnoses, determine if the hospital has received awards from HealthGrades, and learn about survival and complication ratings for a variety of listed procedures. There are large differences in quality between hospitals; there are also large differences in quality within each hospital. Even great hospitals may not be great across the board. It's important to find a hospital that not only performs the best for your problem but performs the best in general. If you get pneumonia after your gallbladder surgery, it's nice to know your hospital has a deep bench of pulmonary and infectious disease specialists. HGs offers this in detail and in user-friendly graphics with discussions and definitions of medical conditions.

Do the research on WNTB and HGs. Find your local hospital. Now you're a health-care consumer. Now you're being your own advocate and have acknowledged the imperative caveat emptor.

14

Abandon Ship!

- When is it time for a trek? When must you journey to strange new hospitals; to boldly go where no neighbor has gone before?
- Crisis care: How to recognize and plan for desperation medicine, shotgun medicine, defensive medicine, and when your doctor "hangs crepe." How do you tell your doctor goodbye?
- Every inpatient needs a backup plan. A fast exit is impossible when you're on your last leg. Learn an Internet search technique that finds the best *closest* hospital and its doctors in case things go bad at St. Wutzsisz.

REGIONAL CARE

You used WNTB and HGs to find the best local hospital. You chose your doctor carefully. There will come a time when you need them both—you're an inpatient at St. Home and Hearth. Despite all your efforts, things aren't going your way; something has gone awry and it's time to get away. Fast. Yes, there is going to be a larger, noisier Medtropolis in your future if you are to have one. There are several clinical inpatient scenarios that require thinking outside the box, especially when you realize that you're now stuck in one. Difficult problems, or the complications suffered during the care of common ones, demand a timely "Mayday." It may be that your new diagnosis requires the immediate use of techniques and technologies that are not available at your hospital. You may have used and have now exhausted the local resources. You are no better and are getting worse. You have reached the point of diminishing returns and increasing risks. All the tests

and therapies to this point have been sensitive, specific, and safe. They have
failed to diagnose your problem. They have failed to treat your symptoms.
As your problems close in, your doctor feels outgunned and you get "shotgunned." Shotgun medicine is a term every doctor knows and a technique
each has used. It's a close-range blast from both barrels of a doctor's arsenal
that puts you in the midst of a fusillade of tests and treatments. No aim
is required when the aim is to eliminate every conceivable condition that
might be causing your status to deteriorate. This is not defensive medicine.
It's desperation medicine. Desperate times don't call for desperate measures
if it means getting shotgunned. You know you're getting shotgunned when
you are put on "trials of therapy" and are sent off with a pat on the back and
a "let's see if this does the trick." You've become a plaything for the whims
of the increasing number of 'ologists dragooned from their research labs.

On other occasions you've hit the wall—hard. You can't go around it
and are being crushed against it. No one can say why, but, as the days go
by, you experience one setback after another while you anticipate tomorrow's. While you've become weaker and more detached you've failed to
notice that your doctor has become increasingly frustrated, defensive,
and tense.

Tubes and catheters appear and then disappear inside of you. The proliferation of bedside machinery, an expanding phalanx of nurses, and the
extremes of the young intense physicians and the older more wizened ones
collectively represent the malignant blooms of a failed medical venture. It
will be during these times that your family witnesses the simultaneous decline of your health and your prospects for regaining it. Is it time for them
to sound the alarm?

HANGING CREPE

It's time to sound the alarm. The coda of a desperate but unsuccessful shotgun exercise may lead to another practice known to all doctors and used by
many—hanging crepe. The term comes from the days when placing black
crepe on doors and windows signaled a death in the family. Doctors hang
crepe in anticipation of one. "This approach offers the most pessimistic pre-
dictions and bleak prognoses *presumably* in an effort to lessen the family's
suffering if the patient dies of his illness" (italics mine).[1]

The operant word here is "presumably." More often hanging crepe is a
cold, calculated method to lessen the doctor's suffering that might occur in
a malpractice action. A doctor tries to get it both ways in a "no lose" scenario when he hedges his bets by issuing dire pronouncements. In the event
of a death—"you were, after all, warned—it's not my fault." In the event
of a survival, even one associated with debility, the doctor becomes a hero.

In either case he is less likely to be a defendant. Regardless of blame, it's important to know about this tactic and, more important, to recognize it.

When things start to go wrong you'll see a doctor's body language change from strutting to shrugging. It's accompanied with sighs and a voice now pitched in the lower octaves. Finally, as things get worse, you hear the "we've done all we can," "we've called in everyone we know," "we're leaving no stone unturned," and "we just don't know why. . . ." In an effort to spread the blame some may hear an uncharacteristic physician's entreaty, "can *you* think of anyone you want to be called in?"

As soon as you suspect it, ask your doctor if he is hanging crepe. He'll know what you mean. It is *not* a reliable indicator that all is lost. It *is* an absolute indicator of a loss of confidence—your doctor's. This is when the bad care continues. Desperation medicine gives way to defensive medicine. In a 1975 *New England Journal* article, Mark Siegler confirms the fact that when doctors do all but play the bagpipes and lower the flag to half-staff, there still may be hope! "The odds may be equal or they may actually favor recovery. But in hanging crepe the physician artificially imposes certainty or greatly exaggerates the probability of dying in a situation in which the outcome is uncertain."[2]

This is the time to act quickly. Honest, reflective doctors will hang crepe in a timely fashion or suggest a transfer without the need for clinical gimmicks. Others, self-deluded or fearful of the next doctor's criticism, will never offer or invite alternatives. For them, it's like Time Warner suggesting Verizon provide your high-speed connection. That's when you need your own high-speed connection—out and off to a new hospital.

It's hard to take the reins from the doctor who reigns. It's difficult to be responsible for your own loved one's transfer. But the answer to the question "is there better care out there?" is always "yes." "Is there a better chance for Mom if we transfer her to another facility?" The answer again is always "yes." So . . . "look, we trust you, doc, (even if you don't) and need you to do what's best. We know there are always different doctors with different skills and technology in different hospitals. We're fine with that. It's time to tell us who to see and where to go while there is any hope, otherwise . . ." As your voice trails off and your eyebrows lift, you've left only the faintest residue of an implied threat and dissatisfaction. Right now who cares about fault? Just get your gear together, organize your family, demand every scrap of paper from the medical record, and prepare the lifeboats while the ship is still afloat.

FINDING A HAVEN WITH A MAVEN

The time is short and the odds are long. The transfer should be supervised by the specialist in charge of the offending organ system. By this point in your care you have seen up to a dozen 'ologists. But usually there's only one troublemaker organ (like the heart, lungs, or kidneys) that got you into this mess in the first place. An errant organ will raise a ruckus that eventually involves the whole internal neighborhood. Hearts gone astray will soon involve the lungs, kidneys, and gut. Find the troublemaker's doctor. She's the one to arrange your transfer. Unless you've prepared for this moment (see below) all the decisions that precede your transfer will happen at a level above your skills but still under your scrutiny. This is *not* the time to start from scratch researching any particular doctor, for a particular problem, in a particular region, at a particular hospital.

Standing just a tad too close to Dr. Albee Zeinya, inform him that you expect that an expert at an exceptional hospital will be awaiting your arrival. A "Dear Dr. X" or a "Dear Hospital" referral letter pinned to your paper pajamas won't cut it.

AN ALTERNATIVE STRATEGY—AN INTERNET-BASED SEARCH

You need a transfer and you need it now. So many people come to grief staying too long at their local hospital. So many are then transferred to a facility that makes them pine for the one just left behind. There really should be a limit on what you are willing to accept on blind faith. I offer a plan that allows you to find a doctor and a hospital on your own. The doctor and hospital are chosen for quality but the emphasis is on proximity. Just as it is in real estate, so too for an emergency transfer—it's "location, location, location." Future problems are predictable if you have been treated for multi-organ disease, have an organ that's a real gorgon, or have been previously hospitalized and are left with some debility and difficulty with activities of daily living. This backup then becomes a lifeline. The doctor and hospital that are chosen can also serve as a built-in resource for second opinions. You can obtain the best care on your own or at least be able to offer opinions, alternatives, and the ability to verify the validity of a choice made by others. It must be done in advance but takes only minutes to perform.

An Internet-based search, using trusted hospital rating systems, the hospital's website, and the primary lesson offered in part 3, "Choosing Your Doctor," will provide an invaluable tool when you need someone in place, in a place, just in case. To start, we need a new Internet search priority.

Your first step is finding a site that *ranks* hospitals rather than one that *compares* them. So, so long WNTB. Enter *USNWR*'s 152 top-ranked hospitals and HGs' 269 "distinguished hospitals for clinical excellence."

It's time to make the acquaintance of *USNWR* and HGs. They will point the way to our two criteria—quality and proximity. If they are to be helpful tools you need to become a virtuoso when tickling the keys on these sites' links. Each URL requires a different suite of steps that allows entry into "best hospitals" based on specialty and location.

USNWR chooses its hospitals for their ability to provide advanced technology and support. HGs, in contrast, values more obscure hospitals in smaller cities. HGs "distinction hospitals" are not usually "destination hospitals." They are always fine as "desperation hospitals." An HGs choice is certainly safer than becoming a rolling stone in a hospital that's a complete unknown.

I think that your choice of the doctor and hospital will be at least as good as your own doctor's advice.

Let's set up a scenario that might help navigate these sites.

Search Scenario: "I need a cardiologist. I get chest pains. My doctor says it's angina. I ran into some trouble during my last hospitalization with heart failure. I need a regional backup doctor in the event of an emergency. I need someone that I can trust and who I can get to fast."

Step One: Finding the Hospital

Using USNWR

Each asterisk is a link to make and each hyphen is the new screen that comes up: www.usnews.com*-health*-best hospitals*-search by specialty*-heart and heart surgery*. On this page you'll see *USNWR*'s top heart hospitals. If one is nearby, your search for a hospital is over. There are fifty in the country in twenty-five states and thirty-eight cities. If you live in New York City, Boston, Chicago, Baltimore, or Houston you have multiple choices.

If you need to expand your search then select *search for heart and heart surgery hospitals. Then choose "by zip code" (13323 for Clinton, New York, where I live). The resulting list is of dozens of hospitals and their distance from my zip code. Each includes graphs on reputation, staffing, and survival. I would have to travel 175 miles to the nearest ranked *USNWR* hospital. I'd need a Helivac or a *really* fast ambulance.

Using HealthGrades

HealthGrades.com*-hospital ratings*-New York, and I selected our closest city, Syracuse. Then click on *select a procedure or diagnosis. I chose *coronary interventional procedure; right on top of the screen are a few Syracuse hospitals. St. Joseph Hospital Health Center is the first on the list. It has HGs' three-star rating (average) for survival during and one month after hospitalization. It was awarded five stars (the best rating) for six-month survival. Another click on St. Joe's brings you to HGs' St. Joe's page. Click on *awards and click to link to *patient safety ratings. The result is a mixed picture. But in the six-month survival column St. Joe gets five stars for 4 out of 5 diagnostic/therapeutic categories.

Is St. Joe a *USNWR* heart-ranked hospital? Do the search. We find that although HGs gives this hospital five stars, *USNWR* doesn't even give it a pat on the back. So it is with hospital ratings. What to do? It's off to St. Joseph with the confidence of HGs imprimatur. Of course you want the best of the best, but what you really need now is the "closest of the best"—we just found it.

Step 2: Finding the Doctor

You now have your backup hospital. We know that a good hospital alone is a Headless Horseman. So, getting out of Sleepy Hollow General requires a doctor as good as the hospital you've chosen. To find a doctor we go back to St. Joseph's. Get on St. Joseph Hospital Health Center website—a link away on either *USNWR* or HGs. On St. Joseph's site you want to choose a cardiologist rather than a cardiac surgeon from its physician directory. When in doubt always chose the medical doctor and avoid the surgeon. The cardiologist "physician search" brings up twenty names. Information on each is a link away. Remember that brains are the best predictor of job performance. The more brains the higher the skills. This fact is a settled issue for psychometricians and cognitive scientists. Recall that the recognition of brains requires consulting only one thing—the "writing on the wall"—their diplomas. An elite college, top medical school, and world-class training program are the "trinity for ability" that is the proxy for highly gifted doctor intellects. I soon found a doctor after several dead ends—one who had studied or worked at Georgetown (*USNWR* #23 for national universities), Massachusetts General Hospital (*USNWR* #4 for cardiology and cardiac surgery), and Harvard. 'Nuf said. No other information is needed. That's it—a fifteen-minute task. So get on *USNWR* and HGs. Find the closest ranked hospital for the specialty you need. Get on that hospital website and the physician directory. Go down the list and find one whose ability can be safely inferred from the quality of his educational trajectory that is confirmed on *USNWR*. Make the appointment, size him up. It's okay to tell him why you're there. A yearly visit is the engine for the ethical mandate that requires that he must make himself available to you any time if needed. This information is current for each site's 2010 directory. The data changes each year but the steps to reach your candidate hospitals and doctors don't. Do the work. Being on your last legs is no way to make a fast exit.

This section closes with a wish: "May all your care be local." If you need to go beyond your region it will be for unhappy reasons.

15

Searching for Solutions

- When your doctors have given up—it's not over yet! What to do when the news is bad.
- When is it time to seek the best doctors in our nation's greatest hospitals, regardless of location? Getting over "zip code phobia."
- Some people pass great hospitals on the way to bad ones. How far must you travel?
- What is the single variable that elevates a hospital and its doctors above all others?
- Why some hospitals could save your life while others would fail: "The ability to save"—pulling victory from the jaws of defeat.
- What's more important in your care—a great hospital or the great doctor in it? What is your first priority?
- The surgeries, procedures, and treatments you should NEVER have at your local or regional hospitals.
- If you are going to be put to sleep *for* it, are lying down *during* it, and will stay overnight *after* it, the two questions your surgeon *has* to answer. Learn how to judge the response.
- How to go it alone:
  - Shopping for your very own liver resection.
  - Getting over the "Get my aneurysm fixed? I don't know where to go to get my toaster fixed" fears.
  - Three Internet search techniques that give you better doctors and hospitals than your own physicians' recommendations.
  - Being the smartest and most up-to-date person in the room—at least for a little while.

- The *real* definition of "being your own advocate."
- How $20 can save your life when you're up against the wall.

SCENARIOS

You just received a diagnosis. The resulting shock requires its own recuperation before it's possible to address this terribly existentially threatening news.

There may be a less threatening diagnosis so uncommon your local doctor can't pronounce it, much less treat it—"Acrocephalosyndactylia! If I can't spell it, how can I Google it?"

Many times an established diagnosis proves resistant to all measures. You're forced to deal with the unhappy consequences of an uncontrolled disease state—the perpetual shortness of breath of chronic obstructive pulmonary disease; the painful neuropathy from diabetes; the abdominal pain of refractory Crohn's disease.

On other occasions your medical history is seen as a mystery. You are not reassured by "We checked you out thoroughly, there's nothing wrong. I'm happy for you." Your doctor's confusing his happiness with yours.

Others may suffer from end-stage organ failure—your heart's valves are fused, your cardiac muscle is too far gone, your coronary arteries cannot be approached surgically. You are left to your fate.

It may be that you're too old, too weak, too fat, too thin, too ill, too immunologically, nutritionally, or psychologically compromised to tolerate routine, let alone risky, interventions and therapies—"I wish we could . . . repair that abdominal aneurysm"; ". . . put you on Humira"; ". . . resect that pancreatic tumor, but . . ." There are times when the lack of local resources is assumed to mean that they are absent everywhere.

Finally some patient's problems will suffer no tools held by dilettantes or devoted amateurs. Other doctors try to raise their profile at the low end of a steep learning curve. When you need an advanced procedure or a complicated suite of algorithmically driven medical behaviors, you don't want someone who is "starting an experience."

It's time to expand your search horizons. It's time to go beyond your region. Scenarios like those above and many others that play out each year for several hundreds of thousands of you might require a transregional or transcontinental pilgrimage to a distant medical mecca. If your problem offers nothing more, it offers the time for research. It's time you can spend saving your own life. Never let anyone tell you to go home when you think there is more that can be done. There are dozens of surgical conditions and a host of medical ones that require a concentration of tools and talents so extraordinary, that they must be researched and then sought after. These are the unsettling times when no one opinion can be trusted.

Q&A

What is it that makes these places special? Volume.
How do you find what you need for your specific problem? Research.
Where are these lifesavers? Everywhere—maybe close to home.
Must I do the research alone? Sometimes.

What therapies demand a national APB?—The newest, least invasive interventions that only a handful of doctors perform, or the complex procedures that many do, but only a few do well.

Let's expand on these answers. Before you make a trip online, much less step on an airline, let's make sure you know what makes this exercise so worthwhile and which diseases and interventions benefit from it. Inconvenience, anxiety, and displacement carry a steep price. The reward is measured in the years added to your life and quality of life that you enjoy during those years. Be different. Live longer. Leave your hamlet and be like Hamlet when the "slings and arrows of outrageous fortune" strike.

VOLUMETRICS

There are a lot of conflicting claims over which hospital care-delivery model is best. All offer a combination of better care, safer care, superior outcomes, less mortality, the "ability to save," fewer errors, or a self-touted "culture of safety."

Happily you can ignore the claims. The best hospitals, regardless of their delivery-system model or the promises they make, all share one feature that makes the best stand alone from the rest—*volume*. It's the number of procedures performed and the number of patients treated that are a hospital's and doctor's proxy for quality. The volume-quality premise is accepted by the Institute of Medicine, the National Quality Institute (NQI), the LFG, and hundreds of published studies. Yes, there are criticisms and there are those who would suggest other variables. But *no one* subtracts a hospital's or doctor's volume of cases from the equation. For the reasons I will later list and for the conditions and techniques I will discuss, the questions, "how many of these has this hospital performed?" and "how many of these have *you* done, doctor?" more than any other inquiries provide the final common pathway to the best outcomes. "This relation between high volume and better outcomes is strong and persistent, with approximately 300 studies on the subject having been reported in the English-language literature"[1] The "*why* does volume count?" answer is harder to pin down than the fact that it does. In 2010 Edward H. Livingston and Jing Cao summarized the volume-quality association best: "Procedure volume does not directly affect procedure results; rather, it is a marker for other processes that influence outcomes."[2]

Many procedures, over time and with experience, become high-volume, low-mortality activities. These common interventions usually don't require planes, trains, and automobiles. Examples are colonoscopies, percutaneous coronary interventions, older radiologic and abdominal surgical techniques that are today's state of affairs but not medicine's state of the art. Even so there can be a 2 to 3 percent difference in outcomes depending on where you have them done. Small differences can result in large numbers when such exams are performed hundreds of thousands of times per year.

Volume's effect provides more than an improvement in mortality statistics. Its effect improves important quality of life issues. For example, after radical prostate surgery unpleasant urinary complaints and impotence occur more frequently in low-volume institutions, despite good mortality statistics.

There are a great number of procedures that many do but a few do well. Esophagectomy, pancreatectomy, liver and lung resections, abdominal aortic aneurysms, many cancer and vascular interventions, and HIV treatments are always cited as the high-risk interventions that carry unacceptable mortality at low-volume hospitals. Coronary artery bypass surgery, carotid endarterectomy, bariatric surgery, and organ transplants also demonstrate the benefits of volume.

Finally it's only the high-volume institutions that can offer ultra high-tech low-volume procedures. These state-of-the-art marvels will be tomorrow's routines. For now they are cloistered at large, high-volume centers. These complex medical and surgical interventions benefit from coordinated teams, the absolute mastery of technical sequencing, and fine motor skills and keen depth perception possessed by those with flexible and focused cognitive abilities. They can only flourish in research centers. The laparoscopic, thorascopic, minimally invasive, single port, trans-oral, trans-vaginal, trans-umbilical, percutaneous endovascular, and robotic interventions performed today treat hundreds of thousands of patients for bowel, heart, kidney, stomach, lung, prostate, and vascular conditions. Beating heart, minimally invasive coronary artery and percutaneous nonsurgical cardiac valvular repairs are becoming common at these institutions and are impossible to perform elsewhere.

Surprisingly it's not hard to find a team that minimizes risk through almost flawless performance. The travel time to these institutions and doctors may not be that long.

Doctor versus hospital—who gets the "thank you note"? Is it the hospital or its doctors that makes the difference between your being a surgical candidate or being sent home to your fate? Who's more important to your outcome—the high-volume facility or the high-volume surgeon? It depends. The correct choice can promise a result that is as stark as that between life and death, or as subtle as the postoperative quality of life. In general, high-volume surgeons get better results when working at low-volume hospitals then do low-volume surgeons at high-volume hospitals. Usually the best results occurred when the adjective "high-volume" is shared by both.

The authors of a clinical study that was published by the *New England Journal of Medicine* looked at the national analytic files from the government's Centers for Medicare and Medicaid Services. They evaluated the results for eight high-risk cardiovascular and cancer procedures that a half-million patients underwent during that period. The surgeons get the "thank you note" from a high of 100 percent of the time for aortic valve surgery to a low of 24 percent for lung resections.[3] It makes sense. If the procedure requires advanced surgical skills with a predictably short hospital stay, most of the crucial services are performed by the surgeon (carotid endarterectomy and bariatric surgery). If the procedure will reliably result in a lengthy stay because of the nature of the technique and the high-risk profile of its patients (abdominal aortic aneurysms and major cancer surgeries), then the hospital gets a big share of the credit. It is for these types of problems that you rely on the hospital to provide crucial support services. It's here that the hospital's "ability to save" will save the day and your life, making your journey worthwhile. In October 2009 the *New England Journal of Medicine* noted that even great hospitals' patients get postoperative complications. The study showed on average 1 in 6 patients will develop severe difficulties. What makes these hospitals great is their "ability to save"—to pull victory from the jaws of defeat.[4]

The achievements of these hospitals are more than the quality provided by the sum of its parts. Institutional ethics, pride, teamwork, supervision, and protocols promote an overarching institutional personality that is recognized, not just nationally, but across the globe. These are the gems that adorn the otherwise battered crown of contemporary American medicine.

OKAY, THANKS ALREADY— BUT HOW *MUCH* VOLUME COUNTS?

Many authors use the LFG list as their benchmark. Leapfrog lists seven high-risk surgical procedures with its "recommended annual hospital volume/ (recommended annual surgeon volume)":

1. Coronary artery bypass graft (CABG) ≥ 450
2. Percutaneous coronary intervention ≥ 400

3. Abdominal aortic aneurysm repair $\geq$ 50
4. Aortic valve replacement $\geq$ 120
5. Pancreatic resection $\geq$ 11
6. Esophagectomy $\geq$ 13
7. Bariatric surgery $\geq$ 125[5]

According to Eric Peterson and associates your hospital has to perform at least 150 CABGs to be considered worthy of your care.[6]

Ethan Halm and associates distinguished high-volume vs. low-volume physicians for a variety of conditions.[7] When you need a percutaneous coronary intervention (angioplasty or stent), seventy-five a year isn't enough. Shoot for the doctor who does 140.

Only eight carotid endarterectomies a year? Thirty's more like it.

Shopping for an elective repair of an aortic aneurysm? Two's too few. Ten's enough.

Needing pancreatic surgery is bad enough. Nine = nein. A doctor who does forty-two a year is a pro.

Your prospective surgeon does ten breast cancer surgeries a year? Not for you. Fifty cases performed each year defines high volume and defies bad results.

If you choose a low-volume surgeon for your lung cancer surgery, your mortality rate is ten times higher than it would be if you had chosen a high-volume maestro. Twenty cases per year seem like plenty but you want the doctor who does a hundred.

Almost every observer goes on to suggest that cancer surgery be performed by surgical oncologists. These are cancer surgery specialists. For their respective organ systems they are usually ultra high-volume providers and only work in high-volume hospitals.

Cancer surgeries are amongst the most challenging interventions. In 2007 the volume-quality guru John Birkmeyer offered a guideline. High-volume thresholds for five types of cancer surgeries are listed below.[8]

Bladder cancer: Low volume—3 cases a year. High-volume specialists start at 8 cases but some have 82 bladders under their belts (sorry couldn't resist it).

Colon cancer: 43 cases a year is a low volume. Shoot for the expert with 100–300 cases a year.

Esophageal cancer: 4 cases a year is no experience at all. There are surgeons you can find who perform 15–100 each year.

Pancreatic cancer: For Birkmeyer, 2 cases a year isn't even close. High-volume mavens are those who perform 8 to over 100 cases a year.

Stomach cancer: 7 cases a year doesn't stack up to high-volume surgeons who do up to 135 per annum.

In 2010, Joseph E. Ross et al. weighed in on volume considerations for three common conditions. Heart attack victims did best when the annual hospital volume reached 610 patients. For heart failure, the best results were reached at 500 patients per year, and for pneumonia, 210 cases per year. These numbers defined high volume and best results. Higher numbers per year conferred no additional benefit.[9] Thinking about bariatric surgery? In 2010 it's better to slim down using a hospital with 150–300 cases per year and a doctor who performs at least 150 cases per year.[10] In 2010, an important study revealed that if you are elderly with multiple medical problems you may be better off in a high-volume center for many common as well as complicated procedures.[11]

Even if you're armed with the numbers offered here, it may prove difficult to wrest that information from a doctor, much less his hospital. The high-volume, low-mortality doctors will usually be more than happy to tell you all about themselves, their training, their high-volume numbers, and their outstanding results.

You must ask your prospective surgeon two questions: "How many have you done? How many deaths and complications occurred?" Do not accept national statistics. You already know those numbers from *your* research completed long before the visit. You are only interested in the results for one doctor—the one sitting across from you. The answer to your question is not a discourse. It's a number. No general answers are acceptable for volume—"Gee, a lot. It's hard to keep track." General answers for his mortality and complication rates for your surgery are equally unacceptable— "the vast majority do just great." The dealbreaker answer is, "I've never had a patient complication or mortality for this procedure." If you are going to be put to sleep *for* it, are lying down *during* it, and will stay overnight *after* it, that answer is a lie. All doctors know their volumes as surely as their golf scores. Each doctor lives and suffers through every mortality. Every doctor remembers his complications. Complications do not escape the stamp of memory, they reinforce it. The memories of my failures live in my thoughts and inhabit my dreams. I remember each death and lengthy complication and the names of those who suffered because in medical parlance, "I owned them." How these questions are answered will be as revealing as the answers themselves. Watch the body language. Listen carefully to the tone of their responses.

The accretion of a hospital's case volume occurs for many reasons. Good outcomes promote high referral volume, high referral volume promotes good outcomes. "Quality is volume, volume is quality." Just as "Beauty is truth, truth is beauty," so too for the quality-volume issue, and "that is all ye know on earth and all ye need to know." That's John Keats' "Ode on a Grecian Urn." For the quality-volume conundrum it's the "road to what accretion earns."

WHEN ONLY QUALITY COUNTS—FINDING
YOUR HIGH-VOLUME DOCTOR AND HOSPITAL

The Doctor Search

Despite the nosebleedingly rarified atmosphere these citadels of care project, the resources they require, and the superior outcomes they offer—they're everywhere. As I noted earlier, for local care start with the doctor. Recall that a gifted local doctor can transcend the weaknesses of an underachieving community hospital. There are far more gifted doctors where you live then there are great hospitals. When the tables have turned on your fortunes, you must turn the tables on your search priorities. When the news is bad and you need the best doctor, you must first find the best hospital. It's a big country. In it there are tens of thousands of excellent clinicians perched +2 standard deviations from the mean. There are, however, only several dozen truly remarkable health-care centers. It's encouraging to know that there are wonderful doctors every place you look, but right now you are looking for only one place—the uncommon hospital that delivers uncommon doctors.

Looking for a concert cellist in New York? Don't check the yellow pages. Don't ask around. Don't even go to your local community orchestra. You're going to Lincoln Center, right? That's where the best cellists hang out. It's the same for hospitals. The concentration of the best talents at the best hospitals is not serendipitous. That's why you start at the best hospitals—that's where the best doctors hang out. We've learned that when you're stricken the chances of recovery are dependent first on the talents of the doctor and only then the hospital's. Have both? Priceless.

Top Hospitals

USNWR enjoys an advantage over HGs. *USNWR* hospitals are chosen precisely for patients who have the most difficult and challenging problems that require truly outstanding care. An honor roll hospital must be at least +2 standard deviations from the mean in at least six of sixteen specialties. That's why we'll use the *USNWR* ranking system. You're now looking for "destination hospitals," not HGs' "desperation hospitals." The priority for a regional hospital search is its short distance from home. The priority for a national hospital is its long distance from the mean.

Keeping with our scenario of looking for a cardiologist, we keep in mind that proximity is no longer primary. So off we go to *USNWR* 2010 rankings: USnews.com*-health*-best hospitals*-search by specialty*-heart and heart surgery*-best hospitals heart and heart surgery. Pick amongst the first twenty-five on the list. They are located in fifteen states in twenty cities distributed across our country. Pick the closest city or one with friends and family. Make the choice and then link to its hospital website and, as we demonstrated earlier, check out the cardiologists on the hospital's physician directory. Find the one whose educational trajectory gives you the best chance for success. All of the top hospitals have top websites. Often a doctor's webpage will provide a photograph, inform you of her hobbies, and provide a mission statement and personal data, as well as her publications, awards, and honors. If this doctor turns out to be a poor match you don't need to change hospitals—just doctors. Unlike most health-care facilities there will be plenty of them to choose from. The best teams have the deepest benches. So do the best hospitals.

No one wants to be far from home. But when you are under the cloud of a worrisome problem most of you will travel with your own entourage. When you travel with these Knights Templar that are your family the world becomes your cloister. When you travel to the "bigs" almost all will have facilities for your family. The UCLA's Tiverton House is a 100-room hotel. New York Presbyterian offers guest facilities and a free shuttle. Most of the cities that have the top hospitals may well have a fan club of family and friends already in place. For the sake of what this hospital can deliver, you can make up with your older sister. Sure she has some annoying habits. And how about those facial tics! But she lives in Los Angeles, home to two big-league heart hospitals. You've paid a king's ransom for your daughter's education at Boston College. Well she lives there now. So do two top-ranked cardiology hospitals.

You may not even need to move your watch forward or backward when you arrive at your destination hospital. A high-risk surgery may turn out to be a low-mileage journey. "Access to hospitals for the highest risk procedures can be accomplished without imposing unreasonable travel burdens on most patients. Most patients required to have surgery at a higher-volume center would add fewer than 30 minutes to their travel times. Travel times for many patients would actually decrease. . . . Many patients travel past a higher-volume center to undergo surgery at a low-volume hospital."[12] So take an extra hour. Take five! Get to that great hospital's best doctor.

Disease-Centered Searches: Another Way of Finding the Right Doctor in the Right Hospital

Do you need a successful neurosurgery without the surgery? How about a nice transcranial magnetic resonance–guided high-intensity focused ultrasound? It's not offered at your friendly local neurosurgeon's office.

Too sick and too old for that aortic valve replacement? Maybe not. It can be performed through a small incision or puncture in your groin. A thin catheter can be inserted into an artery, placing a new valve in your heart without incisions or sutures. You won't find *that* around the block.

This list can go on and on. There are alternatives to the "go home and die" decrees that are given (hopefully more tactfully) to many previously thought too ill, inoperable, or at excessive risk for extreme interventions. These procedures are also the "get home and back to work faster and safer" options to the healthy who want the best possible proven technologies provided by experienced, undisputed leaders in their fields. The doctors who perform them are pioneers. In several years they will be found in most mid- to large-size communities. How to find one now?

Got twenty bucks? Where do you start both your research and your search? There is only one site—UpToDate.com (UTD). It is simply the undisputed best source for the most current medical information. It benefits from evidence-based clinical data but doesn't turn away from expert opinion, consensus, and high-quality observational studies. This site is a definitive end source for hundreds of thousands of doctors, hospitals, and medical education centers. All for $500 a year. What? You don't need it for a year? You don't have $500? How about $20? Twenty dollars offers a one-week full-access pass to UTD. For our purposes it will also point us to those doctors who have "written the book" on whatever ails you. So, if you have three things—a big problem, a few minutes to research it, and $20—you can find the doctor and the hospital more likely to be of help than your own doctor's referrals.

When AAA Isn't Your Auto Club

You have an abdominal aortic aneurysm (AAA). It's a bulge on the wall of the aorta—the main artery that supplies blood from your heart to every organ in your body (except the lungs). If the wall weakens it can rupture, an event only 30 percent survive. The surgery that prevents this catastrophe is elective and requires experience. It's on everyone's list of surgeries that require high-volume doctors in high-volume centers. Anything less can triple your mortality. There are, however, minimally invasive options for its repair. An increasing number of surgeries have newer, less invasive little cousin techniques you may never have heard of. You never needed to, but now you do. That $20 UTD pass allows you to learn about aneurysms, minimally invasive procedures, and a lot of information that's important to know when facing a major decision. You'll want to read about an endovascular procedure. This intervention places a stent through a blood vessel that is then positioned across the site of the weakened arterial wall, thus shoring it up. It's performed through small punctures or incisions on both sides of the groin. The pros and cons of each method are learned on this UTD search. What else do you get? *Experts.* In the UTD search box enter "abdominal aortic aneurysm" or any keyword that's relevant to your problem. The portals to UTD's articles will appear. Each article is relatively free from arcane medical cant. Choose "natural history and management of abdominal aortic aneurysm." When you're looking for an expert, you can start with the entry's authors or its section editors. Those who are chosen to write or edit these sections are doctors who are at the top of their game. Their bios are a link away. For surgical conditions, look for professors or associate professors of surgery (not medicine). One of the section's authors of the AAA chapter is a surgeon. He is from the Hospital of the University of Pennsylvania. That's a good start. It's a member of *USNWR*'s Best Hospitals Honor Roll. Link to the hospital website and go to the physician directory. Either search for the doctor's name in the directory or find him in the Surgery Department listings. Now do the research on his training. It's always on his page on the hospital website. Note that he's trained at elite centers. He is the chief of the Vascular Surgery service. Note that his area of interest is in AAA repair and aortic aneurysm stent placement. He was recognized by *America's Top Doctors* in 2007, 2008, and 2010. He's got it all (except 2009), so make the call. Sometimes you won't be able to find the author or authors at the institution from which the section was written. These elite doctors are fast climbers and quick jumpers. They are stars on the rise or czars who have risen to chair new departments and share their techniques. You can Google their names to find where they've landed—perhaps closer to home.

This search technique has given you a diagnosis that you can research, in depth, and a doctor who wrote the book and who also works in a hospital of national renown. Isn't it worth the trip?

An Alternative Search Technique on UTD

This one is more difficult but provides a different tier of clinicians. These are the men and women who pioneer new procedures that others only write about. They don't summarize the data for others to read—they provide it.

You've been told you have a cancer in your left kidney. The good news—it's localized, stage I. If you go to UTD and search kidney cancer, eight articles appear. Choose "Overview of the Prognosis and Treatment of Renal Cell Cancer." Read about your problem, the staging process, and the reassuring 95 percent five-year survival for stage I. On this site you read about minimally invasive surgeries for kidney cancer. You want more information. There's an article that might be just for you—"Radiofrequency Ablation and Cryoablation for Renal Cell Cancer." All the discussions on UTD have footnotes that are linkable. Each link brings you an abstract of the original source material. The abstract summarizes the original article's results and includes the information on the hospital its authors work from. See the link to the reference on radiofrequency ablation and select it. In front of you will be the précis of a current article describing the authors' experience with over one hundred of these procedures. The authors are from the department of urology at the Mayo Clinic. Get on *USNWR* and note it's on their Best Hospitals Honor Roll list and is ranked #1 in the country for kidney disorders and #3 in urology. From *USNWR*, link to the hospital's website and search for the authors of this article. On the directory you will find several of them. One is Harvard- and Mayo-trained and has a list of publications a foot long. Enough said. Make the call. This guy makes Lance Armstrong look like a slacker. If you are elderly with multiple comorbidities, this, or another minimally invasive technique, may be your best chance and perhaps your only chance. If you're healthy it's nice to know you're in good hands.

It's daunting to go shopping all by yourself for your esophagectomy, hepatectomy, pulmonary lobectomy, or your robotic "this" or laparoscopic trans-whazzis "that." When the stakes are high you will have to pull them up to find a place that saves your life or makes it longer or more comfortable.

Making medical decisions and choices that take you far afield without the professional help of your own doctor may seem unrealistic. "Get my aneurysm fixed? I don't know where to go to get my toaster fixed." But sometimes it is wise to have the survival skills of a Bear Grylls. On his television show *Man versus Wild* he tells us, "I'll show you how to survive in places you wouldn't last a day." We watch him, other Brits, Canadians, and Australians on television (why no Americans?) deal with cruel conditions. Someday you may need to deal with your own cruel condition. However unlikely it is that a survivalist's environment will be encountered in your suburban existence, someday it will be your own body that becomes an unsafe environment that threatens your existence. You may need survivalist skills when your problems become as punishing as any jungle, desert, or mountaintop. Your chance of being a survivor drop off dramatically if, when accepting a doctor's referral, you take your orders and march off dutifully without skills, tools, or questions.

These searches are survival tools and at the very least prevent you from becoming a passive third-party recipient of others' advice. Even for routine care it's not wise to be an empty vessel for others' plans.

How often do you hear the call to "be your own advocate"? It's now a television catchphrase or becomes a cliché like "tell the doctor about all your medications." Rubbish! How often are you told *how* to be your own advocate? Here's how. You can at least confirm the validity of your referral. You can offer your own personal research and let your own family doctor explore and evaluate your choices. When it's your life that's on the line your doctor should be online or on the line to verify *your* choices. With today's information access technologies enabled by Internet-based search engines, you can be the smartest person in the room. Your "genius" status is for a limited amount of data and for a limited period of time. But for that data and during that time you are someone to be reckoned with. Your own doctor's plans and repertoire lie within his own boundaries and are influenced by his own biases. We've discussed each doctor's unique perimeters and parameters. There are times you must be ready to journey beyond those limitations. Sure, leave a trail of bread crumbs to find your way back. But don't be afraid. You haven't left your computer screen, much less your home. Yet. Yes, a trip may be expensive. And yes, you can and should keep using these techniques to look for resources as close to home as possible. There are other ways to search for solutions but none should reflexively bow to the whims of your family doctor's referrals. There is no method he will employ that enjoys the rigor of *USNWR* methodology and the advice I offered in chapter 7. There is no other method that places before you the information and experts found on UTD. Aside from the $20 for the week pass, it's all free. While doing your laps on your laptop you may run into a dead end here and there. But I think it is less likely you'll experience a personal one if you use these search techniques while partnering up with your own doctor.

A patient's reach should exceed his doctor's grasp, else what's an Internet for?

V

HOSPITAL DANGERS AND HOW TO PREVENT THEM

16

Hospital Dangers: Introduction

- Will you, your child, or parents be hospitalized this year? It's more likely than you think.
- Are hospital-wide error rates in line with aviation's record?
  - Some examples of error rates in common procedures and treatments.
  - Why a hospital's 99.9 percent proficiency rate is not *nearly* good enough.
- Dying while "healthy" in our hospitals: low mortality mortalities.
- How many Americans die, become injured or debilitated, or suffer psychological trauma in hospitals?
  - It's *many* more than you've been told. What is being done about it?
  - Why error rates have not improved for years.
  - Why you must play a role when you are, in fact, on your own.

In the words of Virginia Woolf, those who are ill are no longer "soldiers in the Army of the upright." Now deserters, "the whole landscape of life lies remote and far, like a shore seen from a ship far out at sea. . . . To look these things squarely in the face would need the courage of a lion tamer," or "a robust philosophy."[1]

It's time to foster that courage and develop those philosophies before you are sick enough to need them. It's time to categorize the types of danger you will face during your hospital stay. More importantly it's time to predict where, when, and why errors occur and learn how to avoid them at each choke point where they are predictable and preventable.

"Thanks, but really, I'm feeling fine." Most people view a hospitalization as a future vague possibility. Although we are able to project ourselves in an almost limitless number of real-life or wish-fulfilling scenarios, we rarely mull over migraines, obsess about obstructions, or plan for our pleurisy.

You can count on a hospitalization for you or a member of your immediate family to occur . . . soon. How soon? Over 25 million (8% of us) will stay overnight in the hospital in the next year. Twelve percent of seniors, 6% of the middle-aged, 5.5% of young adults, 2% of teens, and 6.7% of our younger children will stay in the hospital in the coming year.[2] So when 9% of your children and up to 18% of your parents face a hospitalization, it *is* time to do more than reflect. A 2009 Deloitte study of a representative sample of 4,000 Americans found that 20% were hospitalized the preceding year. Right now 100,000 of our citizens are fighting for their lives in our country's ICUs. Five million of us will join their ranks this coming year and 14% won't be going home.[3] More than 2% of patients who experience the less-intensive brand of hospital care won't survive it.[4]

Perhaps you are reassured by the highly publicized efforts in your behalf by the Agency for Healthcare Research and Quality (AHRQ), the Leapfrog Group (LFG), and the Institute of Medicine (IOM).

The AHRQ focuses on forty-five core measures that represent the most important indicators of health-care quality. Across these measures the median level of receipt of recommended care is only 59 percent. The annual rate of improvement in care delivered in hospitals is only 3 percent. The majority of patient safety measures showed no improvement during the six-year study period, and overall safety measures declined 1 percent a year.[5]

Not too sick to worry? The AHRQ notes that death rates from low-mortality admissions did not improve between 2000 and 2005. "When patients are admitted and die in the treatment of low risk illnesses or procedures healthcare errors are more likely than in deaths of patients with high risk illnesses."[6] The AHRQ puts the "low mortality" diagnoses death rate at 0.5 per thousand patients. HGs puts it at 1.7 per thousand. Not too bad, right? But based on 20 million non-ICU hospital admissions per year, up to 34,000 of us will die "healthy" in hospitals each year. A large multiple of that number are rescued at the price of debility, pain, and severe psychological trauma.

In 2009, the LFG released its hospitals survey results. Using standards endorsed by the major federal and nonprofit patient safety clearinghouses (the Joint Commission, the Centers for Medicare and Medicaid Services, and the National Quality Forum), the results are equally grim. Only 7 percent of hospitals fully met LFG's medical error prevention standards. Sixty-nine percent of its hospitals did not fully meet ICU physicians staffing standards. For several commonly performed procedures, no hospital ranked above a compliance level of 24 percent with LFG's "Efficiency of Care" standards. Finally, 65 percent of LFG hospitals do not have all the recommended policies in place to prevent hospital-acquired infections (HAI).[7]

Ten years after the IOM publication of *To Err Is Human*, a scathing indictment of our country's medical practices, little appears to have changed. The Consumers Union, an independent, nonprofit information organization, stated in 2009 that "there is little evidence to suggest that the number of people dying from medical harm has dropped since the IOM first warned about these deadly mistakes a decade ago."[8]

In 2010 HealthGrades reported that there has been no improvement in patient safety for three years. Patient safety measurements are frozen on one million incidents per year. In 2010 the *New England Journal of Medicine* waded into this issue and then weighed in on its findings. The authors' conclusion: "we found that harm resulting from medical care was common, with little evidence that the rate of harm had decreased substantially over a 6-year period ending in December 2007."[9] Whatever the source, there is no evidence that medical error and the resulting deaths and injuries have decreased since that landmark report. So, despite task forces, national conferences, governmental oversight, expert panels, editorials, position papers, and public outcry, you are still all but on your own when facing the dangers of hospitalization.

Perhaps overstated? In 2008, *Time* magazine named Peter Pronovost, a critical care researcher and anesthesiologist, as one of the world's 100 most influential leaders. He joined the ranks of the likes of Barak Obama, Bill Gates, and the Dalai Lama. So, when he wrote "performance in virtually every facet of medicine is most often unknown or suboptimal, and the tools to self-monitor performance nonexistent,"[10] you know it's so. Fast-forward to 2010 and Pronovost, having achieved rock-star status in medical circles, seems especially gloomy and a little pissed off. "Despite a decade-long effort to improve safety, there is limited empirical evidence of improved patient outcomes." He notes that an estimated 100,000 patients die of health-care–associated infections, another 44,000 to 98,000 die of other preventable errors, and tens of thousands more die of diagnostic errors or failure to receive recommended therapies. He blames physician arrogance, faulty teamwork, and hospital leaders.[11]

From the moment you arrive until the second you leave—your hospital, any hospital, is the most unsafe environment most of you will ever enter.

Six Sigma is not a college fraternity. But it is a fraternity of businesses and industries. The health-care industry is pledging this "frat house" but its prospects are dim.

Six Sigma is a quality improvement system that demands transformational change to improve product safety and consumer satisfaction. Through its methodologies and technologies, Six Sigma minimizes error rates to razor-thin margins of acceptability. For Six Sigma, a process, product, or performance cannot produce a frequency of error or variation greater than 3.4 instances in one million. Six Sigma rules when even a 99.9 percent proficiency rate is not nearly good enough. In the aviation industry, a 99.9 percent level of achievement translates into twenty-eight commercial airline crashes a day![12] US air carrier's error rates are 0.43 per million (99.999957% error free). In aviation, errors are viewed as inevitable. Despite this, products are protected from flaws and people from harm by strictly standardized protocols. Checklists are inviolate and performance is monitored ruthlessly and frequently. For the medical care industry, errors are passed right along the assembly line until they arrive directly at your bedside. The aviation industry performs exhaustive analyses of its near misses. The health-care industry doesn't examine its head-on collisions.

Twelve years ago Mark Chassin, currently the president of the Joint Commission, asked a question, "Is healthcare ready for Six Sigma quality?"[13]

He noted that, "in healthcare quality, problems frequently occur at orders of 200,000–500,000 per million" (!). Other authors have pointed to laboratory and pathology error rates between 500 and 300,000 per million.[14] When the most basic, even primitive, method of patient identification—the wristband—is noted subject to an error rate of 6,500 per million,[15] it's time to step back in wonder and horror.

Well, all these studies were, after all, ten to thirteen years ago. Have the Six Sigma methods, in light of the IOM's recommendations, taken root in the soil of American medicine? No again. Can the American health-care industry be described as ready for Six Sigma's radical organizational changes, paradigmatic shifts, and systemwide changes? You don't need any more evidence than the fact that in 2009, 50 to 70 percent of doctors don't engage in the single most important behavior that prevents deadly hospital-acquired infections—washing their hands!

Between 2000 and 2005 accidental puncture or laceration during surgery occurred at Six Sigma embarrassment rate of 3,500 per million. Postoperative wound separation—2,800 per million. Foreign bodies left in patients postoperatively occur from 10 per million patients to 1,000 per million.[16]

In 2009, the most recent evaluation of Six Sigma in health care identified only a handful of medical centers that were reliably working toward Six Sigma and other industry standards. The rest were, at least in part, Sick Sigmas. "Furthermore frequently absent was any attention to changes in organizational culture or substantial evidence of lasting effects from their efforts."[17]

Profits of billions per year are more important than achieving 3.4 errors per million per year. Although some correction measures are succeeding, they are often grudging and occur hospital by hospital and state by state. In the absence of a systemwide abhorrence of patient harm, the job of protecting yourself devolves, in part, to you. Hey, you've learned that you can go it alone when obtaining the best possible care. You also need to protect yourself while receiving it. Medical care is so complex, communications so primitive, and preventable errors so common, that if you are in an ICU, "nearly all suffer a potential life-threatening error at some point during their stay."[18] No more need be said when, in 2010, prescription errors on a pediatric unit (using a paper system) occurred at a Six Sigma rate of 130,000 errors per million and administration errors were at 190,000 per million.[19]

Twenty years ago when life (and death) was simpler, each patient in the ICU required 178 separate daily clinical "activities."[20] Since then, in the face of the algorithmic increase in medical complexity, the number of activities per patient has increased proportionately. Proficiency rates in that twenty-year-old study approached 99 percent. (The authors noted 1.7 errors per day while performing the 178 activities.) We have already noted that even a 99.9 percent proficiency rate can result in calamity. Today the rate of competency is certainly lower in light of the greater number of steps carried out by a greater number of personnel performing a greater number of complex tasks in a system almost immune to improvement.

So today, those 1.7 errors per day noted in 1989 are looking pretty good. But those days, almost Amish in their simplicity, are long gone in light of the preceding evidence that the health-care industry that deals with flesh, blood, and bone doesn't reach the competency levels that other industries demand when dealing with nuts, bolts, and bricks. For our purposes it's irrelevant whether adverse events arise from carelessness, from work and scheduling overloads, or as the consequences of any enterprise carried out by fallible humans and their institutions. Errors are not failures in character but of process. While they are not invariably associated with negligence, they are routinely associated with a failure in standards. You can't change these things from your hospital bed. It's not possible. It's not your job. It *is* possible to prevent the errors that will complicate your course, delay your recovery, and cause pain, debility, and even death. This is true despite the fact that most of these activities occur beyond your purview and are performed by personnel, invisible and anonymous. How is this possible? Regardless of the thousands of preceding procedural steps it's actually the distance in steps—from your door to your bedside—that counts. These few paces are the choke point and the final common pathway where error occurs and can be stopped. This section advises you how to avoid and prevent medication error, hospital-acquired infection, and the psychological trauma that, in combination, are inevitable during any hospital stay.

Numbers benumb more than stun. As symbols, they separate us from the human aspect of the event. Most importantly, these deaths and injuries occur behind hospital walls and are hidden from view. How do we make these hidden deaths come alive as the tragedies they truly are? Will it take the medieval cry, "Bring out your dead!" to provoke institutional action or your own individual reaction? Any numbers cited here are expressed in ranges that should be seen as minimum estimates. The lack of transparency wrought by fears of civil actions, the loss of institutional reputations, and privacy issues exists in a system of voluntary reporting. Bureaucratic mazes make each state border and hospital record-room door informational barriers rather than conduits.

There is no single study that reliably addresses iatrogenic events ("deaths by doctor"). Each offers only a tiny eyehole into a galaxy of events and practices, most of which go unreported while others are shielded from public scrutiny.

According to Dr. James Bagian, director of the National Center for Patient Safety of the Department of Veterans Affairs, the "close calls" you don't know about (but your hospital does) are estimated to occur between 10 and 200 times more frequently than the sentinel events that you do know about. Close calls don't count if you're not a Six Sigma industry.[21]

Assuming HGs is correct (93,000–195,000 deaths per year), the numbers who die in hospitals from medical error each year is the equivalent of three jumbo jets crashing every two days.[22] Even the IOM's estimate (44,000–98,000 deaths per year), the lowest in the literature, is the equivalent in carnage to a packed jumbo jet crashing every other day. Our (my) medical care industry is almost immune from accountability and the public has largely grown inured to outrage.

17

Medication Errors

- When, where, why, and how they occur.
- The choke point where most medical errors converge.
- Avoiding medication errors.
- High-risk drugs and dangerous drug combinations: they *can* be avoided.
- Avoiding the wrong pill or the wrong dose of the right one.
- Avoiding the medications you *don't* need.
- Which drugs are you on that your doctor will *never* stop, even when you stop needing them?
- Identity errors—the failed twenty-year struggle to "be yourself." Why can't hospitals give you an accurate identification wristband?

Two million Americans experience harmful adverse drug reactions (ADRs) each year. One hundred thousand die from them.[1, 2] There is near-universal agreement that 30 to 50 percent of these errors are preventable.

When people are hospitalized, the chance of error and injury increases in lockstep with the severity of the illness and the intensity and complexity of the care. Drug reactions account for one in five of all adverse events that occur in the hospital.[3] The percentage of patients who experience medical error ranges from under 1 percent to over 30 percent.[4] Most observers agree that up to 750,000 patients are exposed to a serious ADR each year and that fatal drug-related events are between the fourth and sixth leading cause of death in the United States.[5]

The medical literature's most alarming report is that 6 percent of all in-hospital deaths are due, in part, to a drug-related event.[6]

Other investigators parse the risks in a more accessible fashion by stating that 1 in 4 potentially harmful errors occur per patient per admission[7] and that one actual medical error will occur per patient per day.[8] It can also be stated that in a 200-bed hospital a serious medical error occurs every three hours.[9] This is not a problem limited to the frail and elderly. Your children are not immune to Six Sigma outrages. A company that makes your children's toys may not tolerate over 3.4 errors per million, but our hospitals treat its youngest patients to 1,230–4,700 ADR errors per million.[10]

Everyone agrees that despite the historically high rate of ADRs, the numbers are increasing. One observational study showed that there was a 2.7-fold increase in ADRs and deaths reported to the FDA between 1998 and 2005.[11] These numbers are best-guess estimates. Hospitals are not required to report ADRs. The four major medical agencies responsible for medical error data analysis receive no more than 1 to 10 percent of the total.[12] In the face of this onslaught of error you need to protect yourself. You can. The next section examines the types of medication errors and offers advice on their avoidance.

MEDICATION ERRORS—RECONCILIATION ERRORS

Your doctor doesn't know you. Fewer than one-third of patients are seen in the hospital by their family doctors.[13] Fewer than 25 percent of you know the name of the physician in charge of your care[14] and fewer than half of you know the name of your medications.[15] This is the starting point for medication errors. Enter reconciliation errors. Anytime you offer your medical history and someone else listens, writes, summarizes, dictates, transcribes, or transfers it across different sites of care it's like a game of Chinese Whispers—it changes with each retelling. All it takes are new faces in different places. Reconciliation errors start the moment you walk into the hospital; they follow you in it and tag along home after you've left it. Fifty percent of all medication errors occurred at hospital admission and discharge. A 2010 study revealed that for 470 studied admissions 71.9 percent had one or more unintentional discrepancies.[16] The rest occur when you are transferred from floor to floor. Errors, and the potential for harm, occur at a rate of 1.4 per patient per stay.[17] Medication sleights of hand occur when long-standing medication regimens are incorrectly stopped—"now you take them, and now you don't."

You'll have to reconcile yourself to this fact and do the reconciliation yourself.

Preventing Reconciliation Errors

You need to provide a gold standard medication history to avoid reconciliation errors. Here's how. Ask if the hospital has a clinical pharmacist. A history taken and reviewed by one of these professionals is much less likely to contain medication errors. No clinical pharmacist? That's okay. You can go it alone and provide a gold standard medication history. It assures you that your history will be both received and transmitted accurately. Start off by showing your health-care professional that you are a different type of patient. Tell the staffer that you are aware of hospital admission reconciliation errors.

Never describe your pills. That "beige capsule" could be your blood pressure medication, the Alzheimer's therapy Razadyne, or thirteen other beige capsules on the market today. Never verbally offer the names of your medications. Don't read them off a gold standard list. This makes them susceptible to "soundalike errors" (see below). Don't even spell their names. That's when the classic alphabetical and numerical phonetic errors come out to play. If grandma uses the military alphabet, is "Alpha, Charlie, Tango, Oscar, Sierra" her diabetes medication or is she calling in a SWAT team?

The gold standards are your pill bottles. Medical lists offer what others suppose you are taking (assumed as true) or what you are supposed to be taking (believed to be true). Only your pill bottles document what you are *actually* taking.

Show the nurse each bottle. Await its transcription and then *tell* her to repeat back its name, dose, frequency, and indication (the reason it was prescribed or the condition it's treating) before you offer the next bottle. If lists must be used, they should be offered in decreasing order of reliability:

- Typed by you from your own pill bottle labels.
- Provided from your *one* and *only* pharmacy that handles *all* your prescriptions.
- A computer printout from your doctor's EHR medication form.
- Provided from your doctor's written notes—a dangerous way to go.

Always include your drops, sprays, ointments, patches, over-the-counter drugs, and that alternative holistic medication you ordered from China that your doctor told you not to take.

Provide your own history. Avoid proxies or family members unless you are unable to offer an accurate one. Ask that your orders be written with a ballpoint pen. Felt tip and roller balls make poor quality faxes or "press through" duplicates. These leave you susceptible to illegibility errors.

Upon hospital discharge, inspect your prescriptions. Return faxes or copies and those that are illegible. Ask your doctor to avoid abbreviations and send them back if they are used.

Any medication taken chronically but missing at discharge is likely an error of omission—question it. New medications must be discussed, their indications confirmed, and an educational brochure provided. Don't leave without reading it and asking questions.

This, and all that follows, seems like quite a lot to do . . . right? But it's important to develop your own culture of medical safety, rather than relying on the hospital's. A medical consumer's self-advocacy eventually becomes second nature and will extend to all medical transactions.

DOSAGE ERRORS

Ask if your hospital has a computerized physician ordering system (CPOE). This technology is only found in 17 percent of our hospitals. CPOE prevents many types of medication errors. Poor physician judgment and factual errors are its key targets. CPOE is considered a proxy for a hospital's quality. But even after the CPOE entry getting a drug from your doctor's brain to your waiting vein doesn't end with its prescription. Following this, the formulation must be prepared, dispensed, transported, administered, and monitored. Each step (and there are 80–200 of them)[18] is subject to a number of possible errors. Standard doses are no longer standard. Many must be tailored to your gender, age, race, weight, and kidney function. Error can be made in a drug's frequency, its route of administration, and its dose. You are susceptible to both overdoses and the less well recognized problem of under-dosing.

How can you assure yourself no medication errors occurred along this long and tortuous path to your bedside?

Prevention of Dose and Administration Errors

You can't protect yourself from *any* medication error if you don't know what medications you're on. Someone has to know—many of your doctors don't. The Medication Administrative Record (MAR; it is not a pronounceable acronym—pronounce each letter) is the definitive summary of all your medications. It is the log that verifies both the receipt and timing of each drug you're on. You must have your MAR. It needs to be updated daily. Absent the MAR you become the potential passive recipient of every type of bedside medication error. If this document is denied to you ask for your charge nurse, speak with your doctor, and call the hospital administrator. You own it. HIPAA (this, unlike MAR, is spoken as a word . . . correct pronunciation is a must), by law, requires that you have access to it (see "Complaints" in chapter 19).

When they "give you this day your daily meds" (borrowed from Matthew 6:11), it's best to know you're also following Proverbs 30:8, "feed me with the food that is my portion."

The receipt of your MAR tells you a lot about your hospital before you even read it. If it is a facsimile of a handwritten original you're in one of the majority of U.S. hospitals that still use and rely on an ancient technology. Your chance for medication error is higher because of illegibility issues, transcription errors, and the lack of built-in safety technologies found in computerized and electronic (eMAR) systems. The Joint Commission shares your pain. A non-computerized MAR is "often in places where the physician cannot readily find it. It is often difficult to determine whether and when a medication was given; to find all the antibiotics currently being given, a practitioner might have to go through several pages . . . inaccuracies of a variety of types are frequent."[19] Whether the MAR is handwritten or computerized, it is a valuable document.

Whenever one of my patients went south (an unexpected turn for the worse) the first place to look for the answer was the MAR. A prime reason for a change in a patient's fortunes is a change in medication, a new drug interaction, a side effect, or a dosage change or error.

Medicine has its own "too many chefs" dilemma. Many doctors have access to your order sheet. Many are pharmacologically profligate and not all will routinely review your MAR before picking up their pens—the most dangerous medical instrument in the hospital. When you have your daily MAR you will know more about what medications you're taking than most of your doctors. Show every physician who comes through your door the MAR. This prevents them from ordering unnecessary duplicate medications or new agents that produce overlapping side effect profiles with your existing ones. Any new drug can also cause dangerous interactions with the rest.

If you have a bar-coded ID bracelet, your eMAR is electronically based. Good news. eMARs provide a real-time network between physicians, nurses, pharmacy, the lab, and your bedside. As reported in 2010, they prevent up to 87 percent of medication errors.[20] Fewer than 2 percent of hospitals have a comprehensive electronic format that includes the two pillars of medication safety, CPOE (preventing prescribing errors) and eMAR systems (preventing administration errors).

Inspect your pills, read the labels on the IV bags. Do it with a smile. After this leave your nurse alone. Don't interrupt his job once you've done yours.

You need to know enough to feel safe. "Knowing enough" is not a boundary. You can also know more and be able to comment on your drug regimen. Although it's not possible to be a partner in your personal pharmacopeia, you can participate and ask questions. The computer is the most important single tool you'll need. If you're reading this book, and there is evidence that you are, you're not the type to shut off your brain, close your eyes, and open your mouth when your meds arrive. You are a medical consumer, not a passive consumer of medicine.

Many hospitals, including our two local community hospitals, offer WiFi. This enables mobile laptop Internet connectivity. No WiFi? No problem. In 2010 Virgin Mobile introduced a no-commitment, unlimited portable hot spot plan that can fire up several computers in your hospital room for forty dollars a month. You can cancel it anytime. Forty bucks too much? Then buy ten days of access for ten bucks (for 100 MB of access—about ten webpages per day). Your hard-earned money is best spent avoiding hard-learned lessons. Computers can be used in any room, including the ICU. The computer connects you to information. The most important portal is your UpToDate.com one-week pass. Use it to educate yourself about each drug you're taking. You'll learn about why you're on it, how it acts, typical dosing ranges, warnings, advisories, and common and uncommon side effects with their percentage incidence. Your medication's contraindications, routes of administration, compatibility, investigational and off label uses, interactions, dietary considerations, and monitoring parameters are right on your screen. "Sound-alike" medications and "look-alike" medication issues are addressed. And that's just the beginning. UTD has a drug interaction tool that allows you to enter each drug you are using to determine if there is a chance for any significant interaction. Every test you're sent for can be researched for its safety, sensitivity, and whether it is being ordered appropriately. The computer allows you to enter another site, drugs.com, and use its "Pill Identifier" link to verify the identity of each of your pills.

Look-Alike and Soundalike Drugs (LASAs)

Many drugs that are entirely different from each other have packaging that appears almost identical. Packaging for wildly different doses of the same drug often look dangerously alike.

Many pills are indistinguishable from each other and their faint, small-type imprints don't help distinguish one from another. There are almost 3,000 round white pills on the market. Do you think that your pink rectangular pill is unique? There are thirteen of them. Almost 600 preparations have some version of the numbers one and five on their surfaces.

Medications don't just look alike—they sound alike. Prednisone, an anti-inflammatory, has twelve soundalike cousins.

Twenty-five thousand LASA errors were reported to two of the four voluntary drug-reporting systems in a four-year period.[21] This number is ludicrously low in light of the previously noted fact that reporting is voluntary. Reports of compliance rates fall under 1 percent in some studies.

The FDA is slow to correct existing LASA medications. They are only grudgingly addressed after multiple reports of damage occur, when the media becomes interested, or when lawsuits are filed.

The actor Dennis Quaid's twins aren't identical but their heparin dosage vials were. The twins recovered from an overdose of 1,000 times the prescribed amount. Look-alike, soundalike errors, so disastrous, shouldn't be so predictable, so easy to make, and so resistant to reform.

Preventing LASA Errors

To repeat, on admission don't verbally offer your medications' names. Show your medication bottle or your carefully prepared lists. Log onto your computer—find the list of LASAs that create the greatest risk for medication error. Find it on the Joint Commission website—jointcommission.org— and in the search box enter LASA. If you are on one of the LASA medications, inform your doctor and nursing staff. Tell them to tag your MAR. It serves as a warning to all who view it. If you have a trade name soundalike (Celexa/Celebrex) tell the staff to enter these meds' names using their generic names and vice versa.

Ask if there are soundalike patient names (Smith/Schmidt) on your unit. If so, get your chart tagged.

Instruct nursing to both show you your arriving medications and to intone each name, dose, and indication. Question any medications that don't look or sound familiar.

LASA errors will wilt under the lights of an accurate, confidently offered history and your bedside vigilance.

HIGH-RISK DRUGS

Some therapeutic agents are just more dangerous than others. Risky drugs given alone and especially in combination can cause ADRs with a high degree of likelihood. A study in 2009 noted that 53 percent of deaths caused by ADRs were caused by a combination of nonsteroidal anti-inflammatory medications (NSAIDs) such as Naprosyn, Aleve, or Motrin, with antiplatelet drugs like aspirin and Plavix and corticosteroids like prednisone.[22]

When high-risk patients are treated with high-risk drugs, or a member of a high-risk drug family, it's possible to predict the likelihood of an ADR. Most reports agree on the identity of the risky drug families—sedatives, narcotics, gastrointestinal and cardiovascular drugs, anti-seizure agents, and antibiotics.[23]

Preventing High-Risk Drug Errors

If, as an outpatient, you can't list your medications and are on over a dozen pills, several of which are the "high-risk" variety mentioned earlier, you are at high risk. *And* if you have had a dozen trips to the doctor in the previous year *and* used a relative to supply the preadmission medication list you can pretty much count on one.[24]

INTRAVENOUS DRUG DANGERS

Intravenous agents produce high drug blood levels more rapidly than when orally administered. They reach their cellular targets in hearts, lungs, brains, and kidneys much more quickly and in higher concentrations. Their use presupposes more serious problems in more compromised patients. For all these reasons, ADRs for intravenous agents will be more common and more severe. Patients in intensive care units stay an average of four to five days. During that time each patient will experience three IV medication errors. Most errors are for late or missed doses but 25 percent are for the wrong medication, dose, or route of administration.[25]

The IV agents most prone to administration errors with subsequent harm and death are vasopressin (for low blood pressure), insulin, blood thinners, electrolytes (e.g., potassium, calcium), antibiotics, sedatives, and narcotics.

Preventing Intravenous Drug Dangers

IV medications are lifesaving when you need them. At the very least ask that they be stopped when no longer needed. Fifty percent of patients on IV antibiotics can be switched to the oral route in two to three days. The risks of ADRs, fluid overload, electrolyte imbalance, and infection should prompt the question, "Can we avoid the IV, doc?" Many agents can be given orally, nasally, by injection, or by tube (nasal and rectal) and can be as effective and, therefore, preferable although not delightful alternatives. Blood levels comparable to those with IV administration can be reached using alternative routes for a variety of antibiotics, acid blockers, anti-nausea agents, analgesics, and antipsychotics.

My law firm, "Bunchak, Reapes, and Oapes," has asked me to remind you that all medical advice should come from your on-site physicians.

IDENTIFICATION ERRORS: BEING YOURSELF

There is no step more basic, no fact more important, and no safety measure more obvious than "being yourself" when in the hospital. The staff must know who you are. And if you think that wrong-patient, wrong-site surgeries are a thing of the past you'd be wrong too. A 2010 *Archives of Surgery* article noted a continuing "high frequency of surgical never events."[26]

Wristband identification would seem to be an intuitive, foolproof solution to potential medical identity errors. What speaks more of institutional intransigence, inertia, and incompetence than the two decades' struggle that has still failed to end wristband errors?

When you're not feeling yourself and not "being yourself" you will be susceptible to every error a hospital can dish out. How will bar codes, retinal scanning, and digital fingerprint technology succeed when hospitals still don't know how to strap on a wristband and guarantee you it contains accurate information?

Wristband errors range between 5.5 and 16 percent for hospitalized patients. In a 2002 study, wristband errors occurred at a Six Sigma–busting rate of 6,500 per million. Missing wristbands accounted for 71 percent of the errors. Incorrect or conflicting information made up the rest, except for the final, most egregious error—patients wearing the wrong wristband (1 percent of wristband errors).[27]

A 2009 study continued to show poor hospital compliance. Wristband safety was found in only 23 percent of surveyed hospitals.[28]

Preventing Identity Errors

Get a wristband. Read it. Confirm that it's yours and that it's accurate. Make sure that it fits and can't be removed except by scissors. The wristbands may need to be updated, changed, or moved due to local swelling, rashes, or IV placement. You want it to be changed if its information degrades with hospital wear and tear.

Do not allow your wristband to be removed until its replacement is onsite, reviewed for accuracy, and secured in place. Only then can the first be cut off.

No medication or examination or delivery of *any* service should occur without the staff first inspecting your wristband. Don't wait for the inspection—hold up your arm with wrist cocked. Put it at the eye level of anyone who does anything for you, with you, or to you—even the chaplain. When I was hospitalized at St. Elizabeth Hospital the nuns and priests roamed the wards like hall monitors. Even without the "H" (for Hebrew) on modern wristbands, they knew I was Jewish. I was nonetheless comforted when they dropped in and prayed with me. From my window I could see four stone crucifixes perched atop green tile peaks and arches, each sharply outlined despite their staggered display and the long depth of field across the roofline. It took four days for the rabbi to find me—"Hey Rabbi, no sweat, the nuns have me covered. Have you seen these beautiful crucifixes?"

SHROUD MEDICATIONS

The best way to avoid ADRs is to avoid drugs when possible. Many are not necessary. Ask your doctor to periodically review and prune your medication list. Do it as an outpatient. The authors of a 2010 study discontinued 311 medications in sixty-four patients with no adverse results. Eighty-four percent reported an improvement in their health.[29] Some of my most productive times with patients were spent describing, not prescribing. Alternatives to the easy path to a prescription pad provide safer therapies to your problems. Sleep, appetite suppression, tobacco cessation, anxiety reduction, pain relief, and the reduction of a host of somatic symptoms ranging from headaches to irregularity can be achieved without pills, much less dangerous ones. Many patients are on polypharmaceutical regimens that grow by accretion. Many are fossils prescribed by doctors now long gone or long gone in your care. It is common today for patients to have several doctors. A 2010 research survey demonstrated that "no one caregiver feels responsible for the patient's total medicine use."[30] When doctors inherit patients and their drug lists, there is an unwritten rule that some drugs can never be stopped. This "never stop" list includes digoxin, blood thinners, antidepressants, blood pressure medications, and psychotropic and sedative agents. These medications sound familiar. They are the high-risk medications referenced earlier. Unless you inquire, these pills will be all but placed under your shroud on the off-chance you may need them in the afterlife. Their cumulative effects promote sedation, constipation, imbalance, weakness, and poor concentration and vision. The results are infections, loss of appetite, dementia, falls, fractures, and nursing home addresses. These, in turn, promote more prescriptions.

Enter the Prescribing Cascade. When a medication causes a side effect, rather than stopping the first drug, a second is added to deal with the problem. An example: Alzheimer's drugs are given for dementia. Many cause urinary incontinence. Instead of being viewed as a side effect of the first medication, the incontinence is viewed as a new problem (frequent in Alzheimer's patients), which leads to a second drug. The drugs typically started for the incontinence not only cancel out the benefits of the Alzheimer's drug, they also can increase dementia and start their own cascade of side effects that in turn require more medications. The result: an increasingly demented patient on an increasing number of medications.[31]

The average senior in America today takes twice to three times the medications they require.[32] Almost 40 percent of those over sixty take five or more prescription drugs daily, according to the most recent 2010 report from the US Department of Health and Human Services.[33]

THE DRUG NOT TAKEN: MAKING ALL THE DIFFERENCE

When going to the hospital, bring in a pared-down drug list. Tell the invading hoards to put down their pens—you want only what you need. On hospital admission most patients get "PRN meds," or drugs to be taken "as needed." These are given at the request of the patient. They are then, by definition, unnecessary. Other doctors preemptively prescribe "bed and board" medications. They are routine and are also, therefore, unnecessary. "PRN" and "bed and board" medications' main purpose is to avoid late-night nursing calls to your doctor. The list need not be repeated—they are the members of each and every "risky medication" family. They include "convenience medications" that are convenient for nursing. These are the chemical restraints that keep you in bed, the sedatives that keep you quiet, and the binding gastrointestinal agents that keep you off the bedpan—all to no one's benefit but the staff's. Tell your doctor—"no 'PRNs,' no 'bed and boards,' and no 'convenience' medications, please. If I need something I will let you know."

18

Hospital-Acquired Infections

- Why you should stop worrying and learn to love your bugs.
- The era of the super drugs is over . . . enter the era of the super bugs. What have too *many* free antibiotics and too *few* free-range chickens wrought?
- The biofilm. The myth of "99.9% effective" disinfectants and the birth of zombie bugs.
- What the Dutch know that we don't and why it's killing us.
- Handwashing—the doctors most likely to infect you are the least likely to wash their hands.
- Preventing the preventable: *your* role in preventing surgical site infections, ventilator-associated pneumonia, blood-borne infections, and urinary tract infections.
- Who's been sleeping in my bed? Why private rooms are a must; how the previous occupant of your room can sicken or kill you.
- Your hospital room—over 50 percent of its surfaces are *never* thoroughly cleaned. How to clean them in thirty seconds for thirty cents.

THE TWO FBIS

You don't know it but the United States has two FBIs. The first is the Federal Bureau of Investigation (FBI) and the second is our Centers for Disease Control. It's our "Federal Bureau of Infection"—the "FBI." The FBI and "FBI" each have a ten-most-wanted list. The FBI's is for dangerous criminals. The "FBI's" is for the dangerous microbes that cause hospital-acquired infections (HAIs). These are the infections that you catch while you are in the hospital and are, by far, the most common complication that you will face when there.

The FBI says it best. Members of both lists are a "particularly dangerous menace to society"[1] and are published according to the "FBI" because each is a danger "for which regular, frequent and timely information regarding individual cases is considered necessary."[2] The FBI "always gets its man." It has apprehended 463 of 494. The "FBI" never gets its man. Instead the bugs grow stronger, becoming "super bugs"—the multiple drug–resistant organisms (MDROs) that shrug off an increasing number of antibiotics. When an antibiotic comes to arrest them, these bugs just chew them up with enzymes, spit them out with pumps, close their doors with stronger barriers, or just change their locks and deny them access.

Millions of patients meet them each year. A hundred thousand die as a result. It's even worse. These numbers are minimums because super bugs are in a "witness protection program." Only twenty-six states are required to report them to the authorities. HAIs are at least the sixth-leading cause for death in the United States, logging in between accidental deaths and diabetes mellitus.[3]

Despite initiatives launched by health-care organizations, professional associations, federal and accrediting bodies, legislators, regulators, insurers, consumer advocacy groups, and media campaigns, their numbers have only increased over the last several decades. In 2009 the "FBI" noted no changes in HAIs[4] but in 2010 noted some improvements.[5]

When you are *colonized* by dangerous bacteria their presence in your body does no damage. You become a reservoir for those little stinkers. If you are a colonized health-care worker (HCW) you will pass them along to patients. Patients pass them along to each other and back to non-colonized HCWs and then into the community to their children and pets. This round-robin eventually causes infections. *Infections* start when colonization turns into rebellion. Insurrectionist and resistant bugs take advantage of a compromised host, invading and damaging vital organs.

Staphylococcus is a human groupie. It lives in our nostrils and on our hands. When it becomes a super bug it becomes methicillin-resistant staph aureus (MRSAs) and is the "FBI's" #1 most wanted. In the 1990s, MRSA was found in 20 percent of our hospitals. That number has tripled. In an average year, MRSA sends at least seven million Americans to the doctor, forces 369,000 into the hospital, and kills almost 19,000. Vancomycin-resistant enterococcus (VREs), the second-most wanted, used to be a happy symbiont colonizing our digestive tracts. It's now a resistant disease-causing pathogen. It used to colonize 1 percent of hospital patients. It's now 15 percent. MDROs have escaped the confines of our hospitals where they were born. Set loose, they now wander freely in our community. In 2009, MRSA was the leading cause for skin and soft tissue infections seen in

United States' emergency rooms. A playground scrape that used to need a kiss and a Band-Aid now poses a reason for concern if it becomes infected. These former boo-boos now cause more frequent hospitalizations that require more potent antibiotics. This puts the patient and the community in jeopardy—the patient must take toxic antibiotics that in turn expose the community to the emergence of even more MDROs.

"Our Gang"

We should be able to live in harmony with our micro faunal friends. The microbes living in our bodies facilitate digestion, ramp up our immunity, activate enzymes that manage metabolism, and prevent cancers, autoimmune disease, allergies, and asthma. Healthy bacteria help defend us from external pathogens that can cause disease. "Our" bacteria, with their power to multiply logarithmically, deny these pathogens a beachhead from which they would launch an invasion. Members of "our gang" are not just in us. In a real way they are part of us. They possess hundreds of times the genetic material of our own DNA and interact with our genes in a way that regulates our cells' development and shapes their biology. Ninety percent of us are them (by cell count). Some investigators in 2010 viewed humans as "holobionts," the sum of our human and bacterial parts. They viewed the holobiont, not just our own genes, as the unit of evolutionary selection.[6] They really are "our gang." So, what's not to like?

Why do we hate them so? Americans have confused the admirable state of cleanliness—being free of visible unwanted soil and contaminants—with the state of surgical sterility—being free of *all* microbes. Since we can't make our bodies and environments sterile lunar landscapes, we settle for the myth of a life led antiseptically. This view is foisted on us by those who sell disinfectants, deodorants, and environmental and biological decontaminants. This antimicrobial campaign causes us to be repulsed by our own bodies, our breath, and our emanations. We try as best we can to kill each bacillus "within-us." We are afraid to live in our own homes, depicted on TV ads as crawling with vermin-sized microbes. From Clorox to chloramphenicol and from Listerine to Levaquin, business is up, but our defenses are down. In 2010 it was shown that some disinfectants encourage the growth of bacteria and enable their resistance to antibiotics.[7] The overuse, misuse, and abuse of antibiotics has selected out highly efficient and evolved organisms that are more likely to infect and that put up a tougher fight when they do. These bacteria and their infections were born and are most frequently found where antibiotics are used the most irrationally—in our hospitals.

There lives in our environments a perpetual, impregnable biofilm. It's a matrix of microorganisms (you can call it slime) that adheres to every surface, whether a countertop or a body part. TV commercials for antiseptics   •

promise a 99.9 percent kill rate for bacteria, viruses, and spores. First, that's unlikely, and second, even if true, the 0.1 percent that *do* survive represent a huge number of bugs that resuscitate the biofilm in minutes. Bacteria evolve many thousands of times more rapidly than humans. A new generation will populate your counter in under ten minutes. Bugs marinating in antibiotics, most often in hospitals, but increasingly in your homes, cause bacteria to become resistant. When they emerge they are stronger and, frankly, they act like they're a little pissed off.

The colonization of HCWs ends in infection for patients whose diseases have broken down their natural barriers and decreased their immunocompetence. Sick people become easy targets.

The era of super drugs is over—enter the era of the super bugs. There are very few new antibiotics coming down the pike to rescue us. The "FBI's" bad cops—antibiotics—too dangerous to be kept on the job, are being reenlisted. These brass-knuckle thugs have been set loose on today's resistant perps—and you. We continue to feed these bugs their favorite snacks—broad-spectrum antibiotics (BSAs). The year 2010 was a banner one for their prescription.[8]

The best way to keep an antibiotic effective is *not* to use it. BSAs are used with abandon. They cut a wide swath through bacterial populations and are often prescribed for no valid reason. This practice of shooting blind continues the cycle of resistant infection. Patients on BSAs are particularly vulnerable to the emergence of resistant bugs.

When we take antibiotics for every cold and cough and give millions of pounds of antibiotics to our livestock, we aren't killing bacteria. We are killing ourselves. Too many free antibiotics and too few free-range chickens and livestock are the unlikely and unlucky pairing of events that have turned our hospitals into petri dishes brimming with biologic agents of mass destruction.

Our health-care workers have been transformed into Typhoid Marys and Martys. From our barnyards to our backyards, from our doctors to our children, we have closed the circle and created a cycle—a cycle of perpetual cross-contamination for resistant infections in the United States.

Why in the United States? HAIs are preventable. In Northern Europe fewer than 5 percent of staph infections are caused by MRSA. Here it's over 60 percent. No, the "ten most wanted" bugs didn't pack their bags, forge their passports, and immigrate to the United States from Northern Europe. In Denmark, Holland, Finland, and Belgium they were killed on sight. In Holland, every infection control behavior and technique that demonstrates *any* evidence of efficacy is employed. Health-care workers who become MRSA carriers are temporarily furloughed and subjected to rigorous de-colonization regimens. Other hospitals prevent cross-contamination by segregating MRSA-positive employees, requiring that they care only for MRSA-positive patients. Entire floors close with the first sign of a unit-wide

MDRO outbreak and are not reopened until the source is found, decontaminated, or decolonized. All incoming patients are screened for MRSA with nasal swabs. If they test positive they will be segregated, isolated, and decolonized. The Netherlands sends these bugs to the netherworld—only 2 percent of all staph infections are MRSA.

What are the exotic behaviors and high-tech initiatives that the United States must employ to achieve parity with European rates? To what extremes must we subject HCWs and patients? We have to wash our hands, provide a clean environment and barrier precautions (masks, gloves, and gowns), identify colonized patients and staff, and use antibiotics properly. That's it? That's it! Europe's success is testimony to the fact that HAIs are largely preventable.

There are, however few, some hospitals here at home that have all but eradicated MRSA and VRE. This fact proves it's not Northern European altitudes but Six Sigma attitudes that succeed. Some of our hospitals are even moving in on the "third-most wanted" bug, Clostridium difficile (C. diff), which currently infects 1 percent of hospitalized patients, sickens thousands, and kills hundreds each day.[9]

Why is it then that the doctors and nurses who attend you, the surfaces you touch, the beds you sleep in, the water you drink, and the disinfectants you're cleaned with continue to cause infection rather than prevent it? The answer: In the United States almost every method the Europeans use is subjected to endless analysis, debates, further studies, and inertia. Those methods that are employed are neither monitored nor enforced. Compliance with the basic rules of handwashing, cleanliness, isolation techniques, and antibiotic use is lacking. Hospitals in 2010 are still not fulfilling or consistently complying with infection control guidelines.[10]

Handwashing

Let's get down and dirty (literally) on a topic we are all familiar with—handwashing. Handwashing is universally acknowledged as the single most important behavior that prevents the spread of HAIs throughout a hospital. Poor compliance in handwashing technique and frequency is the leading cause of HAIs.[11]

Handwashing is one of the very few infection control behaviors that is both unanimously recommended and backed by multiple high-quality scientific studies. Easy, cheap, safe, and effective, it's ignored by most—yes, most HCWs.

Before you organize and march to your hospitals' gates with pitchforks and flaming torches, let's look for a moment at your own habits. The American Society of Microbiology found that 97 percent of women and 92 percent of men claimed they washed their hands after using the toilet.

Seventy-five percent and 58 percent actually do. Other studies claim only 20 percent of us do. When you wash, do you scrub your palms, the back of your hands, between your fingers, and under your nails? Do you do it for twenty seconds? Are your hands then thoroughly rinsed and dried? That biofilm is tough. You need to scrub it off to effect an even temporary antiseptic status. It's not a rinse and run affair. Do you lather up before *and* after preparing food? Before *and* after eating it? Do you scrub each time you touch your pet or use your own toilets? Half of us don't clean our toilets more than once a week. C'mon, of course we don't do it all. Well, what you do at home is, after all, your business, but all this is good to think about. Handwashing is neither as quick nor as easy as it seems. But it's also your business to demand it of your HCWs. There are no good reasons for compliance rates so low that they are called "dismal," "disgraceful," and "inexplicable" in the medical literature.

Yes, the CDC does list fourteen individual steps for medical handwashing. Yes, soap and water handwashing compliance by a unit's nursing staff requires sixteen hours of total nursing time per shift. Alcohol-based regimens require a total of three nursing hours per shift.[12] Yes, handwashing is demanded so frequently and must be performed so thoroughly, skin irritation and infections result. So, when something that is seen as easy and, therefore, routinely expected turns out instead to be a time-consuming skill and a rule-based activity, what then of the other mandated behaviors, previously mentioned, that are far more labor intensive and complex?

Handwashing compliance rates for doctors hover between 30 and 55 percent and are rarely cited as being above 57 percent. Amongst health-care workers, doctors are the most resistant to change. The specialists most likely to bring their dirty hands to you rank the lowest in compliance.[13] In 2010 it's still more likely that your guests will wash their hands when leaving a restroom than will your doctor.[14]

Nurses fare better with handwashing compliance. The great unknown are the legions of staff who collectively interact with you the most—housekeeping, dietary, radiology, phlebotomy, transport, and nursing aides and the rest, who, despite being hard-working, are low on the hospital's food chain. Especially disturbing is the opinion voiced in 2010 that "healthcare providers are probably driven to wash their hands by their need to protect themselves more than their patients."[15] With all this in mind, there is the need to take things, other than soap, into your own hands.

PREVENTING HAIS

Four distinct clinical syndromes account for 80 percent of all HAIs: Surgical site infections (SSIs), ventilator-associated pneumonia (VAP), catheter-associated bloodstream infections, and catheter-associated urinary tract infections.

We have learned that infection control in your hospital's world resembles that in the Third World. You must improve your odds.

Handwashing Advice

"Did you wash your hands?" This is *not* the way to start off. A doctor or staffer who responds "No" is guilty of a grave medical lapse. If he didn't wash and then lies to you he's also guilty of a grave ethical lapse. Either way the question raises his defenses and his hackles. If you didn't witness a handwashing ritual then assume it didn't happen—don't ask.

Doctors will improve their handwashing compliance if the cleaning solution is available. That's your solution too. When they, or anyone, approach your bedside give them notice of your intent. Hold out the bottle of sanitizer with a big smile. As you squirt them say, "I know how busy you are and I am sure you've already done this a million times today. But I'm terrified of those infections I've been reading about. I hope you're okay with this." That's it. Easy, pleasant, and effective.

Sterile gloves placed over contaminated hands are *not* a substitute for clean hands. Soap and water is best for C. difficile spores. These are walled-in organisms that live on surfaces for months. They can be a remnant from the room's former occupant or be passed from roommate to roommate. Twenty to fifty percent of inpatients are colonized with C. difficile. If you arrived without it your chances of getting colonized are one in five.[16] Ask the nurse manager if anyone on the unit is on "enteric precautions." That means contact precautions for stool and that means C. difficile. Look for doorway precaution signs. If so, all you can do is ask that entering personnel use soap and water rather than sanitizer. Tell them why.

Got hang-ups? Before hospitalization, download and print up a few handwashing posters from http://www.hibigeebies.com/resources/hand washing_poster.pdf. Hang them up. One goes over your room's entrance-way and the other over your bed.

Preventing SSIs

Tens of millions of you will have a surgical or an invasive nonsurgical technique performed this year. Five hundred thousand of you will get an SSI.[17] If you do, you'll spend an extra week in the hospital, be more likely to be readmitted, and be two to ten times more likely to die as a result.[18, 19, 20] SSIs are considered preventable and many are non-reimbursed Medicare "never events."

Prevention? Handwashing, antibiotics, skin preparation, and barriers. Handwashing has been covered. Using the correct antibiotic one hour before surgery and stopping it twenty-four hours later is the only SSI prevention technique that's both strongly recommended and backed by multiple high-quality studies. The surgical trifecta of the right drug, given and stopped at the right time, is no sure thing. Each year at least 100,000 patients are left needlessly vulnerable to SSIs. Hundreds of hospitals have been tagged as poor compliers for SSI prevention.

Which surgeries require prophylactic antibiotics? All of them. It used to be thought that a "clean surgery" did not require them. Clean surgeries are elective; do not involve inflamed, infected, or traumatized tissue; and don't enter the respiratory, gastrointestinal, or urinary tract. Recently, clean surgeries for breast cancer, hernias, joint replacements, and intravascular procedures were placed on the "need antibiotics" list. Most recently almost *all* surgeries were suggested as antibiotic-worthy in light of the fact that surgical glove perforations and tears occur in 8 to 50 percent of operations and put patients at risk for contamination.[21] There is no current consensus regarding this suggestion but it's worth a discussion with your surgeon, especially for a surgery that will last two hours or longer.

When you are waiting for surgery make sure you're not waiting for your antibiotics. Two hours before gate-time, start asking.

Skin-Prep

Hair removal should be avoided unless its presence interferes with the surgery. No depilatories and no razor blades. If it's necessary, only electric razors are allowed. It must be done no earlier than a couple of hours before surgery. Bathe in chlorhexidine 4 percent (Hibiclens) at home or, if in the hospital, for two days preceding the surgery. On the morning of the operation neither wash nor dry it off. Insist on this ritual. Ask for mupirocin, a nasal ointment that may decrease postoperative staph infections. These are safe, cheap, and easy—words not often heard in medicine nowadays. You may be told that chlorhexidine and mupirocin are not officially recommended by the "FBI." That's true. But that's why we get infections while the Europeans don't. In 2010 and 2011 scholarly articles have appeared that support these suggestions.[22, 23, 24, 25]

Creating Barriers

When you are post-op, no one should get near you without hand cleaning. When your dressings are changed the staff must be capped, gloved, gowned, and masked. No subtlety is needed here. Tell them to create a barrier or create a distance by leaving your room.

In these times when you go home quicker and sicker, it's also good to know that up to 84 percent of SSIs are detected after hospital discharge. Remain wound-vigilant for several weeks.[26]

Pneumonia—BYOB

Pneumonia contracted in the hospital is usually ventilator-associated pneumonia that affects respirator-dependent patients. Three hundred thousand patients a year get them and 25 percent will die as a result.[27] Why? Pathogenic MDROs colonize most of these sick patients' saliva. After intubation with breathing tubes, saliva pools in the very back of the throat, gets inhaled, and causes infection.

Your strategy is to make sure your relative or friend gets the low-tech, highly effective VAP-prevention behavior—toothbrushing. So BYOB— bring your own brush. Simple brushing with regular toothpaste, tap water, and Colgate PerioGard oral rinse (our friend chlorhexidine) cuts the rate of VAP by 50 percent. It must be performed by a nurse or respiratory therapist who suctions away the residual water and oral rinse. Twice a day and a minute in duration—it should be routine. It's not.

Some breathing tubes have built-in suction ports. Most don't. Either way, the CDC wants you to make sure your relative at least receives manual deep throat suctioning every four hours.[28] Your charge should be in a heads-up, feet-down position (say "reverse Trendelenburg, please") to prevent pooling. That's it—you've done your job—toothbrush, suction, positioning.

Blood-Borne Infections

These are the most deadly HAIs. They typically arise from large-bore catheters that are placed through the skin and threaded into large veins near the heart. Call them "central venous catheters" (CVCs). MDROs and other pathogens run on an express track to the bloodstream provided by the puncture, the catheter, and breaches in its tubing. CVC blood-borne infections have tripled in the last three decades.[29] Each year five million patients get them, 250,000 become infected, and up to 35 percent of those will die because of it.[30] Dr. Peter Pronovost developed a CVC checklist that prevented the staff from relying on memory. The list included steps for handwashing, barrier protection, and chlorhexidine site cleaning. The list advises avoiding the groin as the CVC's entry site and protocols for its early removal. As a result, in just eighteen months and in only one state (Michigan), 1,800 lives were saved. Despite this, doctors skip steps a third of the time[31] and only half of our hospitals have all the recommended practices and policies in place for placement technique and monitoring.[32]

You already know about handwashing, chlorhexidine, and barrier precautions. Your job is limited but important. Before you make your demand—"Will you be following Dr. Pronovost's checklist?"—it's good to be sure the CVC is needed. They are most frequently placed to monitor the fluid status in critically ill patients with heart, kidney, and liver disease, to infuse caustic drugs and nutritional fluids, as well as to position leads for a temporary cardiac pacemaker and to monitor cardiac output. They are *not* needed solely to administer fluids or blood products or to provide a handy port for venous access for blood sampling. Even when the peripheral veins are difficult to access it's better to use them. Every shift has its resident IV-access expert. Ask for them: "Who's your local pro?" If necessary ask for an anesthesiologist to place a peripheral IV line. When a CVC is needed, experience counts. The task is often relegated to trainees—not for you.

Yes it *is* your job to ask for chlorhexidine-impregnated catheters. It's okay to demand proper catheter care. The dressing should be transparent and changed once a week using sterile technique. Look for loose, soiled, or damp dressings. Demand daily chlorhexidine baths. If blood must be drained for lab sampling it must be performed by a nurse using sterile technique. Each breach of the rubber stopcock provides the opportunity for bugs to slip inside along with the needle.

As a general rule for all patients, blood should be drawn once a day unless blood chemistries demand frequent monitoring. Ask if you are on a routine blood drawing schedule. Routine is a bad word. Tell (don't ask) your doctor to discontinue this order because she'll likely forget you're on it and you'll be stuck needlessly for days on end. Ask if urine and fingersticks are adequate alternatives for blood sugar monitoring. Each consult's "by the way," or "sudden inspiration," should not lead to an immediate blood draw. It can wait till the next day's morning bloodletting. You should ask if each subsequent draw could be delayed until then. If the answer is no—ask why. It's always okay to say "no!" until someone explains the rationale for any activity that you question.

Urinary Tract Infections

The most frequent HAIs are urinary tract infections. They are caused by urinary catheters—you can call them Foleys. These tubes are placed through the urethra to the urinary bladder. Foleys turn urinary aqueducts into infections' viaducts. Thirty million Foleys go into people each year. Twenty-five percent of you will get one. Six hundred thousand become infected.[33] The chances are pretty good—up to 50 percent—that you never needed it in the first place.[34, 35] But even if you did it's kept in too long 58 percent of the time.[36] They are painful, embarrassing, and restrict mobility. Count on the fact that the more unnecessary a Foley was in your care, the longer you'll keep it because your doctor has forgotten you have one and no one will remind him.[37]

Protocols have been established that inform the staff you have a Foley. They include scheduled reminders of how long it has been in and suggest when it's time to remove it. Despite this, few hospitals use them. It's your job.

The vast majority of hospitals don't use all of the recommended safety practices that prevent urinary infection—antimicrobial catheters, bedside bladder ultrasounds (which decrease the need for Foleys), or alternatives to indwelling Foleys (external condom catheter for men and "as needed, in and out" catheterization). In 2008, a national survey[38] found that there was no single national, widely used strategy in place to prevent catheter-associated urinary tract infections despite a wealth of evidence and infections. You again are utterly on your own. So unnecessary are these infections, Medicare won't pay hospitals for the expense of their treatment.

Suggestions

First make sure you need one. They are *not* for urinary incontinence. Sometimes, unforgivably, the skin on the thighs and lower back have, through negligence, been allowed to break down so severely the catheter may be needed to allow time for healing. If you or your charge is incontinent prevent this with frequent in-bed turning, cleaning, barrier creams, and linen changes. Demand that quilted pads be placed underneath incontinent patients and make sure you demand that a bedpan or commode is offered every two hours.[39]

Foleys are not needed to check the bladder for residual urine. That's what the bedside bladder ultrasound is for. Catheters are needed if the bladder is obstructed, for palliative end-of-life care, for some neurological diseases, and preoperatively for some, but very few, surgical procedures. They are needed in the critically ill for whom the exact measurement of daily urine output is critical for safe fluid and electrolyte management. Such patients often have CVCs.

So ask questions and say "no thanks" unless and until someone gives you a good reason for your soon-to-be-inserted Foley catheter.

If you do need one, ask for an antimicrobial catheter impregnated with silver or antibiotics.[40] It must be placed by experienced staff and performed under sterile conditions. Monitor the Foley and collection system. The collection bag should never touch the floor. It should not be raised to the level of your torso to prevent backwash. This happens most frequently while you are in transport. The Foley and bag is a closed system and should not be opened or disconnected. Most importantly, remind your doctor every day that you have one and that you want it removed. Follow these suggestions and the chances are you'll never get a Foley or it'll be out before it turns on you.

Clean Rooms

Who's been sleeping in my bed? After you've checked into a hotel room what are the first things you should do? Remove and store the bed covers and blankets. Boil the glasses and scrub the toilet. You should avoid sitting on any upholstered surface without the barrier protection of your clothing. You know these areas are cleaned rarely, if at all, and never meticulously. And that's just a hotel room! When you check into a hospital room it's even more important to wonder and worry "who's been sleeping in my bed?" In a word, your room is dangerous. It's not only occasionally visibly dirty but even "clean" rooms are bacteriologic playgrounds for some of the toughest bugs on the block. Private rooms are a must if for no other reason than they are easier to clean. In 2011 it was found that changing an ICU to all private rooms cut the infection rate by more than half.[41] Private rooms are, well, more private. They also speed your recovery (see chapter 19).

The CDC doesn't recommend the routine eradication of bacteria on your rooms' surfaces. For the "FBI," it's neither feasible nor proven to decrease HAIs. Many disagree, but just watch the staff. Doctors and nurses will use almost any part of their anatomy, other than their hands, to open doors, turn on lights and faucets, and open garbage bins. They flush toilets with the bottoms of their shoes, leaving behind God-knows-what for *your* next bathroom journey. Even when pumping out hand sanitizers, they cover the dispensing hand with their uniforms.

Visibly clean rooms mean almost nothing. Seventy-five percent of hospital rooms harbor pathogens after routine cleaning.[42] That's bad enough, but fewer than half of your rooms' surfaces are *ever* thoroughly cleaned.[43] Amazingly, if you are in isolation because you have an infection it's even less likely your room will be cleaned. Handwashing is crucial, but it's sobering to realize that its effect may last no longer than it takes for the HCW to touch your room's doorknob, the sink's tap, the privacy curtain around your bed, or the bedside railing surrounding it. It's not just the staff that brings bugs to your bedside. The surfaces that surround you do too.

Another independent risk factor for colonization and potential infection, aside from the staff and surfaces, are the other patients. John Paul Sartre was correct. "Hell is other people," if only in the hospital. Other patients produce what's called colonization pressure. The more patients with whom you co-exist, the more likely you'll be colonized or infected.[44]

Some hospitals don't routinely isolate MRSA-positive patients. Few perform universal screening for it. If your roommate has a "contact precaution" alert over the bed or is approached by HCWs in full-body barrier suits, complain and get yourself out—right away.

The ghosts of patients past are in your room. You have a 40 percent increased risk of picking up MRSA or VRE hitchhikers if your bed's prior occupant had either.[45] Livestock pens, enclosures, runs, and holding rooms are cleaned more frequently and stringently and are monitored for compliance more compulsively than is your hospital room.[46, 47] The reigning hospital cleanliness guru, Philip C. Carling, says it all when he lists items in hospital rooms and the percentage frequency they are cleaned.[48]

The do-not-touch zones are hard to avoid but the percentage of the time they are cleaned may lead you to wear gloves. Telephones (50%), chairs (48%), toilet doorknobs (28%), toilet handholds (28%), and room doorknobs (23%). When leaving the bathroom you'll have to figure out a way to turn off those lights. They are only cleaned 20 percent of the time. As recently as 2010, Carling et al. wrote "recent studies . . . have shown disinfection cleaning can be improved on average more than 100% over baseline."[49]

In light of the above and because "there is no doubt that surfaces can act as a source of pathogens which can give rise to nosocomial infections,"[50] you are, once again, on your own.

So BYOBs—your brains, brooms, bleach, bactericides, buckets, barriers, and blood pressure cuffs. That brain you brought along tells you that every room is in need of your family's daily attention. A broom with moistened bristles will clean the visible bacteria-laden dust. Bleach and bactericides clean your room—the doorknob, sink, and toilet handles, bedrails, bed stands, telephones, and light switches. A simple solution of 1/2 cup of Clorox bleach to 1 quart water is an inexpensive environmental germicide that kills bacteria, viruses, and fungi. The bucket is needed to completely immerse your cleaning cloth. Scrub a little to upset that biofilm. Too much? You do it at home for less reason. Why not spend a few cents and even fewer minutes going over your loved one's room surfaces? If the hospitalization is brief and doesn't involve surgery and if the patient has no open wounds or punctures it's okay to take a pass. If the stay is a higher-risk venture then get your designated sitters to roll up their sleeves, put on gloves, and get to work. Bring brooms, not blooms. Yes, cleaning the room will never eliminate microorganisms. "Regardless, an argument can be made to decrease the microbial burden through regular and thorough cleaning."[51]

You know this is a job best done by family.

Gloves, masks, protective eyewear, and body barriers are easily obtained at any home health center. Patients should don their gloves when using the commode, toilets, bedpans, and when going for a stroll. On gurney journeys wear a mask and gloves. It may help prevent MRSA and C. difficile colonization and, just as importantly, warns HCWs to employ their own hygiene techniques if for no other reason than to protect themselves.

The last barrier is a disposable apron. At a nickel a throw and torn from a roll, they belong in your doorway. If the staff don't put on a gown upon their arrival you should ask them to. Sixty-five percent of lab coats and uniforms will pick up MRSA when its occupant just leans over the bedside of a

MRSA carrier. In light of this the otherwise ever-complacent AMA is thinking about making the white coat as much a reliquary as the doctor's little black bag. If all you can manage is draping a disposable gown over your exposed skin it may to do some good. It can't harm and it does alert the staff that someone is taking standard industry-wide precautions seriously.

BYO blood pressure cuffs, stethoscopes, and tourniquets. All of these items are inexpensive and available at drugstores and home health centers. Anything that will be shared with *every* other patient on your unit should be obtained for your personal use; particularly if your stay is a high-risk venture. Up to 100 percent of stethoscopes and blood pressure cuffs are contaminated with a variety of bugs.[52] Fifty percent of HCWs have either never cleaned their stethoscopes or do so only monthly.[53] In pediatric ICUs, single-use cuffs have eliminated a variety of bacterial infections and entire families of bacterial contaminants.[54] The people who draw your blood will be happy to give you a new personal-use tourniquet.

Eccentric? No, patient-centric. These things are a reminder to all who care for you that you care about yourself.

19

Isolation

- Isolation rooms: adding injury to insult. When you are infected and then isolated your care will decrease and your complications increase. Why?
- Consolation in isolation. Finding peace and a measure of calm.
  - Your computer, music, aromatherapy, tasty food (and how to get it), and looking fine when you don't feel so fine.
- Enough already! Complaining—the how, when, why, and to whom. Giving it teeth.

Isolation is the cornerstone for the containment of infectious diseases that injure or kill on a mass scale. HAIs are such infections. Universal screening of entering patients, followed by well-known and successful protocols for MRSA carriers, will slash the rates of MRSA infections by 70 to 90 percent.[1, 2, 3]

Isolating patients with MRSA is already mandatory in some US centers and is being debated in others. In June 2009 a bill was introduced to Congress that would make universal screening mandatory nationwide. What might be seen as a patient's civic responsibility to contain infection may become civil law.

CIVIL ISOLATION AND ITS DISCONTENTS

Isolation, as it's practiced in the United States today, has its problems. Doctors are half as likely to enter isolation rooms and less likely to examine its patients when they do. Those on isolation are less likely to have their vital signs monitored. Nursing and physician daily progress notes are less frequent and less detailed.[4, 5] Patients are eight times more likely to experience a variety of failures in supportive care.[6] This leads to a twofold increase in preventable adverse events compared to patients in the hospital's general population. An increase in delirium, falls, bedsores, deep vein thromboses, and more have been reported.[7, 8] Isolation rooms are less frequently cleaned—almost one third of their *air samples* are MRSA positive.[9, 10, 11] This phenomenon has been called a fecal cloud. Think about that when I ask you to clean your loved ones' rooms. Patients in contact isolation are *more* likely to get infections.

The psychological damage resulting from current isolation practices is predictable. Patients feel imprisoned, neglected, depressed, and anxious. Stigmatized, isolation patients have their diagnoses prominently posted on their doors. Some isolation rooms lie behind red-painted lines warning (and warning away) staff and visitors. Isolation has become a hospital's mark of Cain. Mistreated patients are treated like miscreant prisoners and are the embodiment of Susan Sontag's premise in her book *Illness As Metaphor*.[12]

Patients in isolation aren't the only ones subject to emotional tolls. Twenty percent of coronary artery bypass patients suffer an episode of major depression during their hospitalization.[13] Fifty percent of all postoperative patients demonstrate some type of depressive symptomatology.[14, 15] I don't know about you, but I've been hospitalized twice for periods longer than a few days and I cried once during each confinement. Now I may not have the sunniest disposition on the block, but historically it takes quite a bit to turn on my faucets. It's not just the illness, it's the entire experience.

Consolation in Isolation

Every patient's hospital life is an isolating experience. Even with a lot of visitors and a designated sitter you're still the horizontal one in pajamas who's not going home to the family dinner tonight. While in the hospital, we turn again to Ambrose Bierce's *Devil's Dictionary*'s definition of "alone": "adj., In bad company."[16] This still holds even when in the midst of good company.

Yes, despite this you should isolate yourself. All patients are better off in single rooms. If you're on contact precautions and have no choice, the poor care and psychological trauma can be prevented. I'll show you that there can be consolation even in isolation and perhaps a measure of peace.

Single rooms are private. Important conversations and sensitive examinations are more likely to be held in single rooms. The staff is more likely to use their handwashing skills when seeing one patient rather than repeating the task between two or more. There is less clutter, making the room easier to clean. Your room becomes more inviting to your designated sitter and guests. Visitation rules changed in 2011. Now, same-sex domestic partners can visit and stay overnight. In semi-private rooms you will still need your roommate's permission. Without it your partners will have to retreat to visitors' lounges for the long night's journey into day. Single rooms free you from the distractions of a roommate's crew. Sleep is therapeutic. Single rooms are quieter. When you turn off the lights they're darker. During the day they're brighter. In a single room you're never on its windowless dim side. Patients exposed to sunlight ask for fewer analgesics and sleep-aids, are less depressed, and get home more quickly.[17]

There is less colonization pressure when you touch no one and no one touches you. Just having your own bathroom should seal the deal. Tell your M.D./advocate to help keep your medical insurer at bay by providing a medical necessity note. Single rooms are an evidence-based predictor of higher-quality care and better clinical results. That's enough reason to get the note.

If you're in a semi-private room you must never tolerate the chance that your roommate's unfortunate problems can become yours—draining wounds, incontinence, or contact precautions mean a transfer, pronto.

Yes, if you are on contact precautions you've been singled out for a single room. There is no need to pay the price of poor care and psychological trauma promised for isolation patients. Inform your doctor and charge nurse that you are aware of the poor care issues I raised earlier for those on contact isolation. Tell them to get the sign off your door and replace it with a "routine contact precautions—visitors welcome" sign. Tell them that your diagnosis posted on the door is a violation of your HIPAA rights. Tell them you expect their visits to be appropriate to your needs, not their fears. Ask that housekeeping arrive forthwith for a thorough room cleaning as you guide them to the room's trouble spots. Ask after their names. Tell them you'll see them tomorrow. Bring doughnuts. For that matter, have your family invest in doughnuts and pizza now and then for each of the unit's three shifts. Staffers are terribly overworked and dedicated. They skip meals for you on a regular basis. Your kindnesses and kind words are noted—they're strangely rare.

Bed and Bored: Any hospital room can cause boredom and isolation. However even in a semi-private room, surrounded by roommates, their families, reruns of *The Real Housewives of New Jersey*, and the dulcet musical stylings of the Wu Tang Clan, you can still establish your own space, gain a degree of peace, and keep yourself busy. You can isolate yourself logistically if not geographically. You may even be fortunate enough to bring down the barriers of your privacy curtain and find a pleasant soul with whom you can exchange hospital war stories.

Whether in a single or semi-private room, bring earbuds and eyeshades . . . you'll sleep better.

Computer Therapy

The medical benefits provided by a computer were referenced earlier. As important, your computer allows you to view videos, movies, or TV shows of your choice and on your schedule. The anticipation of a personally chosen movie or show provides a fillip to any day, relieving boredom and distracting you from your anxieties.

Your computer can connect you to Caringbridge.com. The site enables you to create a website and journal. Messages and photos can be shared with friends and family. It's free, private, and without advertisements. Creating a network allows you to remain engaged and in touch with your fan club, particularly helpful when you're afield.

Music Therapy

Your computer is a portal to the all-important benefits of music. Rather than listening to movies or music that become part of the ambient din, headphones in your ears and a monitor near your eyes separates you from it. In thirty years of hospital practice I don't recall ever seeing a patient using headphones. That this advice seems at least somewhat novel is remarkable. Music is therapeutic. It lowers the blood pressure, pulse, respiratory rate, and pain levels. In 2011, music's euphoric effect was traced down to its chemical and subcellular levels.[18] Music stimulates dopamine in the brain's pleasure centers. Prokofiev over Prozac!

Pandora.com and www.last.fm each provide free streaming Internet music. They allow you to create channels of your favorite artists and genres. Turn on, tune in, and drop out. It's a psychologic, non-psychedelic benefit of your computer.

Odorant Therapy

Good smells are hard to come by in hospitals. Import your own. Floral and herbal oils relieve stress, facilitate sleep, and may fight depression and block inflammatory pathways.[19] Scientific reinforcement comes from animal models that demonstrate odorants' effect in decreasing stress hormone levels and down modulating blood pressure, pulse, and respiratory rates. The first cranial nerve that mediates the sense of smell runs on a unique express track right to the pleasure centers in your brain. But even if the oils are aromatherapy or New Age baloney, they still smell good in a place that needs good smells. Oils and reed diffusers are inexpensive and easy to find online. Or just bring in a Glade Plug-in. Your home health company stocks the infelicitously named "Fecal Odor Eliminators" that sadly will come in handy sooner or later.

"Photo" Therapy

Make sure there are lots of photos displayed of you in your thirties and forties—the age of most of your healthcare workers. It's all about making personal links. Radiologists who see photos of you while reading x-rays about you provide longer and more meticulous readings.[20] These one-dimensional representations reveal more about your three-dimensional life than almost anything else.

McNugget Therapy

Hospitals laden with dietary protocols deny you the simple pleasure of food. Food is comfort. Food is fuel. The low-sodium, low-fat diets that are routinely ordered are usually unnecessary. Do you need dietary restrictions? Can you get outside food? Pizza over Prozac!

Pajama Therapy

"In war, truth is the first casualty"—Aeschylus. In the hospital, it's your pride. Fight it. Keep up appearances. Reject the gowns with faulty ties and snaps that have been worn by hundreds before you. When you look better you'll feel better and be treated better. Your wardrobe is a social strategy, valuable in uncertain times. Get on Amazon and buy a few brand-new poly-cotton, velcro closure, modesty preserving gowns. Those that open on your side are the best. Get a new robe for extra coverage. A new floor-length comfy cotton robe with side pockets won't set you back much but it will set you apart.

Smile with your head up and with your hands on your hips. It projects a sense of self all will recognize and defer to. When caring for loved ones, don't allow them to go unshaven, un-coiffed, and exposed. Dry shampoo is a must for bedridden patients. Don't let your loved ones fade into their sheets.

Complaints—Get Heard

Errors that are unaddressed require that you express dissatisfaction. When you do complain, pick your targets carefully. No, it's not the poor food, the depressing ambience, or the lack of premium cable on television. It's time to register a complaint based on a problem you feel interferes with your recovery or safety.

How to start? "I am not a complainer. I am someone with a complaint." This is the best lead-off a phrase when it's time to object to unsafe practices, medication errors, unanswered questions, or unwashed hands. Single-issue complaints, placed without drama, rancor, or personal attacks, have the best chance of succeeding. If your problem is a personal one with a staffer speak to the staffer. If your complaint fails or is based on a unit- or hospital-wide problem, start at the unit level and work your way up the hospital food chain. The charge nurse is the unit's shift leader. The nurse manager is the registered nurse administrator for your unit. The social worker is contacted to start a grievance. The hospital's chief operating officer is reached to voice your intent to file with the state and federal agencies. Register your dissatisfaction as soon after an incident as possible.

Know names. You'll never get far when you identify an anonymous party by describing their distinguishing physical characteristics. "I'm complaining about that doctor, you know—the skinny beanpole with the big nose, gray beard, and funny eyeglasses?"

When you've reached the top of the hospital's hierarchy and have failed to obtain a satisfactory response it's time to demonstrate to the hospital's chief operating officer that your intent has teeth. Your knowledge and the availability of the tools that will affect an on-site formal action often obviate its need. "I don't want to be in a position that forces me to file with the Quality Improvement Organization, the Joint Commission, or our state agency. But I really need to know that this problem is being taken seriously." Your computer should be open on your lap, fired up and ready to go.

When it's time to file, complain and be heard: Using your hospital's "patient's rights policy," cite a specific infraction if possible. Medicare patients should go to the website www.ahqua.org and link at the QIO (Quality Improvement Organization) locator for your state's Medicare administrator. You can find your QIO by calling 1-800-Medicare. Medicare addresses issues of inappropriate, unnecessary, or delayed care; medication errors; and discharge issues.

The Joint Commission is a non-profit independent organization that certifies hospitals and addresses unsafe practices, quality of care, patient rights, infection control, and medication safety. Go to www.jointcommission.org/GeneralPublic/Complaint to download and file your grievance. Call the Joint Commission consumer complaint line at 800-994-6610 or e-mail them at complaint@jointcommission.org. File with your state's agency, http://hospitalcomplaint.com/stateagencies.html, via their provided telephone number.

Premature Discharge

If you feel you're being discharged too early, speak first with your doctor. The hospital discharge planner is the person to whom you state your intent to file with the Joint Commission. You cannot be discharged until the appeal has been adjudicated, usually two to three days. People with private insurance policies should phone their company and file their grievance over the phone or receive the information to perform it online.

Be nice, be courteous, but be persistent.

BACK TO THE FUTURE

Several months ago I found a time capsule. It was a 1998 publication from the Joint Commission. Its authors offered what they thought the medical landscape would look like ten years hence. Reading the book for the first time, now twelve years later, we are at that point in time where their prophecies intersect with today's realities. Their dreams encased in this time capsule are castles—castles in the sky. Their prophecies were of an era created anew by system-wide transformational behaviors empowered by informatics and seamless networks of communication and data sharing. They, unlike the classical Cassandra, saw the future optimistically but like her were ignored.

Many still toil toward a promised era. Medical messianism is still alive and well. But until that day arrives our hospitals remain the Miltonian Lost Paradises referred to earlier. It is still the wise person who "pondering his voyage," enters this realm both wary and knowledgeable.

Appendix: Best Medical Websites

In this section I list and briefly describe the most worthwhile URLs for an online medical education. These are not the only resources available but they have been pre-screened and test-driven. These pages, in addition to those mentioned in the text, are authoritative, easily navigable, noncommercial, peer reviewed, timely, durable, and visitor friendly. Each category contains several options. Find one or two that work for you. Too much choice is paralyzing.

USING THE INTERNET FOR MEDICAL SEARCHES TUTORIALS

http://www.vts.intute.ac.uk/tutorial/medicine/?sid=970997&ite mid=12021. This is the most comprehensive Internet tutorial for those seeking to become experts when doing medical research on the web. Just open the page and start from the beginning. It takes an hour and you become an impresario for your own Internet medical experience. There's nothing to it and there's nothing like it.

E-TEXTBOOKS

http://resources.bmj.com/bmj/readers/statistics-at-square-one/statistics-at-square-one. From the *British Medical Journal*, a primer on statistics and probability. Sophisticated but offering important lessons.

http://www.bartleby.com/107/. When a picture is worth a thousand words.

http://www.merck.com/mmpe/index.html. "Old Reliable." A trusted medical encyclopedia.

E-JOURNALS

http://www.nejm.org. The *New England Journal of Medicine*. Many free public-access articles and e-alerts.

http://www.springer.com/medicine/internal/journal/11606. The *Journal of General Internal Medicine*. Each issue has a few free public-access articles. Site is searchable.

http://jama.ama-assn.org. The *Journal of the American Medical Association*; free articles and alerts, and *all original research* is free six months after publication.

http://archinte.ama-assn.org. The *Archives of Internal Medicine*. Many free articles and *all original research* is free twelve months after publication.

The following links are to the other Archive sites that similarly offer free access after twelve months; many offer free access articles in each issue:

http://archsurg.ama-assn.org. *Archives of Surgery*.

http://archpsyc.ama-assn.org. *Archives of General Psychiatry*.

http://archpedi.ama-assn.org. *Archives of Pediatrics and Adolescent Medicine*.

http://archderm.ama-assn.org. *Archives of Dermatology*.

http://archneur.ama-assn.org. *Archives of Neurology*.

http://www.archives-pmr.org. *Archives of Physical Medicine and Rehabilitation*.

http://www.archivesofpathology.org. *Archives of Pathology and Laboratory Medicine*.

http://archinte.ama-assn.org. *Archives of Internal Medicine*.

http://archotol.ama-assn.org. *Archives of Otolaryngology* (head and neck surgery).

http://archopht.ama-assn.org. *Archives of Ophthalmology.*

http://archfaci.ama-assn.org. *Archives of Facial Plastic Surgery.*

http://www.biomedcentral.com/bmcmed. Publisher of 206 peer-reviewed open-access journals.

http://highwire.stanford.edu/lists/freeart.dtl. Lists all journals with open access, most within six months of publication.

GENERAL SEARCH ENGINES

http://www.searchmedica.com. From our friends across the pond. A full-service search engine. It delivers only the most clinically reputable content, intended for practicing medical clinicians. By registering you'll get free searching tips to make finding medical information faster.

http://www.labtestsonline.org. Peer-reviewed, noncommercial, and patient-centered. Search lab tests, conditions and diseases, and screening guidelines.

http://www.healthfinder.gov. Your tax dollars well spent. So use it! All-purpose medical search site from the most trusted sources.

http://www.thecochranelibrary.com/view/0/index.html. The US repository of all things "evidenced based." Plain language and summaries that outline the "best evidence."

http://www.library.nhs.uk/Default.aspx. The British evidence-based search engine. God bless the Queen.

http://www.modernmedicine.com. Modern Medicine's homepage. See the search engine. Click recommended medical sites on the search box and get the most reliable resources.

GENERAL INFORMATION SITES

http://www.healthypeople.gov/2020/default.aspx. Be a healthy person. Healthy People 2020 is a comprehensive set of disease prevention and health promotion sites.

http://www.ahrq.gov/sitemap.htm. The Agency for Healthcare Research and Quality (AHRQ) is the health services research arm of the US Department of Health and Human Services. Clinical facts, updated treatment plans, and more. The mighty AHRQ!

http://healthnewsreview.org/index.php. HealthNewsReview.org provides independent expert reviews of news stories in the media. Award-winning crusader Gary Schwitzer holds health and medical journalism accountable by showing you, the consumer, how, why, and when to trust the media's ripped-from-the-headlines medical news reports.

http://www.abouthealthsatisfaction.org. Assesses adult inpatients' perception of their hospital. Patients rate their hospital on a scale from 0 to 10. Satisfaction is not a substitute for quality; it just complements your database in the case of a tie between two hospitals.

http://www.mayoclinic.com. One of the most respected sites for patient-centered information. It's free newsletter is *Housecall*, a weekly general-interest e-newsletter.

www.fda.gov/cder/drugSafety.htm. Worried about your drugs? Consumers and health-care professionals can go to this page on the US Food and Drug Administration's website to find a wide variety of safety information about prescription drugs.

http://www.healthfinder.gov/scripts/SearchOrgType.asp?OrgTypeID=14 &show=1. Lists all 279 American Associations for "This and That" and other professional organizations; each with valuable links and information.

http://blackboxrx.com. Keep an eye on new black box warnings. They pop up like mushrooms on a forest floor. Has your drug been added?

GENERAL INFORMATION

Below is a sampling of some of the larger national professional medical societies. Many societies have sites specifically designed for patients.

- American Academy of Pediatrics (www.aap.org)
- American Society of Anesthesiologists (www.asahq.org)
- American College of Physicians (www.acponline.org)
- Society of General Internal Medicine (www.sgim.org)
- American Society of Clinical Oncology (www.asco.org)

- American Academy of Family Physicians (www.aafp.org)
- American College of Surgeons (www.facs.org)
- American College of Obstetricians and Gynecologists (www.acog.org)

Medline Plus: Supported by both the National Library of Medicine and the National Institutes of Health, Medline Plus (www.medlineplus.gov) offers patients an array of information on health topics, drugs, and current news. In addition, there are interactive tutorials, surgery videos, health information for older adults, and links to clinical trials and health information for older adults.

Centers for Disease Control and Prevention: The CDC (www.cdc.gov) is an excellent patient resource for communicable diseases, preventive care, and public health.

The American College of Physicians Foundation: In conjunction with the American College of Physicians, the ACP Foundation (foundation .acponline.org) offers succinct and clearly described health information for patients.

For cancer patients: There are three websites that can serve as excellent starting points:

- The National Cancer Institute (www.cancer.gov)
- The American Cancer Society (www.cancer.org)
- The American Society of Clinical Oncology (www.cancer.net)

RISK CALCULATORS

http://www.shef.ac.uk/FRAX/tool.jsp. World Health Organization fracture calculator.

http://www.breastcancerprevention.org/raf_source.asp. Breast cancer risk calculator.

http://www.reynoldsriskscore.org/default.aspx. Heart, stroke risk calculator.

http://xrayrisk.com. Calculate your dose of ionizing radiation and estimate the cancer risk from imaging studies, including CT scans, x-rays, and interventional procedures.

http://www.qfracture.org. This is a second risk fracture calculator to help you decide on whether the risks of osteoporosis treatment are commensurate with its benefits. When your risk is calculated, work with your doctor to make the best decision. Many people are overtreated.

http://www.yourdiseaserisk.siteman.wustl.edu. Cancer, diabetes, heart disease, osteoporosis, and stroke risk calculators.

MEDICAL PRONUNCIATIONS

http://medicalpronunciations.com. For the iPhone. Extensive and terrific. What, no Android?

http://www.merck.com/mmhe/resources/pronunciations/index/a.html. Hundreds of diseases with audio pronunciation.

http://www.howjsay.com. It's important to pronounce your medications and medical terms accurately. This site will help.

DRUG INFORMATION

http://dailymed.nlm.nih.gov/dailymed/about.cfm. DailyMed provides information about marketed drugs. This information includes FDA package inserts.

http://www.consumerreports.org/health/best-buy-drugs/index.htm. Exhaustive patient-oriented information about your medications. Search for the drugs that are typically used for many conditions. Alternative treatments, cost comparisons, and effectiveness data are also listed and come from a trusted source.

http://www.rxaminer.com/consult/consult_mydrugs.asp. Register and compare drug prices. Learn tips to reduce expenditures. Alternative generic agents and their cost savings are listed. Search by condition and view second-line therapies with cost comparisons.

http://www.healthgrades.com/drug-ratings. Good information on price, popularity, and side effects for thousands of drugs.

COURSES AND EDUCATION

http://www.medicine.ox.ac.uk/bandolier/learnzone.html. Excellent collection of PDFs on a variety of topics including medical statistics and guidelines.

http://www.modernmedicine.com/patienteducation. Downloads for hundreds of conditions—easily understood and nicely illustrated.

http://www.healcentral.org/healapp/browse?action=browse&pid=C&page
=1&display=25. Searching by your diagnosis' medical subject heading
(MeSH) code is one of the best ways to start a sophisticated search.

http://www.mondofacto.com/courses/medical/introduction-to-medical
-terminology.html. Register for free and learn more about medical termi-
nology than anyone you know.

http://www.pfizer.com/health/medicine_safety/medicine_safety_education
.jsp. Yes it IS from a drug company; it has been vetted and is free of commercial contamination or promotions. Bravo Pfizer!

http://www.mlanet.org/resources/userguide.html. A user's guide to finding and evaluating health information on the web. Tutorials and links to
disease-oriented best sites.

http://www.medpagetoday.com/Medpage-Guide-to-Biostatistics.pdf. Terrific
eleven-page PDF that gets you well on your way to understanding biostatistics.

http://www.drugs.com/pill_identification.html. Endlessly useful way to
identify your pills and those that strangers offer you.

http://www.nlm.nih.gov/medlineplus/webeval/webeval.html. This audio-
visual tutorial teaches you how to evaluate the health information that you
find on the Web. It is about sixteen minutes long.

INTERNET NEWSPAPERS—DAILIES AND PERIODICALS

http://www.theheart.org. Register and get daily e-mails on current controversies in cardiology. You need to know where the debates rage before you
buy into invasive therapies or unproven and dangerous drugs.

http://www.medpagetoday.com. My favorite daily. Videos. Articles with
summaries. This site keeps you up to the minute. Links to the original
source material are always necessary and accompany each article.

http://www.medicalnewstoday.com/newsalerts.php. I used this site. It's
customizable to your interests. But I suggest readers stick to the Editor's
Choice articles that cite the most reputable sources and experts. These offer
the most reliable links. No links . . . no credence.

http://www.jwatch.org. For the money this is a winner. Although it claims to be "by physicians for physicians," you too can sign up for all-site access at $99 a year. Experts survey the medical literature and select the most important research and guidelines. They edit them into easily understood summaries. Also find the most important medical news, drug information, and public health alerts. The online subscription includes fifty-two weeks of complete access to all site content and services. You can sign up for weekly e-mail alerts in four primary care and nine specialty care areas and take advantage of summaries and insights on twenty key medical topics. Physician's First Watch is thrown in. It's a daily e-mail, dedicated to a few medical news stories that doctors (and you) should know about. If you don't want to spend the money, each issue has at least one public-access article.

http://www.cdc.gov/emailupdates/index.html. The Centers for Disease Control and Prevention (CDC) offers a free e-mail subscription service. It takes seconds to apply and choose from dozens of topics for daily or weekly delivery to your e-mail box. Hey, trust it . . . it's the Feds.

http://www.kaiserhealthnews.org. The Kaiser Family Foundation is a nonpartisan, non-profit, private foundation dedicated to producing and communicating the best possible information, research, and analysis on health issues.

http://www.citizen.org/hrg/healthcare/articles.cfm?ID=6146. Public Citizen Health Research Group *Health Letter* brings you critical information about health issues—arming you with up-to-date information so you can make better health-care decisions. Topics include quality of care, insurance, questionable doctors and hospitals, managed care, and the recalls of drugs, devices, and consumer products. Eighteen dollars for twelve issues.

http://www.worstpills.org. Fifteen dollars a year for online access and e-mail updates. Get unlimited access to hundreds of articles on side effects and drug interactions, e-mail alerts with late-breaking safety information, and more.

http://www.yourhealthbase.com. I have the greatest respect for William Ware, Ph.D. Yes, he sells vitamins on his site, but his monthly analyses of controversial medical issues are understandable and well thought out. You will get a worthy education on the medical issues of the day.

THERE *IS* AN APP FOR THAT—
IPHONE AND ANDROID MEDICAL APPS

On Android

Epocrates Rx is a free drug reference that includes OTC medications and drug interactions. Good enough. The Rx Pro version is ninety-nine dollars/ year and adds treatment protocols for infectious diseases and herbal medications. Not for me.

Epocrates Essentials, at a staggering $159/year, includes peer-reviewed disease content, evidence-based treatment options, and interpretation of hundreds of diagnostic and laboratory tests. This outlay makes sense only if you are on the road or away from a computer for protracted periods of time.

MedPage Today is free. It's been mentioned as your doctors' daily newspaper. It should be yours as well.

Skyscape Medical Resources offers Archimedes, a must-have app for medial professionals (and you), as well as drug databases.

American Health Journal is free and offers videos of interviews that educate on medical conditions, health care news, and the ever-vague topic of "wellness."

First Aid (Health Team). Free, highly rated, and loaded with videos and illustrations. Why not? It's free.

On iPhone

Epocrates. The same as above except the alternative medication app is free.

MedPageToday mobile. Free. See above.

Hermes. This is a really nice app that allows you to store your medical records, medications, allergies, and family and physician contacts. At $1.99 it's a steal.

First Aid Lite. Free and helpful for those times you need to know what to do when junior sticks a marble up his adorable little nose.

Medical Radio. Free. Got nothing going on? Tune in and get up to date on the latest and the greatest. Just don't buy into the hype.

A to Z Drug Facts. Free and with a larger database than Epocrates or Medscape.

SayMedicine. Please spend the five dollars. Don't say "Ahh," say Natalizumab. Nothing elevates you more than pronouncing medications and diseases correctly.

RESOURCES MENTIONED IN TEXT

http://www.uptodate.com/patients/about/stories/index.html
http://www.uptodate.com/home/index.html
http://www.usnews.com/sections/rankings
http://www.medpagetoday.com
http://www.healthgrades.com Healthgrades.com
http://www.hibigeebies.com/resources/handwashing_poster.pdf
http://www.caringbridge.org
http://www.hospitalcomplaint.com/stateagencies.html
http://www.consumerreports.org/cro/index.htm
http://www.plosmedicine.org/home.action
http://www.abms.org
http://www.whynotthebest.org.
http://www.hon.ch/HONsearch/Patients/medhunt.html
http://www.nejm.org
http://archsurg.ama-assn.org
http://jama.ama-assn.org
http://www.annals.org
http://www.jfponline.com

Notes

PART I: WAR:
THE BATTLE OF MEDICAL EPISTEMOLOGIES

1. Covell, D. G., Uman, G. C., and Manning, P. R. Information Needs in Office Practice: Are They Being Met? *Annals of Internal Medicine*. October 1985; 103(4):596–99.

2. Davies, Karen. The Information-Seeking Behavior of Doctors: A Review of Evidence. *Health Information & Libraries*. 2007; 24(2):78–94.

3. Doll, W., and Trueit, D. Complexity and the Healthcare Professions. *Journal of Evaluation in Clinical Practice*. 2010; 16(4):841–48.

4. Bernstein, Peter L. *Against the Gods: The Remarkable Story of Risk*. New York: John Wiley & Sons, 1998, p. 7.

5. Steen, R. Grant. Retractions in the Scientific Literature: Do Authors Deliberately Commit Research Fraud? *Medical Ethics*, published online November 15, 2010. doi: 10.1136/jme.2010.038125.

6. Ioannidis, John. Why Most Published Research Findings Are False. *PLoS Med*. 2005; 2(8):e124. doi:10.1371/journal.pmed.0020124. http://www.plosmedicine.org/article/info:doi/10.1371/journal.pmed.0020124 (last accessed 10/19/2010).

7. Barbour, V., et al. An Unbiased Scientific Record Should Be Everyone's Agenda. *PLoS Med*. 2009; 6(2). doi: 10.1371/journal.pmed.1000038. http://www.ncbi.nlm.nih.gov/pmc/articles/PMC2646782 (last accessed 10/19/2010).

8. Robinson, Karen A., and Goodman, Steven N. A Systematic Examination of the Citation of Prior Research in Reports of Randomized, Controlled Trials. *Annals of Internal Medicine*. 2011; 154(1):50–55.

9. Rid, Annette, Ezekiel, Emmanuel, and Wendler, David. Evaluating the Risks of Clinical Research. *Journal of the American Medical Association*. 2010; 304(13):1472–79. doi:10.1001/jama.2010.1414.

10. Hall, M., et al. Community Hospital Oversight of Clinical Investigators' Financial Relationships. *National Institutes of Health.* 2009; 31(1):7–13.

11. Silversides, A. Clinical Trial Participation Poses Ethical, Practical Issues. *Canadian Medical Association Journal.* 2009; 180(5):500–2.

12. Ioannidis, J. Adverse Events in Randomized Trials. *Archives of Internal Medicine.* 2009; 169(19):1737–39.

13. Barrett, Bruce, et al. Echinacea for Treating the Common Cold: A Randomized Trial. *Annals of Internal Medicine.* 2010; 153:769–77.

14. Clinicaltrials.gov. MEND-CABG (MC-1 to Eliminate Necrosis and Damage in Coronary Artery Bypass Graft Surgery Study). Medicure. http://clinicaltrials.gov/ct2/show/NCT00157716 (last accessed 10/19/2010).

15. Miceli, A., et al. Effects of Angiotensin-Converting Enzyme Inhibitor Therapy on Clinical Outcome in Patients Undergoing Coronary Artery Bypass Grafting. *Journal of the American College of Cardiology.* 2009; 54:1778–84.

16. Cardwell, Chris R., et al. Exposure to Oral Bisphosphonates and Risk of Esophageal Cancer. *Journal of the American Medical Association.* 2010; 304(6):657–63.

17. Green, J., et al. Oral Bisphosphonates and Risk of Cancer of Oesophagus, Stomach, and Colorectum; Case-Control Analysis within a UK Primary Care Cohort. *British Medical Journal.* 2010; 341:c4444. doi: 10.1136/bmj.c4444.

18. Cuddihy, R., et al. Effect of Intensive Treatment of Hyperglycaemia on Microvascular Outcomes in Type 2 Diabetes: An Analysis of the ACCORD Randomized Trial. *Lancet.* 2010; 376(9739):419–30.

19. Bluming, Avrum Z., and Tavris, Carol. Hormone Replacement Therapy: Real Concerns and False Alarms. *Cancer Journal.* March/April 2009; 15(2):93–104.

20. Poynard, T., et al. Truth Survival in Clinical Research: An Evidence-Based Requiem? *Annals of Internal Medicine.* 2002; 136:888–95.

21. Spielmans, G., and Parry, P. From Evidence-Based Medicine to Marketing-Based Medicine: Evidence from Internal Industry Documents. *Journal of Bioethical Inquiry.* 2010; 7(1):13–29.

22. Lee, Dong Heun, and Vielemeyer, Ole. Analysis of Overall Level of Evidence behind Infectious Diseases Society of America Practice Guidelines. *Archives of Internal Medicine.* 2011; 171(1):18–22.

23. Kett, Daniel H., et al. Improving Medicine through Pathway Assessment of Critical Therapy of Hospital-Acquired Pneumonia (IMPACT-HAP). The *Lancet Infectious Diseases,* early online publication. January 20, 2011. doi:10.1016/S1473-3099 (10)70314-5.

24. Reed, M. National Clinical Guidelines for the Management of Breast Cancer in Women: Scottish Intercollegiate Guidelines Network. *Clinical Oncology.* 2007; 19:588–90.

25. Survey Report: Clinicians Confident in Ability to Translate Research but Just Barely. *Medical News – Surveys.* October 25, 2009; 12:16.

26. Boyd, et al. Clinical Practice Guidelines and Quality of Care for Older Patients with Multiple Comorbid Diseases: Implications for Pay for Performance. *Journal of the American Medical Association.* 2005; 294:716–24.

27. Davies, Karen. The Information-Seeking Behaviour of Doctors: A Review of the Evidence. *Health Information and Libraries Journal.* 2007; 24(2):78–94.

28. Wright, H. G. *Means, Ends and Medical Care.* Drury University, Springfield, MO: Springer, 2009, p. 168.

29. Gladwell, Malcolm. *Blink: The Power of Thinking without Thinking.* New York: Little, Brown and Company, 2005.

30. Concato, J., Shah, N., and Horwitz, R. Randomized, Controlled Trials, Observational Studies, and the Hierarchy of Research Designs. *New England Journal of Medicine.* 2000; 342:1887–92.

31. Steinberg, E., and Luce, B. Evidence Based? Caveat Emptor! *Health Affairs.* 2005; 24(1):80–92.

32. Ibid.

33. Stolper, E., et al. Consensus on Gut Feelings in General Practice. *BMC Family Practice.* 2009; 10:66.

34. The official website of the Nobel Prize. http://nobelprize.org/nobel_prizes/economics/laureates/2002/kahneman-autobio.html (last accessed 9/24/2010).

35. Choudhry, N., Fletcher, R., and Soumerai, S. Systematic Review: The Relationship between Clinical Experience and Quality of Health Care. *Annals of Internal Medicine.* 2005; 142:260–73.

36. Miglioretti, D., et al. Radiologist Characteristics Associated with Interpretive Performance of Diagnostic Mammography. *Journal of the National Cancer Institute.* 2007; 99(24):1854–63.

37. Davies, Karen. The Information-Seeking Behaviour of Doctors: A Review of the Evidence. *Health Information and Libraries Journal.* 2007; 24(2):78–94.

38. Largent, E., Miller, F., and Pearson, S. Going Off-Label without Venturing Off-Course: Evidence and Ethical Off-Labeling Prescribing. *Archives of Internal Medicine.* 2009; 169(19):1745–47.

39. Hesse, B. W., et al. The Impact of the Internet and Its Implications for Health Care Providers: Findings from the First Health Information National Trends Survey. *Archives of Internal Medicine.* 2005; 165:2618–24.

40. Fox, Susannah. *The Engaged E-patient Population.* Pew Internet & American Life Project. August 26, 2008.

41. WebWatch 2009: An Insight into Usage of the Web in the Health and Medical Sector.

42. Tan, B., Kostapanagiotou, K., and Jilaihawi, A. A Review of Mesothelioma Information on the World Wide Web. *Journal of Thoracic Oncology.* 2009; 4(1):102–4.

43. White, Ryen, and Horvitz, Eric. Experiences with Web Search on Medical Concerns and Self Diagnosis. *AMIA.* 2009; 696–700.

44. Esserman, L., Shieh, Y., and Thompson, I. Rethinking Screening for Breast Cancer and Prostate Cancer. *Journal of the American Medical Association.* 2009; 302(15):1685–92.

45. Welch, H. G., and Black, W. Overdiagnosis in Cancer. *Journal of the National Cancer Institute.* 2010; 102(9):605–13.

46. Esserman, L., and Thompson, I. Solving the Overdiagnosis Dilemma. *Journal of the National Cancer Institute.* 2010; 102(9):582–83.

47. Screening for Breast Cancer: U.S. Preventive Services Task Force Recommendation Statement. *Annals of Internal Medicine.* 2009; 151:716–26.

48. Braddock, C., et al. Informed Decision Making in Outpatient Practice. *Journal of the American Medical Association.* 1999; 282(24):2313–20.

49. Van Leeuwen, P., et al. Balancing the Harms and Benefits of Early Detection of Prostate Cancer. *Cancer.* September 13, 2010. doi:10.1002/cncr.25474.

50. Andriole, G., et al. Mortality Results from a Randomized Prostate-Cancer Screening Trial. *New England Journal of Medicine.* 2009; 360(13):1310–19.

51. Schroder, Fritz, et al. Screening and Prostate-Cancer Mortality in a Randomized European Study. *New England Journal of Medicine.* 2009; 360:1320–28.

52. Hoffman, R., et al. Prostate Cancer Screening Decisions: Results from the National Survey of Medical Decisions (DECISIONS Study). *Archives of Internal Medicine.* 2009; 169(17):1611–18.

CHAPTER 1: THE OFFICE

1. 2009 Survey of Physician Appointment Wait Times. Merritt Hawkins & Associates, 2009.

2. Covell, David G., et al. Information Needs in Office Practice: Are They Being Met? *Annals of Internal Medicine.* 1985; 103:596–99.

3. Isaacs, Stephen L.. The Independent Physician—Going, Going . . . *New England Journal of Medicine.* 2009; 360(7):655–57.

4. Harris, Gardiner. More Doctors Giving Up Private Practices. *New York Times,* March 25, 2010.

5. Physician Placement Starting Salary Survey: 2010 Report Based on 2009 Data. http://www.mgma.com/press/default.aspx?id=33777.

6. DesRoches, Catherine, et al. Physicians' Perceptions, Preparedness for Reporting, and Experiences Related to Impaired and Incompetent Colleagues. *Journal of the American Medical Association.* 2010; 304(2):187–93. doi:10.1001/jama.2010.921.

7. Analysis & Commentary. Accountable Care Organizations: The Case for Flexible Partnerships between Health Plans and Providers. *Health Affairs.* January 2011; 30(1):32–40. doi: 10.1377/hlthaff.2010.0782.

8. Shanafelt, Tait D., et al. Suicidal Ideation among American Surgeons. *Archives of Surgery.* 2011; 146(1):54–62. doi: 10.1001/archsurg.2010.292.

9. Connelly, Julie. Doctors Are Opting Out of Medicare. *New York Times,* April 1, 2009.

10. Levin, D. C., et al. Ownership or Leasing of MRI Facilities by Non-radiologist Physicians Is a Rapidly Growing Trend. *Journal of the American College of Radiology.* 2008 February; 5(2):105–9.

11. Agarwal, R., et al. Trends in PET Scanner Ownership and Leasing by Non-radiologist Physicians. *Journal of the American College of Radiology.* March 2010; 7(3):187–91.

12. Levin, D. C., et al. Ownership or Leasing of CT Scanners by Non-radiologist Physicians: A Rapidly Growing Trend That Raises Concern about Self-referral. *Journal of the American College of Radiology.* 2008; 5(12):1206–9.

13. Berenson, Alex, and Ableson, Reed. Weighing the Costs of a CT Scan's Look inside the Heart. *New York Times,* June 29, 2008.

14. Congressional Committees Ask GAO to Study Effect of Physician Self-Referral of Advanced Medical Imaging on Medicare Spending. April 29, 2010. www.beckers hospitalreview.com.

15. Bylsma, Wayne, et al. Where Have All the General Internists Gone? *Journal of General Internal Medicine*. 2010; 25(10):1020–23. doi:10.1007/s11606-010-1349-2.

16. Baron, Richard J. What's Keeping Us So Busy in Primary Care? A Snapshot from One Practice. *New England Journal of Medicine*. 2010; 362:1632–36.

17. Gilchrist, Valerie, et al. Physician Activities during Time Out of the Examination Room. *Annals of Family Medicine*. 2005; 3:494–99.

18. Wyatt, Jeremy, Batley, Richard, and Keen, Justin. GP Preferences for Information Systems: Conjoint Analysis of Speed, Reliability, Access and Users. *Journal of Evaluation of Clinical Practice*. 2010; 16(5):911–15.

19. Dick III, John D. Predictors of Radiologists' Perceived Risk of Malpractice Lawsuits in Breast Imaging. *American Journal of Roentgenology*. 2009; 192:327–33.

20. Carrier, Emily, et al. Physicians' Fears of Malpractice Lawsuits Are Not Assuaged by Tort Reforms. *Health Affairs*. 2010; 29(9):1585–92.

21. Dick III, John D. Predictors of Radiologists' Perceived Risk of Malpractice Lawsuits in Breast Imaging. *American Journal of Roentgenology*. 2009; 192:327–33.

22. Ostbye, Truls, et al. Is There Time for Management of Patients with Chronic Diseases in Primary Care? *Annals of Family Medicine*. 2005; 3:209–14.

23. Eaton, John, et al. Effect of Visit Length and a Clinical Decision Support Tool on Abdominal Aortic Aneurysm Screening Rates in a Primary Care Practice. *Journal of Evaluation in Clinical Practice*. January 6, 2011. doi: 10.1111/j.1365-2753.2010.01625.x.

24. Bodenheimer, Thomas. Coordinating Care—A Perilous Journey through the Health Care System. *New England Journal of Medicine*. 2008; 358:1064–71.

CHAPTER 2: THE HOSPITAL

1. Westbrook, J. I., et al. Association of Interruptions with an Increased Risk and Severity of Medication Administration. *Archives of Internal Medicine*. 2010; 170:683–90.

2. Lauridsen, Sigurd. Administrative Gatekeeping—A Third Way between Unrestricted Patient Advocacy and Bedside Rationing. *Bioethics*. 2009; 23(5): 311–20.

3. Neily, Julia, et al. Association between Implementation of a Medical Team Training Program and Surgical Mortality. *Journal of the American Medical Association*. 2010; 304(15):1693–1700. doi:10.1001/jama.2010.1506. http://jama.ama-assn.org/cgi/content/full/304/15/1693.

4. Gulshan, Sharma, et al. Continuity of Outpatient and Inpatient Care by Primary Care Physicians for Hospitalized Older Adults. *Journal of the American Medical Association*. 2009; 301(16):1671–80.

5. Glashien, J., et al. The Spectrum of Community-Based Hospital Practice. *Archives of Internal Medicine*. 2007; 167:727–28.

6. Gulshan, Sharma, et al. Comanagement of Hospitalized Surgical Patients by Medicine Physicians in the United States. *Archives of Internal Medicine*. 2010; 170(4):363–68.

7. O'Malley, Patrick G. Internal Medicine Comanagement of Surgical Patients: Can We Afford to Do This? *Archives of Internal Medicine.* 2010; 170(22):1965–66. doi:10.1001/archinternmed.2010.433.

8. Atlas, Steven J., et al. Patient-Physician Connectedness and Quality of Primary Care. *Annals of Internal Medicine.* 2009; 150(5):325–55.

9. Beckman, Howard. On Being a Doctor. Three Degrees of Separation. *Annals of Internal Medicine.* 2009; 151:890–91.

10. Litvak, Eugene, and Pronovost, Peter J. Rethinking Rapid Response Teams. *Journal of the American Medical Association.* 2010; 304(12):1375–76.

11. Kallen, Alexander, et al. Health Care–Associated Invasive MRSA Infections, 2005–2008. *Journal of the American Medical Association.* 2010; 304(6):641–47.

12. Lo, B. Ethical and Policy Implications of Hospitalist Systems. *American Journal of Medicine.* 2001; 111(9):48–52.

13. Sacks, Oliver. *A Leg to Stand On.* New York: Touchstone Books, 1984.

14. Lindenauer, P. K., et al. Outcome of Care by Hospitalists, General Internists and Family Physicians. *New England Journal of Medicine.* 2007; 357:2589–2600.

15. Vasilevskis, Eduard, et al. Cross-Sectional Analysis of Hospitalist Prevalence and Quality of Care in California. *Journal of Hospital Medicine.* 2010; 5(4):200–7.

16. Auerbach, Andrew D., et al. Comanagement of Surgical Patients between Neurosurgeons and Hospitalists. *Archives of Internal Medicine.* 2010; 170(22):2004–10. doi:10.1001/archinternmed.2010.432.

17. Karnon, Jonathan. Model-Based Cost-Effectiveness Analysis of Interventions Aimed at Preventing Medication Error at Hospital Admission (Medicines Reconciliation). *Journal of Evaluation in Clinical Practice.* 2009; 15(2):299–306.

18. Gandhi, Tejal K., and Lee, Thomas. Patient Safety beyond the Hospital. *New England Journal of Medicine.* September 8, 2010; Topics: Health Care Delivery, Quality of Care.

19. Roy, Christopher, et al. Patient Safety Concerns Arising from Test Results That Return after Hospital Discharge. *Annals of Internal Medicine.* 2005; 143:121–28.

20. Bell, Chaim M., et al. Association of Communication between Hospital-Based Physicians and Primary Care Providers with Patient Outcomes. *Journal of General Internal Medicine.* 2009; 24(3):381–86.

21. Moore, C., et al. Medical Errors Related to Discontinuity of Care from an Inpatient to an Outpatient Setting. *Journal of General Internal Medicine.* 2003; 18(8):646–51.

22. Roy, Christopher, et al. Hospital Readmissions: Physician Awareness and Communication Practices. *Journal of General Internal Medicine.* 2009; 24:374–80.

23. Misky, Gregory, Wald, Heidi, and Coleman, Eric. Post-hospitalization Transitions: Examining the Effects of Timing of Primary Care Provider Follow-up. *Journal of Hospital Medicine.* 2010; 5(7):392–97.

24. http://www.theschwartzcenter.org/ViewPage.aspx?pageId=60 (last accessed 1/20/2011).

CHAPTER 3: MEDICAL ON-CALL

1. Yamaguchi, Koji, Kanemitsu, Shuichi, and the Kitakyushu Surgical Study Group. Surgeons' Stress from Surgery and Night Duty: A Multi-institutional Study. *Archives of Surgery.* November 15, 2010. doi:10.1001/archsurg.2010.250.

2. Landro, Laura. Options Expand for Avoiding Crowded ER. *Wall Street Journal*, August 6, 2008.

CHAPTER 4: THE EMERGENCY ROOM

1. Carr, Brendan, et al. Access to Emergency Care in the United States. *Annals of Emergency Medicine*. 2009; 54(2):270–1.

2. American College of Surgeons: Committee on Trauma. www.facs.org/trauma/verified.html (last accessed 10/12/2010).

3. Garwe, Tabitha, et al. Survival Benefit of Transfer to Tertiary Trauma Centers for Major Trauma Patients Initially Presenting to Nontertiary Trauma Centers. *Academic Emergency Medicine*. 2010; 17:1223–32.

4. The National Report Card on the State of Emergency Medicine: Evaluating the Emergency Care Environment State by State, 2009 edition; section 2:2, p. 10.

5. Takata, Glenn, et al. Development, Testing and Findings of a Pediatric-Focused Trigger Tool to Identify Medication-Related Harm in US Children's Hospitals. *Pediatrics*. 2008; 121:e927–e935.

6. Bierce, Ambrose. *The Unabridged Devil's Dictionary.* CreateSpace, December 14, 2009.

7. Krugman, Paul. The Waiting Game. *New York Times*, July 16, 2007.

8. Medical Health Legal Society, Second Division (public record document). Telephone interview with division representative, October 11, 2010.

CHAPTER 5: CHOOSING YOUR DOCTOR: INTRODUCTION

1. Salisbury, Chris, Wallace, Marc, and Montgomery, Alan. Patients' Experience and Satisfaction in Primary Care: Secondary Analysis Using Multilevel Modelling. *British Medical Journal*. 2010; 341:c5004.

2. Birkmeyer, Nancy, et al. Hospital Complication Rates with Bariatric Surgery in Michigan. *Journal of the American Medical Association*. 2010; 304(4):435–42.

CHAPTER 6: COLLEGE AND MEDICAL SCHOOL

1. Riess, Helen. Empathy in Medicine—A Neurobiological Perspective. *Journal of the American Medical Association*. 2010; 304(14):1604–5.

2. Mohammadreza, Hojat, et al. An Empirical Study of Decline in Empathy in Medical School. *Medical Education*. 2004; 38(9):934–41.

3. Dyrbye, Liselotte, et al. Relationship between Burnout and Professional Conduct and Attitudes among US Medical Students. *Journal of the American Medical Association*. 2010; 304(11):1173–80.

CHAPTER 7: BRAINS

1. Saad, Lydia, "Nurses Shine, Bankers Slump in Ethics Ratings." Gallup poll, November 24, 2008.

2. Smith, Charles John. *Synonyms Discriminated*. London: George Bell and Sons, 1893, p. 645.

3. Sweeney, Mark. Wood's Success Starts with Finishing Touch. *New York Times*, April 7, 2008. www.nytimes.com.

4. California HealthCare Foundation, "Just Looking: Consumer Use of the Internet to Manage Care." Harris interactive survey of 1,007 adult Californians from Nov. 5 to Dec. 17, 2007.

5. Sandeep, Jauhar. The Pitfalls of Doctor's Pay for Performance. *New York Times*, September 8, 2008.

6. Tu, Ha T., and Lauer, Johanna. Word of Mouth and Physicians Referrals Still Drive Health Care Provider Choice. Research brief no. 9; December 2008.

7. Terry, Ken. Impaired Physicians: Speak No Evil? *Medical Economics*. 2002; 19:110.

8. Guey-Chi Chen, Peggy, et al. Professional Experiences of International Medical Graduates Practicing Primary Care in the United States. *Journal of General Internal Medicine*. 2010; 25(9):947–53. doi: 10.1007/s11606-010-1401-2.

9. ECFMG. www.ecfmg.org/cert/factcard.pdf (last accessed 10/12/2010).

10. Norcini, J. J., et al. Evaluating the Quality of Care Provided by Graduates of International Medical Schools. *Health Affairs*. 2010; 29(8):1461–68.

CHAPTER 8: COMMUNICATION

1. Engel, Kirsten G., et al. Patient Comprehension of Emergency Department Care and Instructions: Are Patients Aware of When They Do Not Understand? *Annals of Emergency Medicine*. 2009; 53(4):454–61, e15.

2. Suzanne, Audrey, et al. What Oncologists Tell Patients about Survival Benefits of Palliative Chemotherapy and Implications for Informed Consent: Qualitative Study. *British Medical Journal*. 2008; 337:a752.

3. Temel, Jennifer, et al. Early Palliative Care for Patients with Metastatic Non-Small-Cell Lung Cancer. *New England Journal of Medicine*. 2010; 363:733–42.

4. Cykert, Samuel, et al. Factors Associated with Decisions to Undergo Surgery among Patients with Newly Diagnosed Early-Stage Lung Cancer. *Journal of the American Medical Association*. 2010; 303(23):2368–76.

5. Hudak, Pamela L., et al. Older Patients' Unexpressed Concerns about Orthopaedic Surgery. *Journal of Bone and Joint Surgery (American)*. 2008; 90:1427–35.

6. Launer, John. Conversations Inviting Change. *Postgraduate Medical Journal*. 2008; 84(987):4–5.

7. Van Zanten, Marta, et al. Using Standardized Patients to Assess the Interpersonal Skills of Physicians: Six Years' Experience with a High-Stakes Certification Examination. *Health Communication*. 2007; 22 (3):195–205.

8. Morse, Diane, Edwardsen, Elizabeth, and Gordon, Howard. Missed Opportunities for Interval Empathy in Lung Cancer Communication. *Archives of Internal Medicine*. 2008; 168(17):1853–58.

9. Ross, Jennifer T., et al. A Randomized Controlled Trial of a Close Monitoring Program for Minor Depression and Distress. *Journal of General Internal Medicine*. 2008; 23(9):1379–85.

10. Mauksch, Larry B. Relationship, Communication, and Efficiency in the Medical Encounter: Creating a Clinical Model from a Literature Review. *Archives of Internal Medicine*. 2008; 168(13):1387–95.

11. Scheuer, Eberhard, Steurer, Johann, and Buddeberg, Claus. Predictors of Differences in Symptom Perception of Older Patients and Their Doctors. *Family Practice*. 2002; 19(4):357–61.

12. Greer, Joseph, and Halgin, Richard. Predictors of Physician-Patient Agreement on Symptom Etiology in Primary Care. *Psychosomatic Medicine*. 2006; 68:277–82.

13. Barry, Christine A., et al. General Practice Patients' Unvoiced Agendas in General Practice Consultations: A Qualitative Study. *British Medical Journal*. 2000; 320(7244):1246.

14. Lev-Ari, Shiri, and Keysar, Boaz. Why Don't We Believe Non-native Speakers? The Influence of Accent on Credibility. *Journal of Experimental Social Psychology*. 2010; 46(6):1093–96.

15. These are defined by clashing accents borne from two different native languages.

16. Only four of these are free from *any* dialectal differences. The remaining seven encounters are challenged by at least one participant having a different dialect or two parties with different English dialects.

17. Kiemanh, Pham, et al. Alterations during Medical Interpretation of ICU Family Conferences That Interfere with or Enhance Communication. *CHEST*. 2008; 134(1):109–16.

18. U.S. Department of Health and Human Services, Office of Disease Prevention and Health Promotion. 2010. National Action Plan to Improve Health Literacy. Washington, DC.

19. Sheridan, S. L., and Pignone, M. Numeracy and the Medical Student's Ability to Interpret Data. *Effective Clinical Practice*. 2002; 5:35–40.

20. Schwartz, L. M. The Role of Numeracy in Understanding the Benefit of Screening Mammography. *Annals of Internal Medicine*. 1997; 127:966–72.

21. Baker, D., et al. Health Literacy and Mortality among Elderly Persons. *Archives of Internal Medicine*. 2007; 167(14):1503–9.

22. Stamatakis E., et al. Screen Based Entertainment Time, All-Cause Mortality, and Cardiovascular Events. Population Based Study with Ongoing Mortality and Hospital Events Follow-up. *Journal of the American College of Cardiology*. 2011; 57:292–99.

CHAPTER 9: EMPATHY

1. Pollak, Kathryn, et al. Oncologist Communication about Emotion during Visits with Patients with Advanced Cancer. *Journal of Clinical Oncology*. 2007; 25:5748–52.

2. Morse, Diane, Edwardsen, Elizabeth, and Gordon, Howard. Missed Opportunities for Interval Empathy in Lung Cancer Communication. *Archives of Internal Medicine*. 2008; 168(7):1853–58.

3. Kennifer, Sarah, et al. Negative Emotions in Cancer Care: Do Oncologists' Responses Depend on Severity and Type of Emotion? *Patient Education and Counseling*. 2008; 76(1):51–56.

4. Arora, N. K., and Gustafson, D. H. Perceived Helpfulness of Physicians' Communication Behavior and Breast Cancer Patients' Level of Trust over Time. *Journal of General Internal Medicine*. 2009; 24(2):252–55.

5. Levinson, W., Gorawara-Bhat, R., and Lamb, J. A Study of Patient Clues and Physician Responses in Primary Care and Surgical Settings. *Journal of the American Medical Association*. 2000; 284(8):1021–27.

6. Mohammadreza, Hojat, et al. An Empirical Study of Decline in Empathy in Medical School. *Medical Education*. 2004; 38(9):934–41.

7. Cheng, Y., et al. Expertise Modulates the Perception of Pain in Others. *Current Biology*. 2007; 17(19):1708–13.

8. Kearney, Michael K., et al. Self-care of Physicians Caring for Patients at the End of Life. *Journal of the American Medical Association*. 2009; 301(11):1155–64.

9. Warren, Lynne. *Encyclopedia of 20th Century Photography*. New York: Routledge, 2005, p. 841.

10. Broyard, Anatole. *Intoxicated by My Illness*. New York: Ballantine Books, 1992.

CHAPTER 10: STYLE

1. Shakespeare, William. *The Merchant of Venice*.

2. Sequist, T. D., et al. Quality Monitoring of Physicians: Linking Patients' Experiences of Care to Clinical Quality and Outcomes. *Journal of General Internal Medicine*. 2008; 23(11):1784–90.

3. Kahn, Michael W. Etiquette-Based Medicine. *New England Journal of Medicine*. 2008; 358(19):1988–89.

CHAPTER 11: SECOND OPINIONS

1. Campbell, Eric G. Doctors and Drug Companies—Scrutinizing Influential Relationships. *New England Journal of Medicine*. 2007; 357(18):1796–97.

2. Axona, Anthony, et al. Ethical and Legal Implications in Seeking and Providing a Second Medical Opinion. *Digestive Diseases*. 2008; 26(1):11–17.

3. Newman, Erika A., et al. Changes in Surgical Management Resulting from Case Review at a Breast Cancer Multidisciplinary Tumor Board. *Cancer*. 2006; 107(10):2346–51.

4. Schuhmacher, C., et al. Good Advice Is Precious: The Second Opinion from the Point of View of an Interdisciplinary Cancer Therapy Center. *Deutsche Medizinische Wochenschrift*. 2007; 132(17):921–26.

5. Lehnhardt, M., et al. Importance of Specialized Centers in Diagnosis and Treatment of Extremity-Soft Tissue Sarcomas. Review of 603 Cases. *Der Chirurg*. 2009; 80(4):341–47.

6. Briggs, G. M., et al. The Role of Specialist Neuroradiology Second Opinion Reporting: Is There Added Value? *Clinical Radiology*. 2007; 63(7):791–95.

7. Elixhauser, Anne, and Andrews, Roxanne M. Profile of Inpatient Operating Room Procedures in US Hospitals in 2007. *Archives of Surgery*. 2010; 145(12):1201–8. doi:10.1001/archsurg.2010.269.

8. http://cancercenters.cancer.gov/cancer_centers/cancer-centers-list.html (last accessed 10/19/2010).

9. http://www.nccn.org/members/network.asp (last accessed 10/19/2010).

CHAPTER 12: CHOOSING YOUR HOSPITAL: INTRODUCTION

1. Scott C., et al. Performance of Top-Ranked Heart Care Hospitals on Evidence-Based Process Measures. *Circulation.* 2006; 114:558–64.

2. 2008 Update on Consumers' Views of Patient Safety and Quality Information—Kaiser Family Foundation.

3. Krugman, Paul. "Keeping Them Honest." *New York Times,* June 5, 2009.

4. Finlayson, S. R., et al. Patient Preferences for Location of Care: Implications for Regionalization. *Medical Care.* 1999; 37(2):204–9.

5. Americans as Health Care Consumers: Update on the Role of Quality Information; Highlights of a National Survey. http://www.ahrq.gov/qual/kffhigh00.htm (last accessed 10/19/2010).

CHAPTER 13: STAYING LOCAL

1. Kowalczyk, Liz. Report Lauds Community Hospitals: Quality of Care Is on Par with Teaching Facilities While Costs Are Lower. *Boston Globe,* November 18, 2004.

2. Yasaitis, Laura, et al. Hospital Quality and Intensity of Spending: Is There an Association? Hospitals' Performance on Quality of Care Is Not Associated with the Intensity of Their Spending. *Health Affairs.* 2009; 28(4):w566–w572.

3. Hospital Survey on Patient Safety Culture: 2009 Comparative Database Report. www.ahrq.gov (last accessed 10/19/2010).

4. Ross, J., et al. Hospital Remoteness and Thirty-Day Mortality from Three Serious Conditions. *Health Affairs.* 2008; 27(6):1707–17.

5. Wennberg, John, et al. Inpatient Care Intensity and Patients' Ratings of Their Hospital Experiences. *Health Affairs.* 2009; 28(1):103.

6. Montalescot, Gilles, et al. Immediate vs. Delayed Intervention for Acute Coronary Syndromes: A Randomized Clinical Trial. *Journal of the American Medical Association.* 2009; 302(9):947–54.

7. Cantor, W., et al. Routine Early Angioplasty after Fibrinolysis for Acute Myocardial Infarction. *New England Journal of Medicine.* 2009; 26:2705–18.

8. Brown, D. L. Measuring Outcomes of Coronary Artery Bypass Surgery: What Is Important and to Whom? *Archives of Internal Medicine.* (2010); 170:1189–90.

9. Neugeboren, Jay. In Matters of the Heart, Luck Can Make All the Difference. *New York Times,* February 9, 2009.

CHAPTER 14: ABANDON SHIP!

1. Siegler, M. Pascal's Wager and the Hanging of Crepe. *New England Journal of Medicine.* 1975; 293(17):853–57.

2. Ibid.

CHAPTER 15: SEARCHING FOR SOLUTIONS

1. Kizer, Kenneth. The Volume-Outcome Conundrum. *New England Journal of Medicine.* 2003; 349(22):2159–61.

2. Livingston, Edward, and Cao, Jing. Procedure Volume as a Predictor of Surgical Outcomes. *Journal of the American Medical Association.* 2010; 304:95–97.

3. Birkmeyer, J. D., et al. Surgeon Volume and Operative Mortality in the United States. *New England Journal of Medicine.* 2003; 349(22):2117–27.

4. Gahferi Amir, Birkmeyer, John, and Dimick, Justin. Variation in Hospital Mortality Associated with Inpatient Surgery. *New England Journal of Medicine.* October 1, 2009; 361(14):1368–75.

5. http://www.leapfroggroup.org/media/file/FactSheet_EBHR.pdf (last accessed 10/19/2010).

6. Peterson, Eric D., et al. Procedural Volume as a Marker of Quality for CABG Surgery. *Journal of the American Medical Association.* 2004; 291:195–201.

7. Halm, Ethan A., Lee, Clara, and Chassin, Mark R. Is Volume Related to Outcome in Health Care? A Systematic Review and Methodologic Critique of the Literature. *Annals of Internal Medicine.* 2002; 137:511–20.

8. Birkmeyer, John D., et al. Hospital Volume and Late Survival after Cancer Surgery. *Annals of Surgery.* 2007; 245(5)777–83.

9. Ross, Joseph, et al. Hospital Volume and 30-Day Mortality for Three Common Medical Conditions. *New England Journal of Medicine.* 2010; 362:1110–18.

10. Birkmeyer, N. J. O., et al. Hospital Complication Rates with Bariatric Surgery in Michigan. *Journal of the American Medical Association.* 2010; 304:435–42.

11. Bilimoria, Karl, et al. Risk-Based Selective Referral for Cancer Surgery: A Potential Strategy to Improve Perioperative Outcomes. *Annals of Surgery.* 2010; 251(4):708–16.

12. Birkmeyer, J. D., et al. Regionalization of High-Risk Surgery and Implications for Patient Travel Times. *Journal of the American Medical Association.* November 26, 2003; 290:2703–8.

CHAPTER 16: HOSPITAL DANGERS: INTRODUCTION

1. Woolf, Virginia. *On Being Ill.* Ashfield, MA: Paris Press, 2002, p. 8.

2. Adams, P. F., Barnes, P. M., Vickerie, J. L. Summary Health Statistics for the U.S. Population: National Health Interview Survey, 2007. National Center for Health Statistics. *Vital Health Statistics.* 2008; 10(238).

3. Gawande, Atul. Annals of Medicine: The Checklist; If Something So Simple Can Transform Intensive Care, What Else Can It Do? *New Yorker,* December 10, 2007.

4. Mortality Measurement in the EMR Era: What Real Time Lab and Clinical Data Can Contribute to Precision and Prediction. http://www.ahrq.gov/qual/mortality/Escobar.htm (last accessed 10/19/2010).

5. Patient Safety Indicators Overview. AHRQ Quality Indicators. February 2006. Agency for Healthcare Research and Quality, Rockville, MD. http://www.quality indicators.ahrq.gov/psi_overview.htm (last accessed 10/19/2010).

6. AHRQ Publication no. 090001, March 2009. www.ahrq.gov/qual/qrdr08 .htm (last accessed 10/19/2010).

7. http://www.leapfroggroup.org/media/file/leapfrogreportfinal.pdf (last accessed 10/19/2010).

8. U.S. Health Care System Fails to Protect Patients from Deadly Medical Errors. May 19, 2009. http://www.consumersunion.org/pub/core_health_care/011324 .html (last accessed 10/19/2010).

9. Landrigan, Christopher P., et al. Temporal Trends in Rates of Patient Harm Resulting from Medical Care. *New England Journal of Medicine.* 2010; 363:2124–34.

10. Mathews, Simon C., and Pronovost, Peter J. Physician Autonomy and Informed Decision Making: Finding the Balance for Patient Safety and Quality. *Journal of the American Medical Association.* 2008; 300(24):2913–15.

11. Pronovost, Peter J. Learning Accountability for Patient Outcomes. *Journal of the American Medical Association.* 2010; 304(2):204–5. doi:10.1001.jama.2010.979.

12. National Air Traffic Controllers Association. http://natca.unionlaborworks .com/index.aspx (last accessed 10/19/2010).

13. Chassin, M. R. Is Healthcare Ready for Six Sigma Quality? *Milbank Q.* 1998; 76(4):565–91.

14. Witte, David, et al. Errors, Mistakes, Blunders, Outliers, or Unacceptable Results: How Many? *Clinical Chemistry.* 1997; 43:1352–56.

15. Sevdalis, Nick, et al. Closing the Safety Loop: Evaluation of the National Patient Safety Agency's Guidance Regarding Wristband Identification of Hospital Inpatients. *Journal of Evaluation in Clinical Practice.* 2009; 15(2):311–15.

16. Zhan, Chunliu, and Miller, Marlene R. Excess Length of Stay, Charges, and Mortality Attributable to Medical Injuries during Hospitalization. *Journal of the American Medical Association.* 2003; 290(14):1868–74.

17. Vest, Joshua, et al. A Critical Review of the Research Literature on Six Sigma, Lean and Studer Group's Hardwiring Excellence in the United States: The Need to Demonstrate and Communicate the Effectiveness of Transformation Strategies in Healthcare. *Implementation Science.* 2009; 4:35.

18. Pronovost, P. J., et al. Defining and Measuring Patient Safety. *Critical Care Clinics.* 2005; 21:1-19.

19. Ghaleb, Maisoon, et al. The Incidence and Nature of Prescribing and Medication Administration Errors in Paediatric Inpatients. *Archives of Disease in Childhood.* 2010; 95:113–18.

20. Gopher, D., Olin, M., Donchin, Y., et al. The Nature and Causes of Human Errors in Medical Intensive Care Unit. Presented at the 33rd annual meeting of the Human Factors Society, October 18, 1989, Denver, Colorado.

21. Bagian, James. Online NewsHour: VA Hospital Takes Steps to Avoid Medical Mistakes. February 7, 2005. http://www.pbs.org/newshour/bb/health/jan-june05/ errors_2-7.html (accessed 10/19/2010).

22. Leape, Lucian L. Error in Medicine. *Journal of the American Medical Association.* 1994; 272(23):1851–57.

CHAPTER 17: MEDICATION ERRORS

1. U.S. Health Care System Fails to Protect Patients from Deadly Medical Errors. Consumersunion.org, May 19, 2009.

2. Adverse Drug Reactions: How Serious Is the Problem and How Often and Why Does It Occur? http://www.worstpills.org/public/page.cfm?op_id=4 (last accessed 10/19/2010).

3. Brennan, T. A., Leape, L. L., Larid, N., et al. Incidence of Adverse Effects and Negligence in Hospitalized Patients: Results of the Harvard Medical Practice Study. *New England Journal of Medicine.* 1991; 324:370–76.

4. Davies, E. C., et al. Adverse Drug Reactions in Hospital In-Patients: A Prospective Analysis of 3,695 Patient-Episodes. *PloS ONE.* 2009; 4(2):e4439. doi:10.1371/journal.pone.0004439. http://dx.plos.org/10.1371/journal.pone.0004439 (last accessed 10/19/2010).

5. Lazarou, Jason, Pomeranz, Bruce, and Corey, Paul. Incidence of Adverse Drug Reactions in Hospitalized Patients: A Meta-analysis of Prospective Studies. *Journal of the American Medical Association.* 1998; 279:1200–5.

6. 6 of Every 100 Patients Die in Hospital Due to Adverse Drug Reaction. Official website of the *Journal of Anaesthesiology Clinical Pharmacology.* http://www.joacp.org/index.php?option=com_content&task=view&id=190&Itemid=58 (last accessed 10/19/2010).

7. Pippins, J. R., Gandhi, T. K., Hamann, C., et al. Classifying and Predicting Errors of Inpatient Medication Reconciliation. *Journal of General Internal Medicine.* 2008; 23:1414–22.

8. NQF Safe Practices for Better Healthcare 2009 Update. Webinar: Medication Safety—Complex Issues for All. Safe Practices 17–18. Hosted by NQF and TMIT.

9. From the Pharmacy to the Bedside: Preventing Medication Errors with Barcode Technology. Web Seminar. June 10, 2009. http://www.healthdatamanagement.com/web_seminars (accessed and attended 9/30/2010).

10. Takata, G. S., et al. Development, Testing, and Findings of a Pediatric-Focused Trigger Tool to Identify Medication-Related Harm in U.S. Children's Hospitals. *Pediatrics.* 2008; 121(4):e927–e935.

11. Moore, Thomas, Cohen, Michael, and Furberg, Curt. Serious Adverse Drug Events Reported to the Food and Drug Administration, 1998–2005. *Archives of Internal Medicine.* 2007; 167(16):1752–59.

12. To Err Is Human: To Delay Is Deadly. Consumers Union, May 2009. http://www.safepatientproject.org/safepatientproject.org/pdf/safepatientproject.org-ToDelayIsDeadly.pdf (last accessed 10/19/2010).

13. Sharma, Gulshan, et al. Continuity of Outpatient and Inpatient Care by Primary Care Physicians for Hospitalized Older Adults. *Journal of the American Medical Association.* 2009; 301(16):1671–80.

14. Arora, Vineet, et al. Ability of Hospitalized Patients to Identify Their In-Hospital Physicians. *Archives of Internal Medicine.* 2009; 169(2):199–201.

15. Cumbler, Ethan, Wald, Heidi, and Kutner, Jean. Lack of Patient Knowledge regarding Hospital Medications. *Journal of Hospital Medicine.* 2010; 5(2):83–86.

16. Chan, Amy Hai Yan, et al. Effect of Education on the Recording of Medicines on Admission to Hospital. *Journal of General Internal Medicine.* 2010; 25(6):537–42.

17. Pippins, J. R., et al. Classifying and Predicting Errors of Inpatient Medication Reconciliation. *Journal of General Internal Medicine.* 2008; 23:1414–22.

18. Ibid.

19. DeMichele Cousins, Diane, ed. Medication Use: A Systems Approach to Reducing Errors, The Joint Commission, 1998, p. 65.

20. Poon, Eric, et al. Effect of Bar-Code Technology on the Safety of Medication Administration. *New England Journal of Medicine.* 2010; 362:1698–1707.

21. Kohn, Linda, Corrigan, Janet, and Donaldson, Molla. To Err Is Human: Building a Safer Health System. Institute of Medicine. 2010.

22. 6 of Every 100 Patients Die in Hospital Due to Adverse Drug Reaction. Official website of the *Journal of Anaesthesiology Clinical Pharmacology.* http://www.joacp .org/index.php?option=com_content&view=article&id=190&catid=1 (last accessed 10/19/2010).

23. Moore, T. J., Cohen, M. R., Furberg, C. D. Serious Adverse Drug Events Reported to the Food and Drug Administration, 1998–2005. *Archives of Internal Medicine.* 2007; 167:1752–59.

24. Pippins, J., et al. Classifying and Predicating Errors of Inpatient Medication Reconciliation. *Journal of General Internal Medicine.* 2008; 28(9):1414–22.

25. Valentin, A., et al. Errors in Administration of Parenteral Drugs in Intensive Care Units: Multinational Prospective Study. *British Medical Journal.* 2009; 338:b814.

26. Stahel, Philip F., et al. Wrong-Site and Wrong-Patient Procedures in the Universal Protocol Era: Analysis of a Prospective Database of Physician Self-reported Occurrences. *Archives of Surgery.* 2010; 145(10):978–84. doi:10.1001/archsurg.2010.185.

27. Howanitz, Peter J. Continuous Wristband Monitoring over 2 Years Decreases Identification Errors: A College of American Pathologists Q-Tracks Study. *Archives of Pathology and Laboratory Medicine.* July 2002; 126(7):809–15.

28. Sevdalis, Nick, et al. Closing the Safety Loop: Evaluation of the National Patient Safety Agency's Guidance regarding Wristband Identification of Hospital Inpatients. *Journal of Evaluation in Clinical Practice.* 2009; 15(2):311–15.

29. Garfinkel, Doron, and Mangin, Derelie. Feasibility Study of a Systematic Approach for Discontinuation of Multiple Medications in Older Adults. *Archives of Internal Medicine.* 2010; 170(18):1648–54.

30. Moen, Janne, et al. GPs' Perceptions of Multiple-Medicine Use in Older Patients. *Journal of Evaluation in Clinical Practice.* 2010; 16(1):69–75.

31. Gill, Sudeep, et al. A Prescribing Cascade Involving Cholinesterase Inhibitors and Anticholinergic Drugs. *Archives of Internal Medicine.* 2005; 165:808–13.

32. Peterson, Melody, quoting A. Relman, *Our Daily Meds: How the Pharmaceutical Companies Transformed Themselves into Slick Marketing Machines and Hooked the Nation on Prescription Drugs.* New York: Farrar, Straus and Giroux, 2008, p. 7 (paperback).

33. Gu, Qiuping, Dillon, Charles, and Burt, Vicki. Prescription Drug Use Continues to Increase: U.S. Prescription Drug Data for 2007–2008. NCHS Data Brief no. 42. September 2010.

CHAPTER 18: HOSPITAL-ACQUIRED INFECTIONS

1. http://www.fbi.gov/wanted/topten/tenfaq.htm#14 (last accessed 10/19/2010).

2. Summary of Notifiable Disease, United States, 2001. http://www.cdc.gov/ncphi/od/ai/annsum/2001/01bg.htm (last accessed 10/19/2010).

3. Klevens, R. M., et al. Estimating Health Care–Associated Infections and Deaths in U.S. Hospitals, 2002.

4. National Healthcare Quality Report, 2009. http://www.ahrq.gov/qual/nhqr09/nhqr09.pdf (last accessed 10/19/2010).

5. Lucado, J., et al. Adult Hospital Stays with Infections Due to Medical Care, 2007. Agency for Healthcare Research and Quality 2010; statistical brief #94.

6. Sharon, Gil, et al. Commensal Bacteria Play a Role in Mating Preference of Drosophila melanogaster. *Proceedings of the National Academy of Sciences.* Published online November 1, 2010. doi: 10.1073/pnas.1009906107.

7. McCay, Paul H, Ocampo-Sosa, Alain A., and Fleming, Gerard T. A. Effect of Subinhibitory Concentrations of Benzalkonium Chloride on the Competitiveness of *Pseudomonas aeruginosa* Grown in Continuous Culture. *Microbiology.* 2010; 156:30–38. doi: 10.1099/mic.0.029751-0.

8. Zhang, Yuting; Lee, Bruce Y., and Donohue, Julie M. Ambulatory Antibiotic Use and Prescription Drug Coverage in Older Adults. *Archives of Internal Medicine.* 2010; 170(15):1308–14. doi:10.1001/archinternmed.2010.235.

9. Martinez, Barbara. Gut Reaction: "Good" Microbes under Attack. *Wall Street Journal,* August 18, 2009.

10. Niedner, Matthew. The Harder You Look, the More You Find: Catheter-Associated Bloodstream Infection Surveillance Variability. *American Journal of Infection Control.* 2010; 38(8):585–95.

11. Henderson, D. Managing Methicillin-Resistant Staphylococci. *American Journal of Infection Control.* 2006; 34(5):S46–54.

12. Voss, Andreas, and Widmer, Andreas. No Time for Handwashing!? Handwashing versus Alcoholic Rub: Can We Afford 100% Compliance? *Infection Control and Hospital Epidemiology.* 1997; 18(3):205–8.

13. Pittet, Didier, et al. Compliance with Handwashing in a Teaching Hospital. *Annals of Internal Medicine.* January 19, 1999; 130:126–30.

14. A Survey of Handwashing Behavior (Trended). Prepared for the American Microbiology Society and the American Cleaning Institute, August 2010.

15. Korniewicz, Denise, and El-Masri, Maher. Exploring the Factors Associated with Hand Hygiene Compliance of Nurses during Routine Clinical Practice. *Applied Nursing Research.* 2010; 23(2):86–90.

16. LaMont, Thomas J. Epidemiology, Microbiology, and Pathophysiology of Clostridium difficile Infection in Adults. UpToDate.com. Last literature review version 18.2: May 2010. This topic last updated: June 15, 2010.

17. Anderson, Deverick, et al. Strategies to Prevent Surgical Site Infections in Acute Care Hospitals. *Infection Control and Hospital Epidemiology.* 2008; 29:s51–s61.

18. Surgical Site Infection. Department of Health and Human Services Center for Disease Control and Prevention. http://www.cdc.gov/HAI/burden.html (last accessed 1/20/2010).

19. Consumers Union Report: Almost 100,000 Surgical Patients Didn't Get the Right Infection Prevention Care during Year Studied. ConsumersUnion.org. April 27, 2009.

20. Anderson, Deverick, et al. Strategies to Prevent Surgical Site Infections in Acute Care Hospitals. *Infection Control and Hospital Epidemiology.* 2008; 29: s51–s61.

21. Misteli, Heidi, et al. Surgical Glove Perforation and the Risk of Surgical Site Infection. *Archives of Surgery.* 2009; 144(6):553–58.

22. Wenzel, Richard P. Minimizing Surgical-Site Infections. *New England Journal of Medicine.* 2010; 362:75–77.

23. Evans, H. L., et al. Effect of Chlorhexidine Whole-Body Bathing on Hospital-Acquired Infections among Trauma Patients. *Archives of Surgery.* 2010; 145(3):240–46.

24. Walsh, Edward, Greene, Linda, and Kirshner, Ronald. Sustained Reduction in Methicillin-Resistant *Staphylococcus aureus* Wound Infections after Cardiovascular Surgery. *Archives of Internal Medicine.* Published online September 13, 2010. doi: 10.1001/archinternmed.2010.326.

25. Walsh, Edward E., Greene, Linda, and Ronald Kirshner. Sustained Reduction in Methicillin-Resistant *Staphylococcus aureus* Wound Infections after Cardio-thoracic Surgery. *Archives of Internal Medicine.* 2011; 171(1):68–73. doi: 10.1001/archinternmed.2010.326.

26. Mangram, Alicia, et al. Guideline for Prevention of Surgical Site Infection, 1999. *Infection Control and Hospital Epidemiology.* 1999; 20(4).

27. Gujadhur, Rahul, et al. Continuous Subglottic Suction Is Effective for Prevention of Ventilator Associated Pneumonia. European Association of Cardio-Thoracic Surgery, 2005.

28. Ibid.

29. Kollef, Marin. The Prevention of Ventilator-Associated Pneumonia. *New England Journal of Medicine.* 1999; 340:627–34.

30. Guidelines for the Prevention of Intravascular Catheter-Related Infections. *Morbidity and Mortality Weekly Report.* August 9, 2002; 51(RR10).

31. Landro, Laura. "Superbugs" That Strike the Sickest Patients. *The Informed Patient.* October 1, 2008.

32. Leapfrog Hospital Survey Results. The Leapfrog Group. 2008. http://www.leapfroggroup.org/media/file/leapfrogreportfinal.pdf (last accessed 10/19/2010).

33. Remove that Foley! http://www.apic.org/Content/NavigationMenu/PracticeGuidance/APICEliminationGuides/Foley_2.doc (last accessed 10/19/2010).

34. Jain, P., et al. Overuse of the Indwelling Urinary Tract Catheter in Hospitalized Medical Patients. *Archives of Internal Medicine.* 1995; 155:425–29.

35. Tambyah, P. A., and Maki, D. G. The Relationship between Pyuria and Infection in Patients with Indwelling Urinary Catheters: A Prospective Study of 761 Patients. *Archives of Internal Medicine.* 2000; 160(5):673–77.

36. Jain, P. et al. Overuse of the Indwelling Urinary Tract Catheter in Hospitalized Medical Patients. *Archives of Internal Medicine.* 1995; 155:425–29.

37. Saint, S., et al. Are Physicians Aware of Which of Their Patients Have Indwelling Urinary Catheters? *American Journal of Medicine.* 2000; 109(6):476–80.

38. Saint, Sanjay, et al. Preventing Hospital-Acquired Urinary Tract Infection in the United States: A National Study. *Clinical Infectious Diseases.* 2008; 46:243–50.

39. Prevent Catheter-Associated Urinary Tract Infection. IHI.org. http://www .ihi.org/IHI/Programs/ImprovementMap/PreventCatheterAssociatedUrinaryTract Infections.htm (last accessed 10/19/2010).

40. Ibid.

41. Teltsch, Dana Y., et al. Infection Acquisition Following Intensive Care Unit Room Privatization. *Archives of Internal Medicine.* 2011; 171(1):32–38.

42. Griffith, C. J., et al. An Evaluation of Hospital Cleaning Regimes and Standards. *Journal of Hospital Infection.* 2000; 45:19–28.

43. Carling, P. C., et al. Identifying Opportunities to Enhance Environmental Cleaning in 23 Acute Care Hospitals. *Infection Control and Hospital Epidemiology.* 2008; 29:1–7.

44. Merrer, Jacques, et al. "Colonization Pressure" and Risk of Acquisition of Methicillin-Resistant Staphylococcus Aureus in a Medical Intensive Care Unit. *Infection Control and Hospital Epidemiology.* November 2000; 21(11):718–23.

45. Datta, R., et al. Impact of an Environmental Cleaning Intervention on the Risk of Acquiring MRSA and VRE from Prior Room Occupants. Society of Hospital Epidemiologists of America. 2009; Abstract 2.

46. Animal Cage Washing and Room Cleaning Guidelines for Personal Protective Equipment (PPE) and Biosafety Requirements. http://www.ncsu .edu/ehs/www99/right/handsMan/animal/forms/an_cge_wash.pdf (last accessed 10/19/2010).

47. Establishment of Health Regulations for Concentrated Animal Feeding Operations (CAFOs). http://agebb.missouri.edu/commag/permit/pdf/PlatteCounty .pdf (last accessed 10/19/2010).

48. Carling, P. C. Identifying Opportunities to Enhance Environmental Cleaning in 23 Acute Care Hospitals. *Infection Control and Hospital Epidemiology.* 2008; 29:1–7 (original article).

49. Carling, Philip C., and Bartley, Judene M. Evaluating Hygienic Cleaning in Health Care Settings: What You Do Not Know Can Harm Your Patients. *American Journal of Infection Control.* 2010; 38(5 Suppl. 1):S41–S50.

50. Griffith, C. J., et al. An Evaluation of Hospital Cleaning Regimes and Standards. *Journal of Hospital Infection.* 2000; 45:19–28.

51. Johnston, B. Lynn, and Bryce, Elizabeth. Hospital Infection Control Strategies for Vancomycin-Resistant Enterococcus, Methicillin-Resistant Staphylococcus aureus and Clostridium difficile. *Canadian Medical Association Journal.* March 17, 2009; 180(6):627–31. doi:10.1503/cmaj.080195.

52. Base-Smith, Victoria. Nondisposable Sphygmomanometer Cuffs Harbor Frequent Bacterial Colonization and Significant Contamination by Organic and Inorganic Matter. *AANA Journal.* 1996; 64(2):141–45.

53. Jones, Jeffrey, Hoerle, David, and Riekse, Robert. Stethoscopes: A Potential Vector of Infection? *Annals of Emergency Medicine.* 1995; 26(3):296–99.

54. Myers, Martin G. Longitudinal Evaluation of Neonatal Nosocomial Infections: Association of Infection with Blood Pressure Cuff. *Pediatrics.* 1978; 61:42–45.

CHAPTER 19: ISOLATION

1. Hall, Gerri, and Flayhart, Diane. Approaches to Infection Control: Active Surveillance Culture as a Promising New Tool. *Infection Control Today.* February 1, 2006.

2. Robicsek, Ari, et al. Universal Surveillance for Methicillin-Resistant Staphylococcus aureus in 3 Affiliated Hospitals. *Annals of Internal Medicine.* 2008; 148:409–18.

3. McCaughey, Betsy. Unnecessary Deaths: The Human and Financial Costs of Hospital Infections. 3rd edition. http://www.hospitalinfection.org/ridbooklet.pdf (last accessed 10/19/2010).

4. Siegel, Jane, et al. Management of Multidrug-Resistant Organisms in Healthcare Settings, 2006. http://www.cdc.gov/ncidod/dhqp/pdf/ar/mdroguideline2006.pdf.

5. Henderson, D. Managing Methicillin-Resistant Staphylococci: A Paradigm for Preventing Nosocomial Transmission of Resistant Organisms. *American Journal of Infection Control.* 2006; 34(5 Suppl 1):s46–54.

6. Ibid.

7. Nasraway, Stanley A. Search and Destroy for Methicillin-Resistant Staphylococcus aureus in the Intensive Care Unit: Should This Now Be the Standard of Care? *Critical Care Medicine.* 2007; 35(2):642–44.

8. Kirkland, Kathryn B., and Weinstein, Jill M. Adverse Effects of Contact Isolation. *Lancet.* October 2, 1999; 354.

9. Donskey, C. J. Preventing Transmission of Clostridium difficile: Is the Answer Blowing in the Wind? *Clinical Infectious Diseases.* 2010; 50(11):1458–61.

10. Best, E. L., et al. The Potential for Airborne Dispersal of Clostridium difficile from Symptomatic Patients. *Clinical Infectious Diseases.* 2010; 50(11):1450–57.

11. Sexton, T., et al. Environmental Reservoirs of Methicillin-Resistant Staphylococcus aureus in Isolation Rooms: Correlation with Patient Isolates and Implications for Hospital Hygiene. *Journal of Hospital Infection.* 2006; 62(2):187–94.

12. Sontag, Susan. *Illness As Metaphor.* New York: Farrar, Straus, Giroux, 1988.

13. Freeland, Kenneth, et al. Treatment of Depression after Coronary Artery Bypass Surgery: A Randomized Controlled Trial. *Archives of General Psychiatry.* 2009; 66(4):387–96.

14. Nickinson, Richard, Board, Timothy, and Kay, Peter. Post-operative Anxiety and Depression Levels in Orthopaedic Surgery: A Study of 56 Patients Undergoing Hip or Knee Arthroplasty. *Journal of Evaluation in Clinical Practice.* 2009; 15(2):307–10.

15. Carr, Eloise, Thomas, Veronica Nicky, and Wilson-Barnet, Jennifer. Patient Experiences of Anxiety, Depression and Acute Pain after Surgery: A Longitudinal Perspective. *International Journal of Nursing Studies.* 2005; 42(5):521–30.

16. Bierce, Ambrose. *The Unabridged Devil's Dictionary.* CreateSpace, December 14, 2009.

17. Walch, Jeffrey, et al. The Effect of Sunlight on Postoperative Analgesic Medication Use: A Prospective Study of Patients Undergoing Spinal Surgery. *Psychosomatic Medicine.* 2005; 67:156–63.

18. Salimpoor, Valorie N., et al. Anatomically Distinct Dopamine Release during Anticipation and Experience of Peak Emotion to Music. *Nature Neuroscience.* Published online January 9, 2011. doi: 10.1038/nn.2726.

19. Komori, Teruhisa, et al. Stress Repression in Restrained Rats by ®-(-)-Linalool Inhalation and Gene Expression Profiling of Their Whole Blood Cells. *European Neuropsychopharmacology*. 1995; 5(4):477–80.

20. Turner, Yehonatan, and Hadas-Halpern, Irith. The Effects of Including a Patient's Photograph to the Radiographic Examination. Presented at the Radiologic Association of North America, December 2008.

Bibliography

Abramson, John. *Overdosed America: The Broken Promise of American Medicine*. New York: HarperCollins Publisher, 2004.

Angell, Marcia. *The Truth about the Drug Companies: How They Deceive Us and What to Do about It*. New York: Random House, 2004.

Angier, Natalie. *The Canon: A Whirligig Tour of the Beautiful Basics of Science*. New York: Houghton Mifflin Company, 2007.

Bausell, R. Barker. *Snake Oil Science: The Truth about Complementary and Alternative Medicine*. New York: Oxford University Press, 2007.

Bernstein, Peter. *Against the Gods: The Remarkable Story of Risk*. New York: John Wiley & Sons, 1998.

Best, Joel. *Stat-Spotting: A Field Guide to Identifying Dubious Data*. Berkeley: University of California Press, 2008.

Bierce, Ambrose. *The Unabridged Devil's Dictionary*. CreateSpace, December 14, 2009.

Blastland, Michael, and Andrew Dilnot. *The Numbers Game: The Commonsense Guide to Understanding Numbers in the News, in Politics, and in Life*. New York: Gotham Books, 2009.

Brownlee, Shannon. *Overtreated: Why Too Much Medicine Is Making Us Sicker and Poorer*. New York: Bloomsbury USA, 2007.

Broyard, Anatole. *Intoxicated by My Illness*. New York: Fawcett Columbine, 1992.

Charon, Rita. *Narrative Medicine: Honoring the Stories of Illness*. New York: Oxford, 2006.

Colvin, Geoff. *Talent Is Overrated: What Really Separates World-Class Performers from Everybody Else*. New York: Portfolio, 2008.

de Waal, Frans. *The Age of Empathy: Nature's Lessons for a Kinder Society*. New York: Random House, 2009.

———. *Primates and Philosophers: How Morality Evolved* (The University Center for Human Valued Series). Princeton, New Jersey: Princeton University Press, 2006.

Ekman, Paul. *Telling Lies: Clues to Deceit in the Marketplace, Politics, and Marriage*. New York: W. W. Norton, 1993.

Gawande, Atul. *Better: A Surgeon's Notes on Performance.* New York: Metropolitan Books, 2007.

Gilovich, Thomas, Dale Griffin, and Daniel Kahneman. *Heuristics and Biases: The Psychology of Intuitive Judgment.* New York: Cambridge University Press, 2002.

Gladwell, Malcolm. *Outliers: The Story of Success.* New York: Little, Brown and Company, 2008.

Goleman, Daniel. *Emotional Intelligence: 10th Anniversary Edition; Why It Can Matter More Than IQ.* New York: Bantam Dell, 1995.

Hadler, Nortin. *The Last Well Person: How to Stay Well Despite the Health-Care System.* Montreal: McGill-Queen's University Press, 2004.

———. *Worried Sick: A Prescription for Health in an Overtreated America.* Chapel Hill: University of North Carolina Press, 2008.

Herrnstein, Richard, and Charles Murray. *The Bell Curve.* New York: Free Press, 1994.

Hoffman, Martin. *Empathy and Moral Development: Implications for Caring and Justice.* New York: Cambridge University Press, 2000.

Iyengar, Sheena. *The Art of Choosing.* New York: Twelve, 2010.

Lehrer, Jonah. *How We Decide.* New York: Houghton Mifflin, 2009.

Medication Use: A Systems Approach to Reducing Errors. Joint Commission on Accreditation of Healthcare Organizations, 1998.

Montgomery, Kathryn. *How Doctors Think: Clinical Judgment and the Practice of Medicine.* New York: Oxford University Press, 2006.

Nussbaum, Martha. *The Fragility of Goodness: Luck and Ethics in Greek Tragedy and Philosophy.* New York: Cambridge University Press, 1986.

Pinker, Steven. *The Blank Slate: The Modern Denial of Human Nature.* New York: Penguin Group, 2002.

Pollan, Michael. *The Omnivore's Dilemma.* New York: Penguin Press, 2006.

Relman, Arnold. *A Second Opinion: Rescuing America's Health Care.* New York: PublicAffairs, 2007.

Sacks, Oliver. *A Leg to Stand On.* New York: Touchstone, 1984.

Schulz, Kathryn. *Being Wrong: Adventures in the Margin of Error.* London: Portobello Books, 2010.

Smith, Charles John. *Synonyms Discriminated.* London: George Bell and Sons, 1893.

Sontag, Susan. *Illness As Metaphor.* New York: Farrar, Straus, Giroux, 1988.

Warren, Lynne. *Encyclopedia of 20th Century Photography.* New York: Routledge, 2005.

Woloshin, Steven, Lisa Schwartz, and H. Gilbert Welch. *Know Your Chances: Understanding Health Statistics.* Berkeley: University of California Press, 2008.

Woolf, Virginia. *On Being Ill.* Ashfield, MA: Paris Press, 2002.

Wright, H. G. *Means, Ends and Medical Care (Philosophy and Medicine).* Dordrecht: Springer, 2007.

Wright, Robert. *The Moral Animal: Why We Are the Way We Are: The New Science of Evolutionary Psychology.* New York: Vintage, 1995.

Zuk, Marlene. *Riddled with Life: Friendly Worms, Ladybug Sex, and the Parasites That Make Us Who We Are.* Florida: Houghton Mifflin Harcourt Publishing Company, 2007.

Index

About the Author

Dr. Steven Z. Kussin is a physician and patient advocate. His website, medicaladvocate.com, is a destination for patients to become empowered consumers. His medical advocacy practice will be launched in the summer of 2011. He lives with his family in Clinton and New York City, New York.

CPSIA information can be obtained at www.ICGtesting.com
Printed in the USA
BVOW041545210612

293352BV00001BA/9/P